This book belongs to

Mr. Gaunt.

Lasers in
Facial Aesthetic and
Reconstructive Surgery

LASERS IN
FACIAL AESTHETIC AND
RECONSTRUCTIVE SURGERY

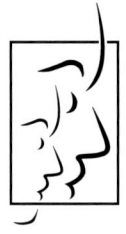

BRIAN S. BIESMAN, MD

DIRECTOR, OCULOPLASTIC AND ORBITAL SURGERY

NEW ENGLAND EYE CENTER

TUFTS UNIVERSITY SCHOOL OF MEDICINE

BOSTON, MASSACHUSETTS

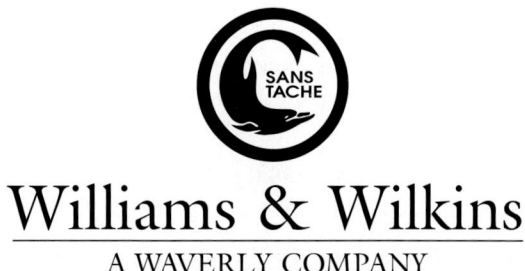

A WAVERLY COMPANY

BALTIMORE • PHILADELPHIA • LONDON • PARIS • BANGKOK
BUENOS AIRES • HONG KONG • MUNICH • SYDNEY • TOKYO • WROCLAW

Editor: Charles W. Mitchell
Managing Editor: Danielle Hagan
Marketing Manager: Adam Glazer
Project Editor: Jennifer D. Weir

351 West Camden Street
Baltimore, Maryland 21201-2436 USA

Rose Tree Corporate Center
1400 North Providence Road
Building II, Suite 5025
Media, Pennsylvania 19063-2043 USA

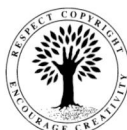

Printed in the United States of America

Library of Congress Cataloging-in-Publication Data

Lasers in facial aesthetic and reconstructive surgery / [edited by]
   Brian S. Biesman.—1st ed.
      p.   cm.
   Includes bibliographical references and index.
   ISBN 0–683–30414–3
   1. Face—Laser surgery.   2. Surgery, Plastic.   I. Biesman, Brian
S.
      [DNLM: 1. Face—surgery.   2. Laser Surgery—methods.   3. Surgery,
Plastic—methods.   WE 705 L342 1999]
   RD119.5.F33L37   1999
   617.5′2059—dc21
   DNLM/DLC
   for Library of Congress   98-21399
                                                                    CIP

The publishers have made every effort to trace the copyright holders for borrowed material. If they have inadvertently overlooked any, they will be pleased to make the necessary arrangements at the first opportunity.

To purchase additional copies of this book, call our customer service department at **(800) 638-0672** or fax orders to **(800) 447-8438.** For other book services, including chapter reprints and large quantity sales, ask for the Special Sales department.

Canadian customers should call **(800) 665-1148,** or fax **(800) 665-0103.** For all other calls originating outside of the United States, please call **(410) 528-4223** or fax us at **(410) 528-8550.**

Visit Williams & Wilkins on the Internet: **http://www.wwilkins.com** or contact our customer service department at **custserv@wwilkins.com**. Williams & Wilkins customer service representatives are available from 8:30 am to 6:00 pm, EST, Monday through Friday, for telephone access.

98 99 00 01 02
1 2 3 4 5 6 7 8 9 10

This book is dedicated to my wife, Didi,
and our children, Adam and Abigail

Foreword

The field of cosmetic laser surgery is evolving faster than any other field of medicine at present. This is due to a variety of economic and social factors. Certainly the media, in its quest to be on the cutting edge of technology in our lives, drives the engine of progress in the field of medicine. This factor, along with the modern era obsession of looking young has pushed the cosmetic surgeon into the arena (sometimes reluctantly) of high tech medicine, and propelled the development of increasingly advanced models of the fountain of youth. Ponce de Leon would be fulfilled in his abortive search for this fabled goal if he could only see where we are today.

Several results have derived from this helter-skelter process. In some instances, the technology is brought to the market place before it has been tested or even fully developed. You can imagine only a few of the problems that this creates. Another effect (beneficial or adverse depending on your opinion) is that the cosmetic physician, a term I use in deference to those practitioners of the art who are not surgeons, is encouraged—if not driven—to keep current on the latest techniques and technology. A plethora of organizations, seminars, publications, and modern soothsayers have been established to fill the information lag created in the field. Yet, what are we to do? Are we to join the effort to keep current in this field or resist the forces that have created this dearth of knowledge?

Dr. Biesman has made it his mission to help fill the void through this volume. Other books are published on the subjects covered herein. Many are outdated almost as soon as they are printed. A part of that information void is filled by this book. Few are written from the perspective of the oculoplastic surgeon editor and the authoritative vision of the contributors he has chosen to accompany him on his mission. Additionally, the authors are recognized to be among the leaders in their respective fields of laser medicine, recognition gained only through diligent dedication to the task of keeping current, or pushing the frontier of knowledge into the wilderness of ignorance. Finally, the reader of this book will find it to be well organized and very readable, with illustrations and help that make it worthy to take its place among the better tomes of laser medicine and surgery.

While it isn't the first book published on the subject, and neither will it be the last, it will provide the reader with the information needed to be well informed about the latest developments in the field of laser cosmetic surgery. Dr. Biesman and his contributors are to be congratulated for this monumental work in the effort to keep us current in the field of cosmetic laser therapy.

Richard O. Gregory, MD
Director
Institute of Aesthetic Surgery
Celebration Health
Florida Hospital

Preface

My interest in laser surgery was inspired during my fellowship with Dr. Albert Hornblass at the Manhattan Eye, Ear, and Throat Hospital. It was under his tutelage that I first performed periorbital incisional surgery with a continuous wave carbon dioxide laser.

Shortly after completing my training, I accepted a position at the New England Eye Center in Boston, MA, under the directorship of Dr. Carmen A. Puliafito, a well recognized clinician and research scientist with a strong interest in lasers. I owe my early access to the next generation of CO_2 lasers to Dr. Puliafito. Although I was intrigued by the new lasers, I did not begin to appreciate the full scope of their clinical applications until I had the opportunity to observe Dr. Sterling Baker in Oklahoma City, OK. Dr. Baker has remained a mentor and a friend, and I am particularly pleased and honored that he has contributed to this text.

In the beginning, as surgeons attempted to learn more about this new laser technology and its clinical applications, information was quickly disseminated via local seminars, national association meetings, and non peer-reviewed journals. Sometime later, articles were printed in peer-reviewed journals, and text books are just now beginning to appear. Due to a lack of clinical experience and long term follow up, some of the early information was incomplete, misleading, and occasionally even incorrect. This is an excellent time to publish a book as enough time has passed since the introduction of the new laser technology that accurate statements about proper surgical technique, wound care, and the true advantages and disadvantages offered by these devices may be made.

This book is designed to give the reader a solid foundation upon which to build both current practice and future learning about lasers and their clinical applications. Through my experiences introducing physicians worldwide to laser surgery, perhaps the most commonly expressed concern is the inability to critically evaluate new equipment or, in other words, to decide which laser is "best." Although laser technology and surgical techniques will undoubtedly continue to evolve, laser physics, laser-tissue interaction, and surgical anatomy are constants that, if understood well, will enable surgeons to evaluate devices and techniques not yet described. Without mastery of these fundamental principles, we are doomed to listen to the most convincing salesperson. I have deliberately emphasized and encourage the reader to become familiar with certain topics throughout the text, which I believe are of paramount importance.

Each procedure is described in a simple yet comprehensive fashion including preoperative patient evaluation, a step-by-step intraoperative approach containing recommended laser settings, postoperative management, and the prevention and treatment of complications. The anatomic and surgical drawings have been created with great care and attention to detail. Surgical "tricks" and "pearls" as well as common pitfalls have been described and illustrated as completely as possible. Every effort was made to choose clinical photographs that are representative of everyday experience, as opposed to a best or worse case scenario, unless otherwise indicated. The text has been referenced completely, and in some chapters exhaustively, with sources representing both an historic as well as a current perspective.

Each of the contributing authors is a skilled and recognized surgeon and teacher who has presented material in an objective and unbiased fashion. Their multidisciplinary backgrounds reflect the broad spectrum of surgeons who have achieved expertise in the discipline of aesthetic laser surgery.

The goal of this text is to provide a guide which will be useful to students, residents, and practicing physicians interested in performing laser-assisted facial aesthetic and reconstructive surgery. It is my sincere hope that the information provided will enhance the understanding and practice of aesthetic laser surgery.

Acknowledgments

This project was conceived in late 1996 when my colleague, Elias Reichel, encouraged me to meet with Beth Barry, then of Igaku-Shoin Publishing Company. For many months I resisted accepting the responsibility and time commitment but, due to Ms. Barry's persistence, I ultimately agreed. Without the help of many faithful and understanding individuals, I would have been unable to bring this project to completion in an expeditious fashion.

I must first acknowledge Didi, my kind, loving and patient wife who endured the countless late nights, early mornings, and weekends I spent alone in the study while she cared for our one-year-old twins. Drs. Allen Putterman and Albert Hornblass instilled in me the importance of making useful contributions whenever possible. Dr. Robert Goldwyn has been a role model as the complete physician and surgeon I someday hope to be. Dr. Sterling Baker has given me many opportunities and continues to be my teacher and friend. Drs. Tina Alster and Jeff Dover have faithfully supported my clinical and academic efforts and I am fortunate to have worked with them.

Dr. Daniel Buerger was a fellow in Oculoplastic Surgery at the New England Eye Center when the manuscript was prepared, and I am indebted to him for his contributions and assistance. My colleague, Dr. Yunhee Lee, is a brilliant and kind individual who carefully reviewed much of the manuscript.

I must thank my assistant, Lauren Parker, for patiently helping with a seemingly endless list of last minute projects, phone calls, opinions, and faxes as this effort drew to a close. Without her influence and help, my practice could not have achieved its current degree of success.

Melissa Visintin is a bright, talented artist and medical illustrator who patiently made countless changes in her work to meet my demands. Her contributions to this manuscript increase its value immeasurably.

Coherent Medical generously provided funding, which was used to help defray art and production costs, and also created some of the artwork needed in Chapter 1. Chris and Dan Palmerton of Buffalo Filter also provided generous support, and for this I am grateful.

Finally, Danielle Hagan, Fran Klass, and Charley Mitchell of Williams & Wilkins worked diligently to make this book a reality.

Contributors

Tina Alster, MD
Director
Washington Institute of Dermatologic Laser Surgery
Clinical Assistant Professor
Georgetown University Medical Center
Washington, DC
Lecturer
Harvard Medical School
Boston, Massachusetts

Sterling S. Baker, MD
Clinical Assistant Professor
Department of Ophthalmology
University of Oklahoma College of Medicine
Oklahoma City, Oklahoma

Brian S. Biesman, MD
Director, Oculoplastic and Orbital Surgery
New England Eye Center
Tufts University School of Medicine
Boston, Massachusetts

Daniel E. Buerger
Clinical Instructor of Ophthalmology
University of Pittsburgh School of Medicine
Active Staff
University of Pittsburgh Medical Center
Pittsburgh, Pennsylvania

Harvey P. Cole, III, MD
Clinical Instructor of Ophthalmology
Emory University School of Medicine
Director
Specialty Surgery Center
Chairman, Atlanta Oculoplastic Surgery
Piedmont Hospital
Atlanta, Georgia

Jeffrey Dover, MD, FRCPC
Associate Chairman
Department of Dermatology
Beth Israel Deaconess Medical Center
Associate Professor of Clinical Dermatology
Harvard Medical School
Boston, Massachusetts

Christine M. Hayes, MD
Assistant Professor
Tufts University School of Medicine
Chief, Surgical Division
Department of Dermatology
New England Medical Center
Boston, Massachusetts

George J. Hruza, MD
Associate Professor of Medicine (Dermatology), Surgery
 (Plastic Surgery), Otolaryngology
Washington University School of Medicine
Director
Cutaneous Surgery Center
Barnes-Jewish Hospital
St. Louis, Missouri

Jemshed A. Khan, MD
Director, Oculoplastic
Clinical Professor of Ophthalmology
Kansas University School of Medicine
Director, Cosmetic Laser Services
Hunkeler Eye Centers
Kansas City, Missouri

Christopher Nanni, MD
Assistant Clinical Professor of Dermatology
George Washington University
Washington, DC

Kenneth D. Steinsapir, MD
Assistant Clinical Professor of Ophthalmology
Jules Stein Eye Institute
UCLA School of Medicine
Los Angeles, California

Walter P. Unger, MD, FRCP (c), FACP
Toronto, Canada

Cynthia Weinstein, MD, MBBS, FACP, FRACP
Member
Australasian College Dermatologist
Member
Australasian College of Physicians
Consultant to Freemason's Hospital
Melbourne, Australia

Contents

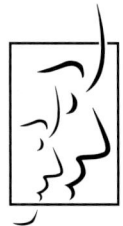

Chapter One

Carbon Dioxide Laser Physics, Laser Tissue Interaction, and Laser Safety

Brian S. Biesman and Jemshed A. Khan

The carbon dioxide (CO_2) laser has been recognized as a valuable asset to the aesthetic surgeon for its role in skin resurfacing and incisional surgery. However, the CO_2 laser surgeon is forced to choose from a bewildering array of lasers, each differing from the next in some way, and must also be capable of making intraoperative laser adjustments so as to achieve the desired tissue effect. To accomplish these objectives, a clear understanding of CO_2 laser physics and the nature of the interaction between CO_2 laser energy and soft tissue is very important.

A laser is a device that generates an intense beam of light: it has several unique characteristics differentiating it from nonlaser light. Laser is an acronym for Light Amplification by Stimulated Emission of Radiation, a concept first described by Einstein. When an atom in its resting or ground state absorbs energy in the form of electromagnetic radiation it may be elevated to a higher energy level or an excited state. Atoms in this condition are relatively unstable and with time will spontaneously revert to their more stable ground state with the concomitant emission of a quantity of energy known as a photon. This process is known as spontaneous emission. The photon released by spontaneous emission may be described as having a wavelength $[\lambda]$ and hence an energy E as $E=(h)(c/\lambda)$ where h is Planck's constant and c is the speed of light. From the theory describing the wave-particle duality of light, a photon may also be considered capable of behaving as a solid particle, which can interact with other electrons in the excited state. Einstein postulated that when an atom elevated to an excited state by irradiation with a photon of a certain energy is irradiated with another identical photon, it will return to its ground state while releasing two waves of light: each with the same direction and energy and traveling together such that their wave peaks coincide identically. This process is known as stimulated emission and the identical light waves produced are known as laser light.

As follows from the theory of stimulated emission, the generation of laser light requires the emission of photons, which must initially be derived by spontaneous emission. The greater the number of atoms in the excited state, the higher the probability that spontaneous emission will occur. When most of the atoms present in a given population are in the excited state, achieved by adding energy from an external source, a population inversion has occurred and laser light may be readily produced. Even a small number of electrons from this population undergoing spontaneous emission emit photons that will interact with excited electrons, each of which will produce two photons that can in turn interact with other excited atoms. In this manner, the process is amplified and a type of chain reaction is produced.

The tube in which the above process occurs is known as an optical or resonator cavity and contains a laser medium. The medium may be gaseous as in the case of carbon dioxide (CO_2), and argon lasers, a solid as in the case of the neodymium:yttrium-aluminum-garnet (Nd:YAG) or erbium (Er):YAG laser, or a liquid as in a tunable dye laser. The energy source used to create the population inversion may be electricity, radiofrequency pulsed energy, high intensity light as produced by a flashlamp or other laser, among others.

The light produced by lasers has special and unique properties that make it useful in a large number of industrial, navigational, and medical situations. As opposed to light produced by any other source, laser light waves are monochromatic, collimated, and coherent. Monochromatism refers to the production of very narrow bands of electromagnetic radiation by any given laser. A laser may produce only one band of light or may produce several bands: each is narrow, distinct, and in the same region of the electromagnetic radiation spectrum. Monochromatism may be used advantageously to achieve specific therapeutic goals in medical laser systems as the various components of our tissues absorb certain wavelengths more highly than others. Hemoglobin, for example, highly absorbs energy with a wavelength of 420 nm while water has absorption peaks at approximately 2900 nm and 10,600 nm. Thus, the property of monochromatism allows us to select the correct laser to accomplish a given task. Collimation refers to the fact that laser light, as compared with light produced by other sources, is highly directional with little divergence as it becomes further from its source. Laser light is thus very intense and may be projected to distant objects such as the earth's moon. The third unique characteristic of laser light is coherence: the peaks and troughs of the waves that comprise the laser beam coincide in an exact way, allowing for the beam to transmit high energies over a great distance.

RADIOMETRY

In order to use lasers to achieve clinical goals successfully and safely, a working knowledge of basic laser surgery terminology is required. Lasers produce energy, which is the capacity to do work. Energy is usually measured in joules (J) and the energy of a laser may be increased only by increasing the number of photons in the beam (1). Power is the rate at which energy is delivered, and is measured in watts (W) where one watt equals 1 J/sec. As power is inversely related to time, increasing the power setting on a pulsed laser only increases the rate at which the pulses are delivered as the energy per pulse remains constant.

Power density, or irradiance, is the rate of energy delivery per unit area of target tissue and is measured in watts per square centimeter (W/cm^2) (2). The power density is calculated by dividing the power by the cross-sectional area of the beam at the place where it hits the tissue (3). As most commercially manufactured lasers do not produce beams with sharply defined borders, the conventional definition of the diameter is a circle which contains 86% of the total power. If a laser produces a beam with a diameter of 1.0 mm at the tissue, and the beam has a power of 20 W, the power density (Pd) is 2000 W/cm^2. If the beam diameter is decreased to 0.2 mm, the Pd increases to 50,000 W/cm^2. Conversely, increasing the spot size decreases the Pd exponentially. Thus, for most effective cutting, the smallest spot size possible is used. In order to effectively vaporize or ablate tissue with a pulsed laser system, a Pd of approximately 150 W/cm^2 is required. This number increases substantially when a continuous wave laser is used. With increasing Pd, the zone of peripheral necrosis at wound edges decreases, although at very high Pd (>1000 W/cm^2), wound edge necrosis will be highly related to irradiation time (4, 5). Power density is maximized when a laser beam is focused, and falls exponentially as the beam is defocused (Figure 1.1). This has an important clinical implication as defocusing the laser by even a small amount can result in subthreshold power densities and unwanted thermal damage.

Fluence, or energy density, is the term used to describe the concentration of energy applied to the tissue. It is expressed as J/cm^2 and is measured by dividing the total energy by the cross-sectional area of the beam at the point where it interacts with the tissue. It is useful to consider the calculation of fluence as (Pd)(exposure time). Once the critical Pd of about 150 W/cm^2 has been produced, tissue effect is proportional to exposure time and not Pd. Thus, the Pd determines the rate of tissue removal whereas the fluence determines how much tissue is removed (6). When treating skin, fluence of not less than 5 J/cm^2 should be applied (7).

BEAM DELIVERY AND PROFILE

The energy produced by the CO_2 and Er:YAG lasers cannot be delivered via a flexible fiber because of technical limitations of the fibers. Instead, the beams are delivered via an articulated arm containing a series of mirrors that "bounce" the beam to its destination. After escaping from the articulated arm, the beam is brought into focus through a lens contained within the handpiece. Some lasers produce a focused beam, which may be transmitted from the optical cavity to the tissue by means of a flexible waveguide, and others use waveguides, which may be

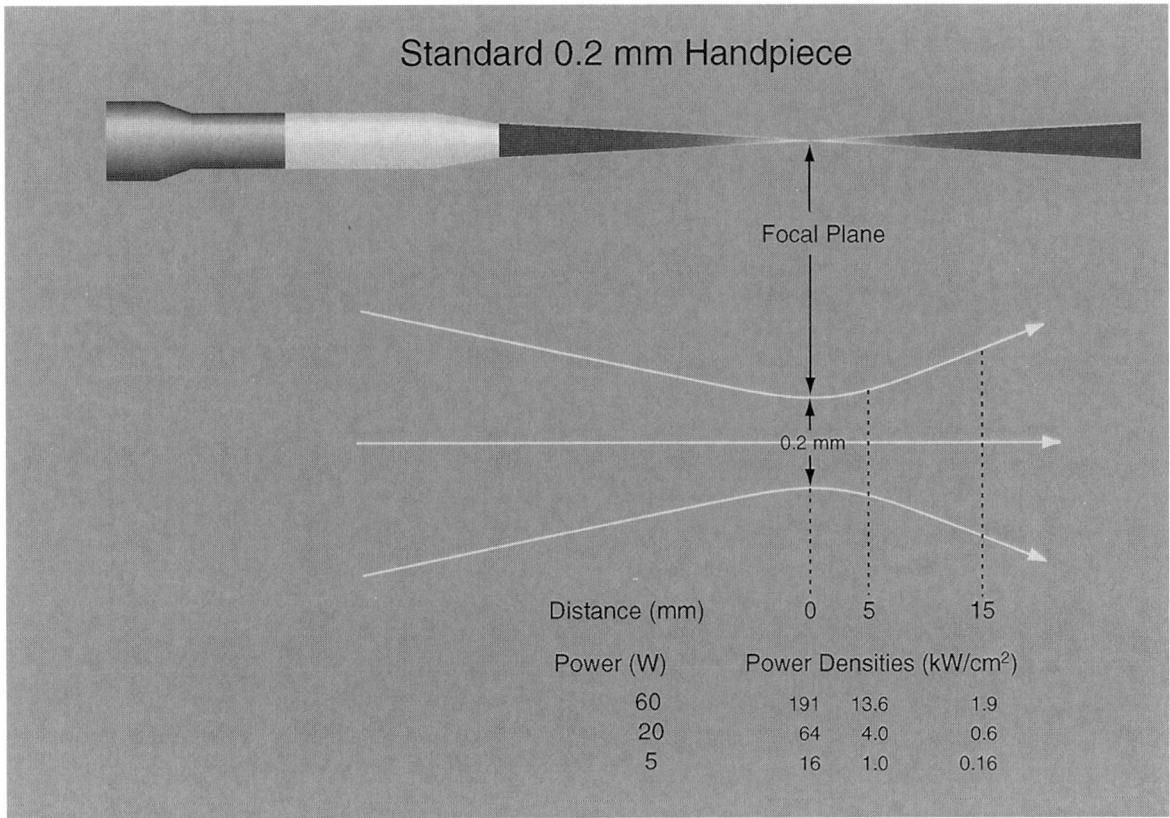

Figure 1.1. Power density falls dramatically as the laser handpiece is moved away from the tissue. This fact underscores the need to keep the laser focused.

attached to the articulated arm for use in endoscopic procedures. Since CO_2 and Er:YAG lasers emit infrared radiation invisible to the human eye, most laser manufacturers include a coaxial aiming beam (usually helium:neon, 632.8 nm). Excessive movement or transportation of the entire laser may misalign the mirrors so that the He-Ne and infrared beams are no longer aligned. Testing the laser on an inanimate object such as a tongue blade before each use is therefore important.

The ideal laser beam is of uniform intensity across its entire diameter and produces a sharply defined uniform burn (8). Such a beam is extremely difficult to produce and the beam profile found most often in commercially produced lasers is known as the fundamental or transverse electromagnetic $(TEM)_{00}$ mode. This beam has a Gaussian energy distribution and produces a burn that is deeper centrally than peripherally corresponding to the energy distribution within the beam itself. This is important clinically because two burns placed immediately adjacent to one another will not produce a uniform burn; rather there will be two hot spots separated by an intervening colder area. Thus, to produce a uniform tissue ef-

fect, some overlap of the laser spots is required. Other more complex beam intensity profiles may be produced which are usually focused to a larger spot size and may produce uneven burns.

BEAM TYPE

The earliest CO_2 lasers produced energy in a nearly constant or continuous fashion and were thus known as *continuous wave* lasers. When operating one of these devices, the laser fired continuously when activated and stopped only when inactivated. While these lasers were effective at cutting soft tissue, they often produced an excessive thermal effect in the tissue surrounding the intended target zone with resultant scarring and unacceptable wound appearance. The transfer of heat to tissue surrounding a laser burn is a time-dependent process with greater tissue heating occurring with prolonged exposure time (9). In circumventing this problem, continuous wave lasers were subsequently modified with mechanical shutters, which were controlled manually or electronically, to limit the time the tissue was exposed to the laser energy. While shorter pulses were produced, the peak power of these pulses remained low and the exposure times were still too long to allow soft tissue surgery to be performed without significant lateral thermal damage.

The next advance in laser technology was the development of "superpulsing," a concept introduced in the 1980s to further limit the time soft tissue was exposed to CO_2 laser radiation while maintaining the parameters required to ablate tissue. Superpulsed lasers produce a controlled train of short duration, high peak power pulses and thus generate high power densities with more precise control of thermal effect on surrounding tissue. When used for incisional procedures, superpulsed lasers may produce less than one third of the thermal damage caused by continuous wave lasers (10, 11). A typical superpulse waveform has a rapid upstroke to peak power, followed by an exponential decay to lower power, before dropping precipitously to zero. The frequency usually ranges from 100–900 Hz and the peak powers produced may be one-to-two orders of magnitude greater than the power produced in continuous wave mode. Superpulsed CO_2 lasers deliver peak powers up to 10 times higher and pulse durations 10-100 times shorter than is possible with continuous wave CO_2 lasers (12-14). A limitation of the superpulsed laser is the relatively small spot size required to deliver sufficient fluence that soft tissue may be ablated.

The latest generation of pulsed lasers use a radiofrequency pulsing device to produce a waveform that does not have as abrupt a decay to a lower power before returning to zero. This results in increased area under the power-time curve and increased energy of the laser pulse. The higher energy pulse can be delivered in a large enough spot size to be clinically more useful for skin resurfacing than the superpulsed lasers. The radiofrequency pulsed lasers thus develop high peak powers, short duration pulses, and larger spot sizes. Many surgeons consider these lasers the current "gold standard" of CO_2 lasers.

As an alternative to superpulsing, another method of delivering CO_2 laser energy in high energy, short duration pulses is to use a computer controlled optokinetic scanner. This allows a continuous wave beam to be applied to the skin so that the exposure time is limited to less than 1ms and the fluence generated is above the 5 J/cm² threshold required for tissue ablation. Produced and developed by Sharplan industries, this device was, and has been, used effectively for skin resurfacing (15, 16). The beam produced by an optokinetically scanned continuous wave laser does not have a Gaussian energy distribution and these laser spots should not be overlapped.

LASER TISSUE INTERACTION

Laser surgery is made possible due to the absorption of electromagnetic radiation by elements within the target tissue with the subsequent conversion of this energy to heat. The beneficial and detrimental effects of laser treatments may be attributed to the heating of tissue. Anderson and Parrish introduced the principle of selective photothermolysis to describe the criteria, which must be met to allow heat induced destruction of specific tissues with the relative sparing of surrounding structures, a "magic bullet" type of effect. These criteria include a laser wavelength that reaches and is preferentially absorbed by the desired target structures, sufficient fluence to reach a damaging temperature in the targets, and exposure duration less than or equal to the time necessary for the target tissue to cool (17, 18). If laser treatments that do not respect these principles are delivered, unwanted thermal damage may occur. The CO_2 and Er:YAG lasers may be used to perform dermatologic surgery effectively and safely as they can be engineered to meet each of the criteria for selective photothermolysis, as outlined in the discussion below. The CO_2 and Er:YAG lasers emit at wavelengths of 10,600 nm and 2940 nm, respectively, placing them in the infrared portion of the EMR spectrum where water is the chromophore or material that acts as an absorptive target (Figures 1.2, 1.3). As the water content of skin is approximately 70%, CO_2 and Er:YAG lasers are well adapted to cutaneous surgery (19). The absorption coefficient of the Er:YAG laser for pure water is approximately 10 times that of the CO_2 laser. The depth to which laser energy penetrates into a given tissue depends on the wavelength and the tissue itself (Figure 1.4A, B). When interacting with normal human skin, the Er:YAG and CO_2 lasers penetrate approximately 1 and 20-30 microns, respectively (20). Despite the very shallow penetration of the laser energy itself, the clinical effects of these devices may extend much deeper because of the deposition of heat that may occur with certain laser delivery systems.

When laser energy is applied to tissue, it may be absorbed, reflected, transmitted, or scattered. Scatter is a change in direction of energy propagation within the skin occurring as a result of interaction with tissue proteins such as dermal collagen. Scatter becomes a significant factor once the dermis has been entered during resurfacing with the CO_2 laser. Reflection occurs at the air-skin interface due to the difference in refractive indices between the air and the skin. Approximately 5% of incident radiation is reflected. Absorption is required for heating of tissue and thus for a laser's clinical effect. It is the primary

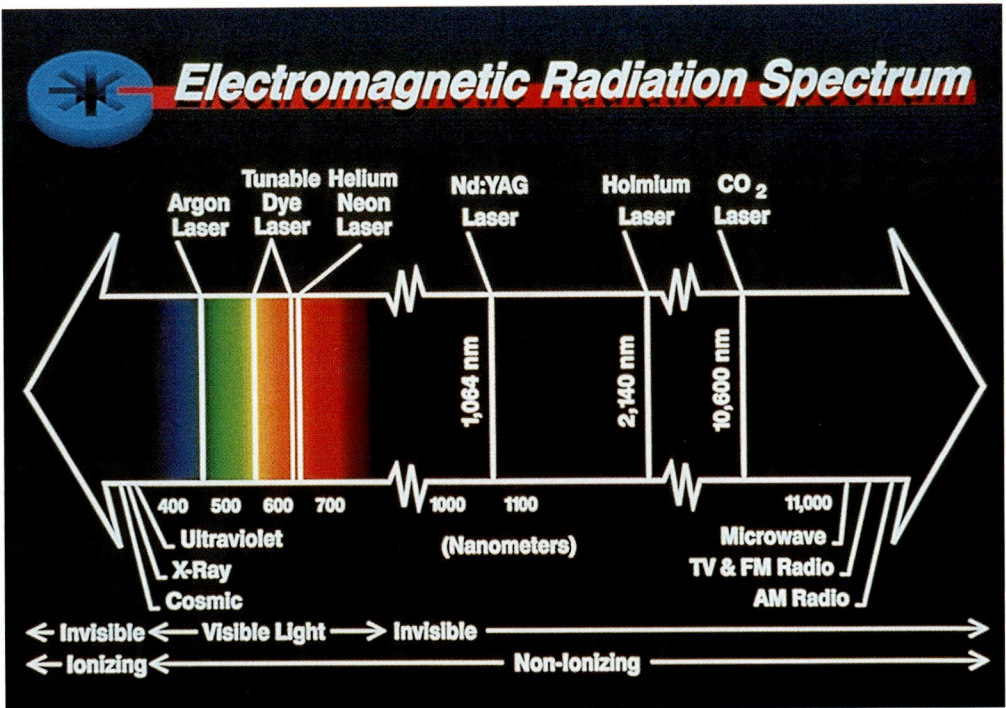

Figure 1.2. The electromagnetic radiation spectrum. Er:YAG and CO_2 lasers emit in the infrared (nonionizing) portion of the spectrum (Figure courtesy of Coherent Medical, Inc.)

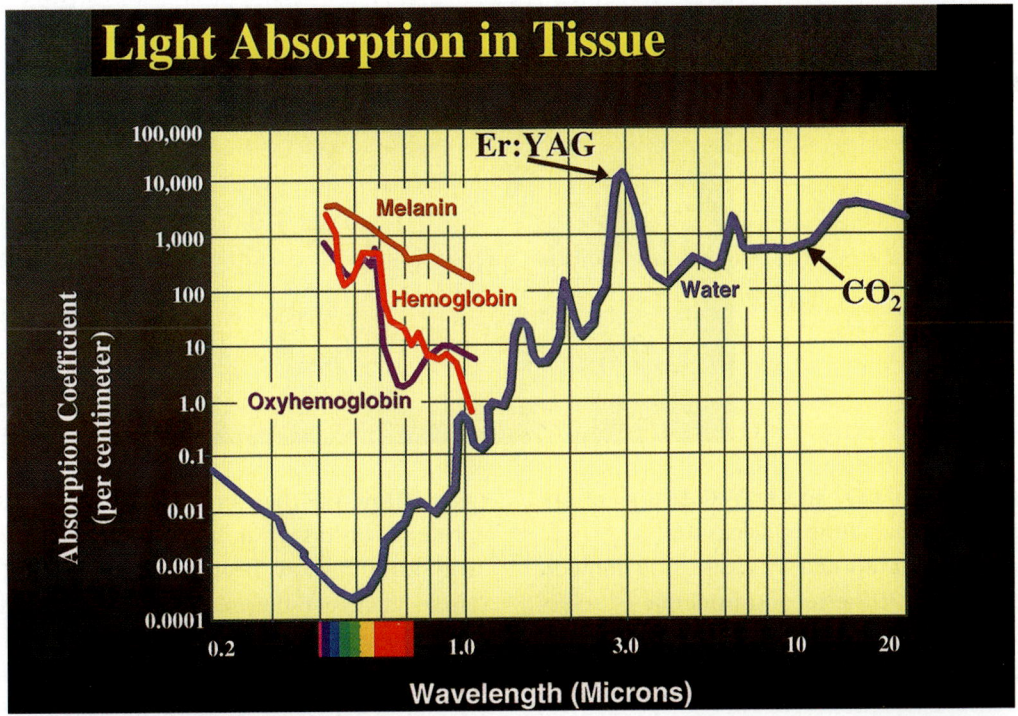

Figure 1.3. Absorption characteristics of major soft tissue components. The absorption of energy by water is nearly 10 times greater at 2940 nm (Er:YAG) than at 10,600 nm (CO_2) (Figure courtesy of ESC Medical Systems)

Figure 1.4. A. Penetration of laser energy into a given tissue is a function of wavelength and the nature of the tissue (Figure courtesy of Coherent Medical, Inc.). **B.** Comparison of tissue effects produced by Erbium:YAG and CO_2 lasers. Using similar fluences, after a single pass in resurfacing mode, the CO_2 laser ablates approximately four times as much tissue as the Er:YAG (Figure courtesy of Coherent Medical, Inc.)

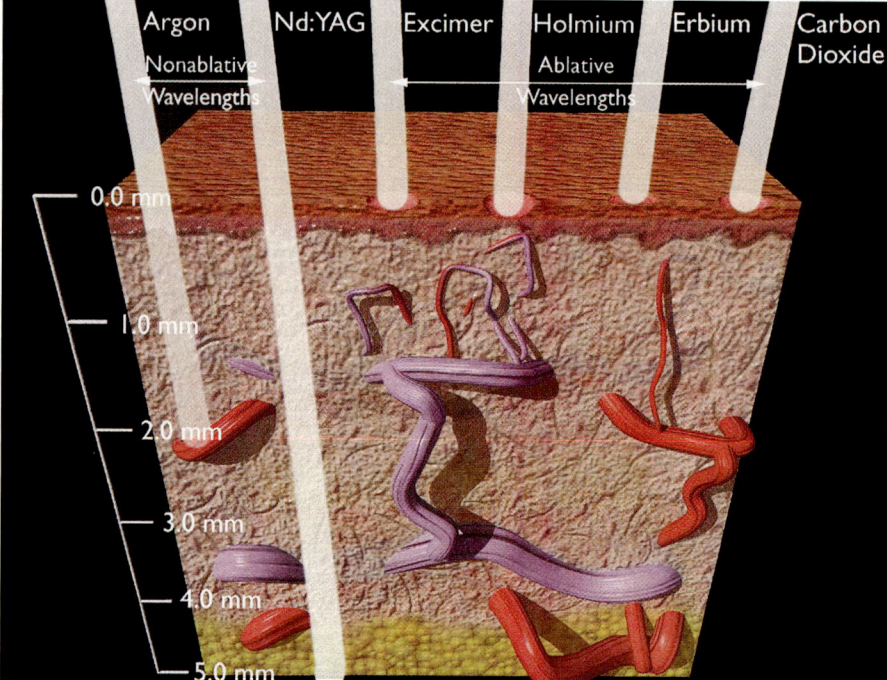

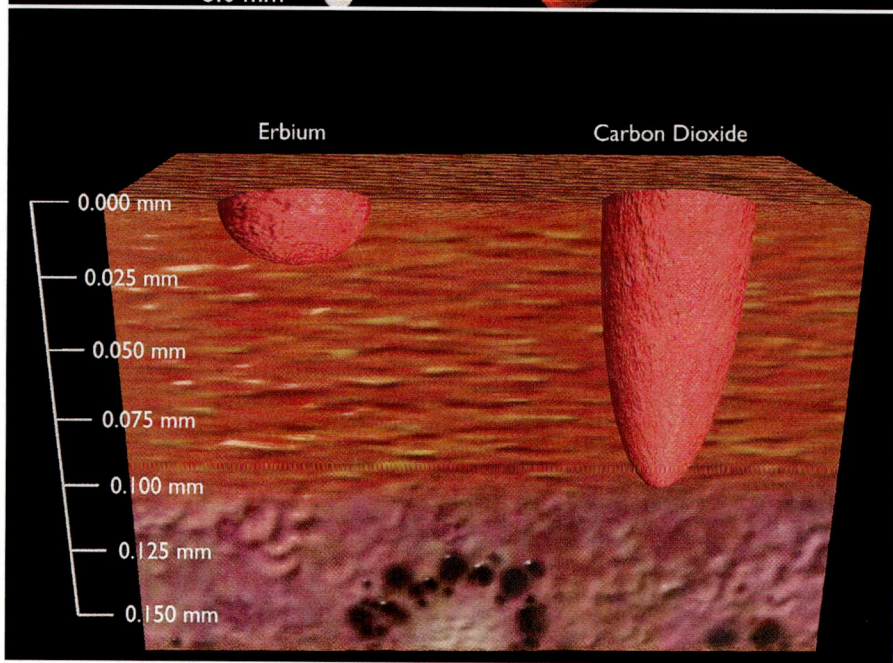

process occurring when CO_2 and Er:YAG lasers are applied to skin and thus bears further discussion.

When laser light is absorbed by tissue, it is immediately converted to heat. If the second principle of selective photothermolysis is violated and tissue is heated slowly or with excessively low power density or fluence, it may become coagulated, desiccated, and finally, charred or carbonized. These carbonized tissues may attain a temperature of several hundred degrees centigrade and act as a "heat sink," conducting heat to the surrounding tissues. As tissue temperature is raised, a sharp demarcation has been observed at 50–60°C with reversible damage occur-

ring below this barrier and permanent denaturation of proteins observed at higher temperatures (21). Thus, with subthreshold heating of tissues by CO_2 or Er:YAG lasers, excessive thermal damage will occur in the irradiated tissue and the surrounding tissues to which heat is conducted. In contrast, if a suprathreshold quantity of CO_2 or Er:YAG laser energy is delivered over a sufficiently short duration of time, vaporization of intra- and extracellular water occurs with minimal heating of surrounding tissues. In this model, tissue temperatures at the site of laser impact do exceed 100°C and conduction of heat to the surrounding tissues is minimized. The important variables in achieving this goal are power density and exposure time. Referring back to the radiometry section, P=E/t where P is power, E is energy and t is time. Solving for E, E=P(t). While the same value for E can be achieved with a high P and low t or vice versa, the tissue effects vary greatly. Thus, energy alone does not predict the effect of laser energy on tissue.

While it has been established that the length of time the energy is in contact with skin (pulse duration) needs to be minimized, how short is short enough? According to the principle of selective photothermolysis, the pulse duration should be shorter than the time it takes for tissue to cool. Tissue cooling is a complex phenomenon which may be simplified by the concept of thermal relaxation time. The thermal relaxation time of tissue is generally defined as the time it takes for a volume of tissue to lose 50% of its heat. From a practical standpoint, if the duration of a laser pulse (or the dwell time of a scanned continuous wave beam) is shorter than the thermal relaxation time of the target tissue, then lateral thermal damage resulting from residual heat will be minimized.

In one sense, the ideal soft tissue laser may be defined as a device that produces complete tissue vaporization with no deposition of residual heat into the surrounding tissue. On the other hand, a controlled, minimal thermal effect may in fact be of clinical benefit. The CO_2 laser may be used for skin resurfacing to ablate epidermal and dermal tissue effectively, but also produces a thermally induced "shrinkage" or remodeling of dermal collagen believed to enhance the procedure outcome in some patients. In contrast, the Er:YAG laser produces energy with

shorter pulses, up to ten times higher pulse powers, and greater absorption by water. As predicted, these features provide for greater tissue ablation with less thermal effect. Clinically, this translates to more superficial ablation with each pass of the laser (a wavelength-dependent phenomenon) with a shortened period of postoperative erythema but with little remodeling of dermal collagen and no hemostatic effect. The definition of "ideal" must be made in the context of the clinical goals and the needs of the patient (22, 23).

When lasers are used to perform incisional surgery, the concept of limiting lateral thermal damage remains important. The goal of laser incisional surgery is to create a zone of thermal damage large enough to ensure a hemostatic incision and small enough to avoid a significant risk of scar formation. As described by Anderson, when the CO_2 laser creates a soft tissue incision, three distinct zones of injury are produced. In the central zone tissue is vaporized and ejected from the wound creating an incision. Adjacent to the incision is a zone of irreversible thermal damage created by conduction of energy and subsequent elevation of temperature above 50–60°C. This zone is recognizable histopathologically as coagulative necrosis. Peripheral to the zone of irreversible thermal damage is a zone of reversible injury where the temperature was elevated by heat conducted from the incision site, but in which the temperature never reached the threshold above which coagulation of tissue proteins occurs (Figure 1.5). The zone of thermal damage is minimized by using a narrow beam, a pulsed delivery system, and by keeping the handpiece focused: a maneuver that

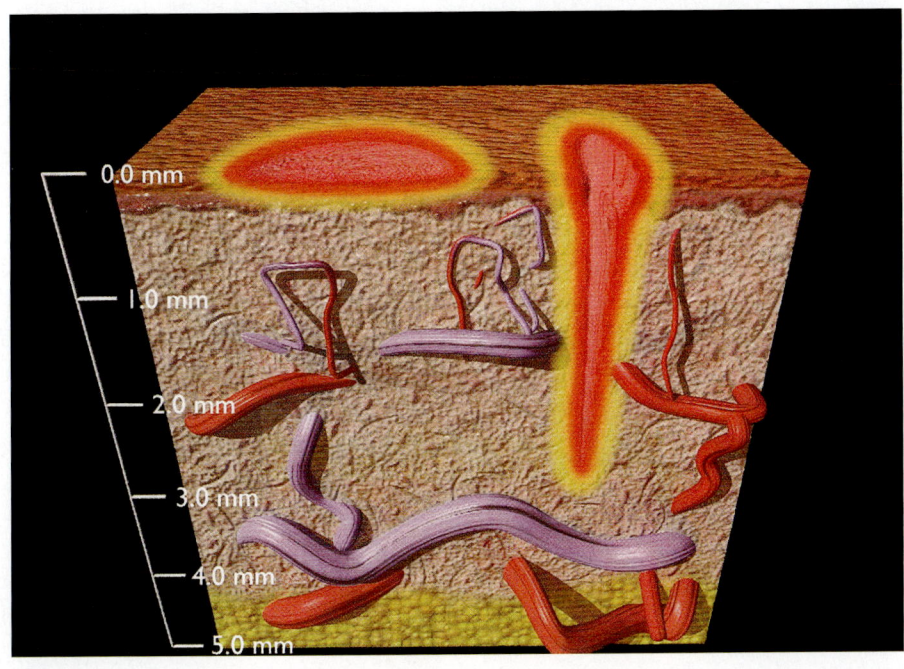

Figure 1.5. Depiction of the effects produced when a CO_2 laser interacts with soft tissue in either resurfacing (left) or incisional (right) mode. In each case the central pink zone represents ablated tissue, the orange zone represents irreversible thermal damage (coagulative necrosis), and the yellow zone represents reversible thermal damage.

beginning laser surgeons sometimes find difficult, but one that can have dramatic effects on the tissue. For example, a 5 W output delivered through a 0.2 mm incisional spot results in a power density of approximately 12,000 W/cm², but if the beam is defocused to a 5 mm spot size, then the power density drops to approximately 50 W/cm² and the zone of thermal damage will increase dramatically in size.

The Er:YAG laser is not yet available with an incisional handpiece although several manufacturers are currently working to develop such a device.

In summary, the general goal of laser surgery is to target a specific tissue, which is then ablated with minimal thermal damage. This goal is best achieved when energy is delivered with high power density for a period of time less than the thermal relaxation time of the targeted tissue. Treatment with low power densities, long pulses, or continuous wave radiation can result in irreversible thermal damage due to coagulation of tissue proteins.

LASER SAFETY

The successful use of lasers demands close attention to laser safety requirements and guidelines. Failure to observe these rules can endanger the patient, surgeon, op-

erating room personnel, and even bystanders. While these potential hazards may be readily avoided, care must be taken to always treat lasers with respect. Laser safety regulations exist at the federal (Occupational Safety and Health Administration Agency [OSHA]), local, institutional, and sometimes departmental levels. Safety standards are also established by the American National Standards Institute (ANSI), a nongovernmental agency, as the American National Standards for the Safe Use of Lasers in Health Care Facilities (Z316.3) (24). A copy of these guidelines should be present in every facility where a medical laser is in use.

As well as instituting a series of general safety measures, each facility storing or using a medical laser should specifically address electrical and mechanical safety, prevention of fires, respiratory protection, ocular protection, and patient safety. Appointment of an individual whose responsibility it is to oversee, enforce and educate others about issues concerning laser safety measures is recommended. Whenever lasers are in use, signs must be clearly marked outside the treatment room. Some highly specialized rooms are equipped with door locks that are activated when the laser is in "active" or "ready" mode. This will clearly prevent individuals from entering the treatment room at an inappropriate or dangerous time, but

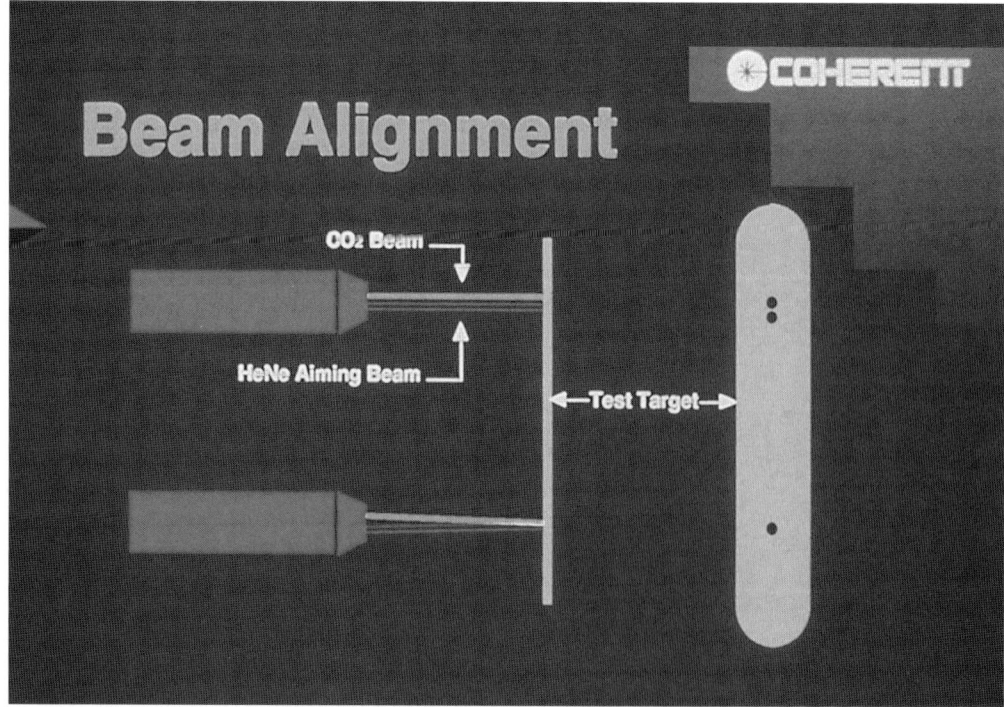

Figure 1.6. A test spot is created on a wet wooden tongue depressor in order to confirm exact alignment of the visible He:Ne aiming beam and the invisible CO_2 laser beam (Figure courtesy of Coherent Medical Laser, Inc.)

may also place personnel within the room at risk in the unlikely event that the laser malfunctions or that a catastrophic event occurs and escape is delayed or prevented. Equipment should be positioned within the treatment room so that the smoke evacuator and laser do not impede the working requirements of the staff. Adequate cooling of the treatment room is important as the lasers generate a large amount of heat even when left in "standby" mode when treatment is not being performed.

Equipment Safety

Lasers are electrical devices that may contain water, gases, or liquid chemicals. These substances may be hazardous, especially if a malfunction has occurred and the possibility of a leak exists. It is recommended that the housing of the laser never be removed by anyone other than an authorized service representative. Whenever concern regarding the function of the unit arises, the power should be turned off and the laser unplugged from its power source. The keys required to start all medical lasers should never be left in the laser itself and must be stored in a safe place. If more than one foot pedal is to be used (different lasers, cautery unit, etc.) make certain that the identity of the foot pedal is clearly established prior to activating the laser. Water or saline on the operating room floor may also interfere with the proper functioning of the footpedal and may cause electrical failure of the laser. As the CO_2 and Er:YAG lasers produce invisible radiation, if an aiming beam is available, always test the laser on an inanimate object such as a moist wooden tongue blade to ensure exact alignment of the aiming beam with the infrared beam (Figure 1.6).

Fire Safety

Surgical lasers can ignite a large number of substances commonly found in the operating room. Surgical drapes, endotracheal tubes, clothing, bed sheets, chemicals used for skin preparation and cleaning, hair, intestinal gas (usually methane), oxygen, sponges, and paperwork, to name some obvious ones. When lasers are in use, none of these substances should be in or adjacent to the surgical field. Wet towels must be used to define the surgical field. Flammable agents must not be used to prepare the skin. Oxygen may be administered so that patients may be sedated, but it may not be flowing when the laser itself is in use. It is particularly important to never let oxygen flow underneath surgical drapes as a pocket of high oxygen concentrations may develop and, if ignited, such pockets may not only ignite but explode. If general anesthesia is required, the safest method of delivering the flammable gas is via a flexible metal endotracheal (ET) tube. Wrapping materials are available and may be placed around plastic ET tubes. Some surgeons prefer to inflate the cuff found at the distal end of the ET tube with methylene-blue-tinted saline so that a leak will be easily detected. This precaution is particularly important if the laser is being used in the oral cavity or nasopharynx. Fire extinguishers should be present and must be inspected annually to ensure their readiness for use (25–30).

Respiratory Protection

The laser plume may deliver hazardous particulate matter to the respiratory tree. Furthermore, the presence of human papillomavirus DNA has been documented in the plume after carbon dioxide laser treatment of warts (31). Reports also indicate a risk of contamination of the operator by human papillomavirus DNA (detectable with the polymerase chain reaction technique) during CO_2 laser treatment (32). These hazards may be reduced by using a smoke evacuator designed for use with surgical lasers, and by donning laser masks. Buffalo Filter produces a small, quiet-yet-powerful smoke evacuator, the instrument of choice of many laser surgeons. Note that a more powerful smoke evacuator such as the Buffalo Filter model 1202, or the recently introduced smaller, but equally powerful, Whisper Turbo, is recommended for use with the Er:YAG laser to accommodate the greater amount of plume generated (Figure 1.7). Laser masks (Tecnol Inc., Fort Worth, TX), unlike general surgical masks, are capable of filtering out contaminants 0.1 microns in diameter at 95% efficiency.

Ocular Protection

The cardinal rule of incisional surgery is to always protect critical underlying structures with a laser-impenetrable shield. Most importantly, the globe must be protected by a laser-impenetrable device whenever periocular incisional or skin resurfacing procedures are performed. The two major options available are metal corneal shields or lid clamps. Most corneal shields are designed to fit behind the eyelids, although some will rest on the lids. The latter

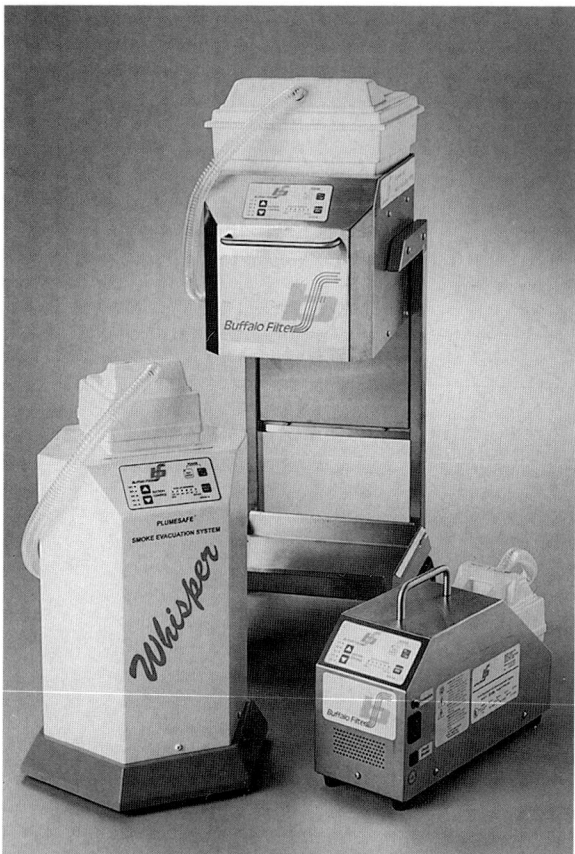

Figure 1.7. The Buffalo Filter family of smoke evacuators. The more powerful 1202 or Whisper Turbo units are required when using the Er:YAG laser due to the greater amount of plume generated. (Whisper Turbo not pictured.)

tion where it is tightened. The David-Baker clamp is available in adult and pediatric sizes (34). When performing lower eyelid blepharoplasty, a metal "bone" or Jaeger plate (Figure 1.10) is used for ocular protection. Any instrument that is placed against the cornea should be inspected carefully to ensure that no burrs, foreign bodies, or other irregularities are present which may injure the ocular surface. For added protection, ophthalmic ointment may be applied to these instruments as well. If these instruments are sterilized chemically, they must be thoroughly rinsed before use. At least one case of severe oc-

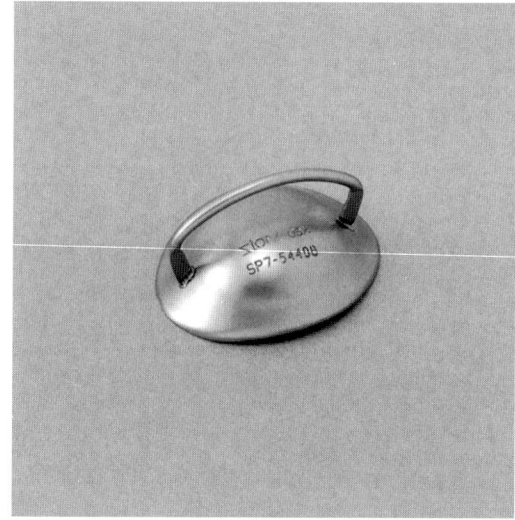

Figure 1.8. Titanium globe protector with unique antirotational posts and eyelash traction bar (Storz Instrument Co., St. Louis, Missouri.)

lenses are more likely to decenter or move, and should not be used when working on the upper face or the periorbital region. Acceptable options include the Cox II shield (Oculo-Plastik, Montreal, Canada), the Stefanovsky shield (Bernsco, Seattle, CA, and others), and the Khan globe protector (Storz, St. Louis, MO). Of special note, plastic corneal protectors may melt when exposed to the CO_2 laser (33) (Figure 1.8). Critics of the metal eye shields argue that they fail to protect the entire superior fornix leaving a portion of the globe vulnerable to injury by the unsuspecting surgeon (34). A potentially safer alternative consists of a large metal blade which is placed between the upper eyelid and the globe and fixed in position by a toothed clamp which is tightened on the upper eyelid. Examples of such devices are the David-Baker (Oculo-Plastik, Byron Instruments, Bernsco) and Khan-Baker eyelid clamps (Storz) (Figures 1.9, 1.10). While these devices offer the advantage of superior protection, they also produce a mild crush injury to the upper eyelid at the loca-

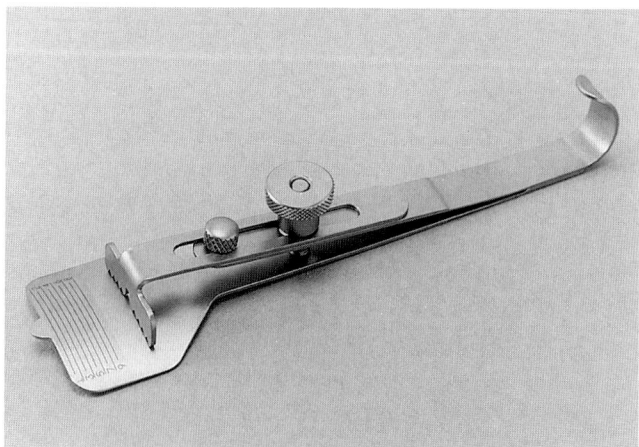

Figure 1.9. A specialized laser eyelid clamp may be used to provide traction and protect the globe (Khan-Baker Laser Eyelid Clamp, Storz Instrument Co., St. Louis, Missouri.)

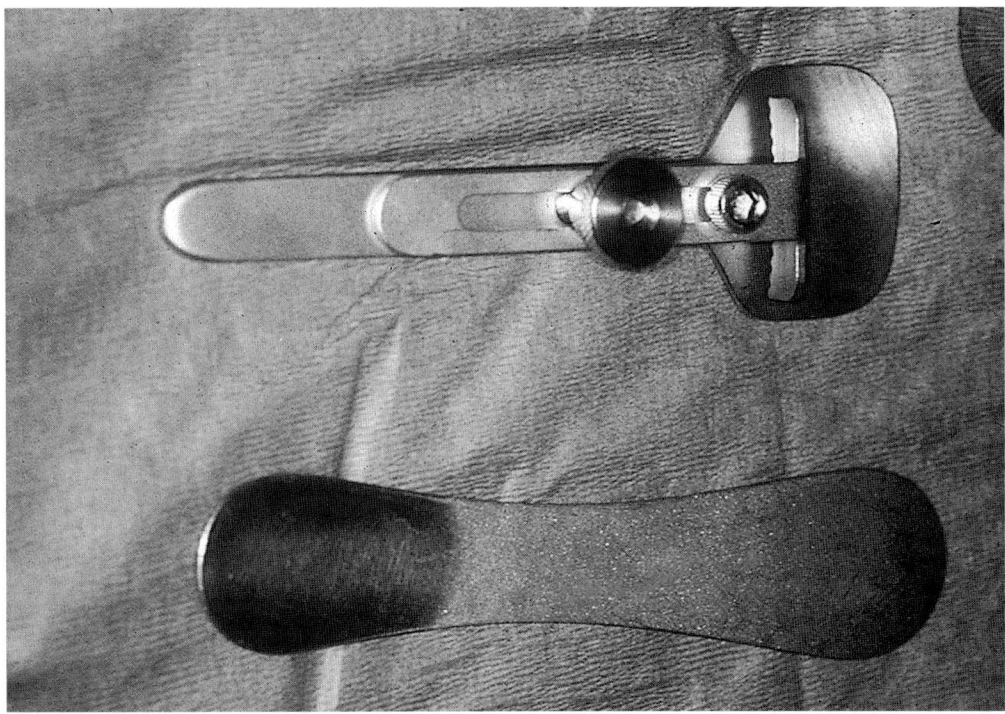

Figure 1.10. David-Baker lid clamp (above) and laser-safe Jaeger plate (below).

ular damage resulting in blindness has been attributed to failure to adequately remove a liquid sterilizing solution from a contact lens that was in place for several hours (Goldwyn R. Personal communication to B. Biesman, September 1996).

When resecting fat tissues or other tissues, a moistened cotton tip applicator, matte-finish Desmarres retractor, metal guard, or hemostat is usually employed to protect distal tissues when transecting eyelid fat pads. Antireflective surfaces reduce the likelihood of injury from reflection of the incisional beam. Hence, most instruments used during a laser procedure do not have a polished surface and are either sand-blasted or anodized to create a matte finish. The cornea may also be burned when performing laser skin resurfacing. The thermal effect of the laser on the cornea can be devastating, especially when using the CO_2 laser. Appropriate eye protection must be used by all personnel within the operating room. Surgical loupes use a double lens system protective against CO_2 and Er:YAG radiation, but laser-safe side shields are recommended. A complete line of laser-safe instrumentation is available from Oculo-Plastik, Montreal, Canada.

Patient Safety

Carbon dioxide laser energy may be reflected off smooth metallic surfaces, but is absorbed by water, biologic tissues, glass, and plastic. All persons within the treatment area should wear protective laser safety glasses. Protective eyewear should be made available outside the door. OSHA standards require posting a sign outside the door indicating that the laser is in use.

WOUND HEALING

Continuous-wave CO_2 laser incisions have less tensile strength than scalpel incisions for the first one to three weeks after surgery, but final wound strength is equivalent (35–37). The delay in wound healing probably results from laser induced thermal injury along the incision edges and the adjacent epidermis. Following injury with a CO_2 skin resurfacing laser, epidermal wounds show a delay of three days in the onset of epidermal migration (38). This delay is believed to result from the eschar of injured tissue that physically impedes epithelialization. Furthermore, injured epidermal cells in the zone of reversible injury may also require time to recover before migrating. The eschar of thermal damage in the dermal and deeper edges of the incision probably impedes healing of the deep wound as well. The efflux of blood-borne macrophages and wound healing factors is reduced because of the laser's hemostatic effect, and further delay is occasioned by the necessity for macrophage influx to clear devitalized tissue. For the aforementioned reasons, eyelid skin sutures are left in longer, usually 7–10 days, in order to avoid wound dehiscence. Another potential risk of laser surgery is an increase in wound infection rates (39). Until the necrotic thermal debris is cleared from the wound, it can act as a nutrient bed for infection.

SUMMARY

Eyelid plastic surgery represents perhaps the most complex surgical laser dissection performed today. Incisional CO_2 laser eyelid surgery may lead the way in revolutionizing the way complex dissection is performed in other surgical fields. In coming years, we may see laser techniques become the accepted norm for eyelid surgery because laser eyelid surgery offers the surgeon rapid and bloodless techniques and benefits the patient with a rapid recovery and diminished swelling and bruising. Though incisional laser surgery holds great promise, one should keep in mind that the laser is merely a tool that simultaneously incises tissue and creates a controlled hemostatic zone of thermal injury. It will not transform poor surgical skills into better surgical results nor does it reduce the need for superb surgical judgement. It is important that surgeons understand how lasers work and how laser energy interacts with tissue so that intraoperative decisions may be made to produce the best possible results while ensuring the safety of our patients and all members of the operating team.

REFERENCES

1. Dover JS, Arndt KA, Geronemus RG, et al. Illustrated Cutaneous Laser Surgery: a practitioners's guide. Norwalk, CT, Appleton and Lange, 1990:2–17.
2. Hobbs ER, Bailin PL, Wheeland RG, et al. Superpulsed lasers: minimizing thermal damage with short duration, high irradiance pulses. J Dermatol Surg Oncol 1987; 13:955–964.
3. Trost MD, Zacherl RN, Smith MFW. Surgical laser properties and their tissue interaction. In: Smith MFW, McElveen JT Jr, eds. Neurological surgery of the ear. St. Louis: Mosby, 1992:131–156.
4. Fuller TA. Laser tissue interaction: the influence of power density. In: Baggish MS, ed. Basic and advanced laser surgery in gynecology. Norwalk, CT: Appleton-Century-Crofts, 1985.
5. Mage G, Pouly JL, Bruhat MA. Laser microsurgery of the oviducts. In: Baggish MS, ed. Basic and advanced laser surgery in gynecology. Norwalk, CT: Appleton-Century-Crofts, 1985.
6. Goldman MP, Fitzpatrick RE. Cutaneous laser surgery: the art and science of selective photothermolysis. St. Louis: Mosby Yearbook, 1994:198–258.
7. Walsh JT Jr, Deutsch TF. Pulsed CO_2 laser tissue ablation: measurement of the ablation rate. Lasers in Surgery and Medicine 1988;8:264–275.
8. Reid R. Physical and surgical principles governing carbon dioxide laser surgery on the skin. Dermatologic Clinics 1991;9:297–316.
9. Fuller TA. Laser tissue interaction: the influence of power density. In: Baggish MS, ed. Basic and advanced laser surgery in gynecology. Norwalk, CT: Appleton-Century-Crofts, 1985.
10. Mihashi S, Jako GJ, Incze J, et al. Laser surgery in otolaryngology: interaction of CO_2 laser and soft tissue. Ann NY Acad Sci 1976;267:264–294.
11. Baggish MS, El Bakhry MM. Comparison of electronically superpulsed and continuous-wave CO_2 laser on the rat uterine horn. Fertility and Sterility 1986;45: 120–127.
12. Fitzpatrick RE, Ruiz EJ, Goldman MP. The depth of thermal necrosis using the CO_2 laser: a comparison of the superpulsed mode and conventional mode. J Dermatol Surg Oncol 1991;17:340–344.
13. Fitzpatrick RE, Goldman MP, Ruiz-Esparza J. Clinical advantage of the CO_2 laser superpulsed mode: treatment of verruca vulgaris, seborrheic keratoses, lentigines, and actinic cheilitis. J Dermatol Surg Oncol 1994;20: 449–456.
14. Dover JS, Hruza GJ. Laser skin resurfacing. Seminars in Cutaneous Medicine and Surgery 1996;15: 177–188.
15. Chernoff WG, Schoenrock LD, Cramer H, et al. Cutaneous laser resurfacing. Int J Aesth Restorative Surg 1995;3:57–68.
16. Chernoff G, Slatkine M, Zair E, et al. Silk touch: a new technology for skin resurfacing in aesthetic surgery. J Clin Laser Med Surg 1995;13:97–100.
17. Anderson RR, Parrish JA. Selective photothermolysis: precise microsurgery by selective absorption of pulsed radiation. Science 1983;220:524.

18. Anderson RR. Laser tissue interactions. In: Goldman MP, Fitzpatrick RE, eds. Cutaneous laser surgery: the art and science of selective photothermolysis. St. Louis: Mosby, 1994:1–18.

19. Warner RR, Morgan NE, Eby TA, et al. Water measurement in biological tissue. In: Romig Ad, Chambers WF, eds. Microbeam Analysis. San Francisco: San Francisco Press, 1986;21:238–240.

20. Green HA, Domankevitz Y, Nishioka NS, eds. Pulsed carbon dioxide laser ablation of burned skin: in vitro and in vivo analysis. Lasers Surg Med 1990;10:475–484.

21. Dover JS, Arndt KA, Geronemus RG, et al. Illustrated cutaneous laser surgery: a practitioner's guide. Norwalk, CT: Appleton & Lange, 1990:15–25.

22. Kaufmann R, Hibst R. Pulsed Erbium:YAG laser ablation in cutaneous surgery. Lasers in Surg and Med 1996;19:324–330.

23. Kaufmann R, Hartmann A, Hibst R. Cutting and skin-ablative properties of pulsed mid-infrared laser surgery. J Dermatol Surg Oncol 1994;20:112–118.

24. American National Standards Institute. American national standards for the safe use of lasers in health care facilities. Standard Z136.3-1996. New York: ANSI Publications 1996.

25. Greco RJ, Gonzalez R, Johnson P, et al. Potential dangers of oxygen supplementation during facial surgery. Plast Reconstr Surg 1995;6:978–984.

26. Lach E. The hazards of using supplemental oxygen. Plast Reconstr Surg 1996;3:566–567.

27. Reyes RJ, Smith AA, Mascaro JR, et al. Supplemental oxygen: ensuring its safe delivery during facial surgery. Plast Reconstr Surg 1995;5:924–928.

28. Pashayan AG, Gravenstein JS. Airway fires during surgery with the carbon dioxide laser. Anesthesiology 1989;71:478.

29. Fontenot R Jr, Bailey BJ, Stiernberg CM, et al. Endotracheal tube safety during laser surgery. Laryngoscope 1987;97(8 pt. 1):919–921.

30. Hirshman CA, Smith J. Indirect ignition of the endotracheal tube during carbon dioxide laser surgery. Arch Otolaryngol 1980;106:639–641.

31. Gloster HM Jr, Roenigk RK. Risk of acquiring human papillomavirus from the plume produced by the carbon dioxide laser in the treatment of warts. J Am Acad Dermatol 1995;32:436–441.

32. Bergbrant IM, Samuelsson L, Olofsson S, et al. Polymerase chain reaction for monitoring human papillomavirus contamination of medical personnel during treatment of genital warts with CO_2 laser and electrocoagulation. Acta Derm Venereol 1994;74:393–395.

33. Riley JR. Safety considerations in the use of the CO_2 laser in facial skin resurfacing. Laser Surg Med 1997;9(supp):61.

34. David LM, Baker SS. David-Baker eyelid retractor. Am J Cosm Surg 1992;9:141–145.

35. Hall RR. The healing of tissues incised by a carbon dioxide laser. Br J Surg 1971;58:222.

36. Buell BR, Schueller DE. Comparison of tensile strength in CO_2 laser and scalpel incisions. Arch Otolaryngol 1983;104:456.

37. Cochrane JPS, Beacon JP, Creasey GH. Wound healing after laser surgery: an experimental study. Br J Surg 1980;67:640.

38. Hashimoto K, Rockwell JR, Epsrein RA. Laser wound healing compared with other surgical modalities. Burns 1973;1:113.

39. Norris CW, Mullarkey MB. Experimental skin incision made with the carbon dioxide laser. Laryngoscope 1982;92:416.

Chapter Two

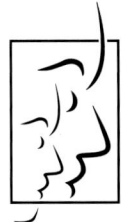

Anatomy of the Eyelid, Forehead, and Temporal Region

Brian S. Biesman

EYELID SOFT TISSUES

The eyelids help to protect the globe from injury and, along with the conjunctiva, play a critical role in maintaining the integrity of the ocular surface. Eyelids blend smoothly with the eyebrows above and the cheeks below and have certain topographical characteristics that bear discussion.

The eyelids are separated by the tarsal plate into orbital and tarsal portions. The upper eyelid crease is formed by the insertion of the anterior portion of the levator aponeurosis into the eyelid skin. Cosmetically important, the upper eyelid also provides an excellent location for eyelid or anterior orbital surgery incisions (1). In the occidental eyelid, the upper lid crease is usually located 8-11 mm above the eyelid margin, and is somewhat higher in women than men. In contrast, the upper lid crease is much lower in the Oriental eyelid due to the low fusion of the orbital septum with the levator aponeurosis (2). In many Oriental patients the upper lid fold will overhang the crease, obscuring it. In the lower eyelid, the crease is less well defined and is formed by the attachment of the orbicularis oculi muscle to the skin. Other folds that may be present in the lower eyelid include the nasojugal fold that slopes inferotemporally from the medial canthus below the lid fold, and the malar fold formed by a prominent cheek, which blends with the nasojugal fold. The upper and lower eyelids become fused at the medial and lateral canthi, and traumatic or involutional disruption of these areas can lead to significant eyelid dysfunction or malposition. The opening between the eyelids is known as the palpebral fissure and averages 10-12 mm in adults: the horizontal distance between the medial and lateral canthi in normal adults is approximately 30 mm (3) (Figure 2.1). The upper and lower eyelids are lined by a double or triple row of eyelashes, short hairs that normally curve away from the eye. Following trauma or other eyelid injury, the lashes may turn toward the globe potentially causing serious disruption of the ocular surface.

The eyelid skin is among the thinnest in the body with little subcutaneous tissue present. Beneath the eyelid skin is found the orbicularis oculi muscle. This muscle is divided into pretarsal, preseptal, and orbital components. The orbital portion blends with the frontalis, procerus, and corrugator supraciliaris muscles of the eyebrow superiorly, and the temporalis and cheek muscles laterally. Medially, the orbital orbicularis fibers arise from the orbital rim (Figure 2.2). The preseptal orbicularis overlies the orbital septum and sends deep fibers to insert on the lacrimal sac (Jones' muscle): the pretarsal orbicularis is just anterior to the tarsal plate, a firm structure composed of condensed collagen that gives structure and support to the eyelids (4). The vertical height of the tarsus is approximately 10 mm in the upper eyelid as compared to 4 mm in the lower lid (5) (Figure 2.3).

At its medial aspect the pretarsal orbicularis splits into superficial and deep heads: the superficial head

15

forming the anterior limb of the medial canthal tendon (MCT) and inserting on the anterior lacrimal crest, and the deep head (Horner's muscle) inserting on the posterior lacrimal crest and contributing to the posterior limb of the MCT. The MCT can play an important role in tightening lax eyelids, especially if a medial ectropion is pres-

ent. Laterally, the pretarsal orbicularis fibers from the upper and lower lids join to form the lateral canthal tendon (LCT). This structure is less well defined than the MCT and inserts onto the lateral orbital tubercle (Whitnall's tubercle), a bony structure several millimeters posterior to the lateral orbital rim. It is important to recognize the normal insertion site of the LCT when performing eyelid shortening procedures as described in Chapter 11. Disruption of either the MCT or LCT will result in marked eyelid malposition and/or canthal deformities. Contraction of the orbicularis muscle results in eyelid closure (6).

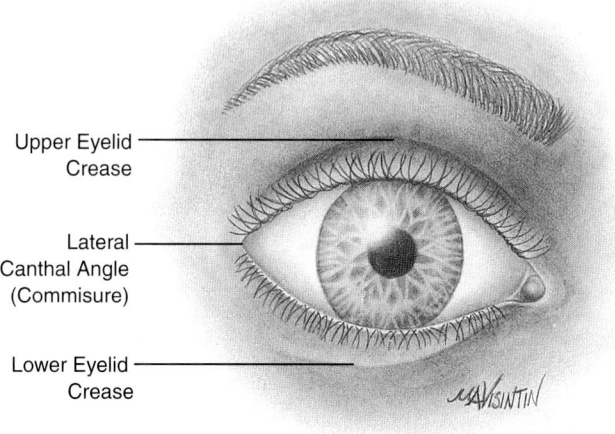

Figure 2.1. Topography and external characteristics of the eyelids. Note the slightly raised position of the lateral canthus, the position of the eyelid margin relative to the corneal limbus, and the position of the eyelid creases. The eyelashes have been omitted from the lower eyelid.

The eyelids are lined by the conjunctiva, a fine, moist mucous membrane that reflects upon itself superiorly and inferiorly, thus forming the superior and inferior fornices before extending onto the globe. It provides a surface conducive to normal ocular function, and disruption of this surface due to trauma or disease can have serious ocular sequelae.

Deep to the orbicularis muscle lies the orbital septum. The septum is a tough fibrous structure that arises from the arcus marginalis at the orbital margin and extends toward the tarsal plates, separating the orbital contents from the eyelids. In the upper eyelid, the orbital septum fuses with the levator aponeurosis prior to their combined insertion onto the anterior surface of the tarsus. In the occidental lid this fusion occurs several mil-

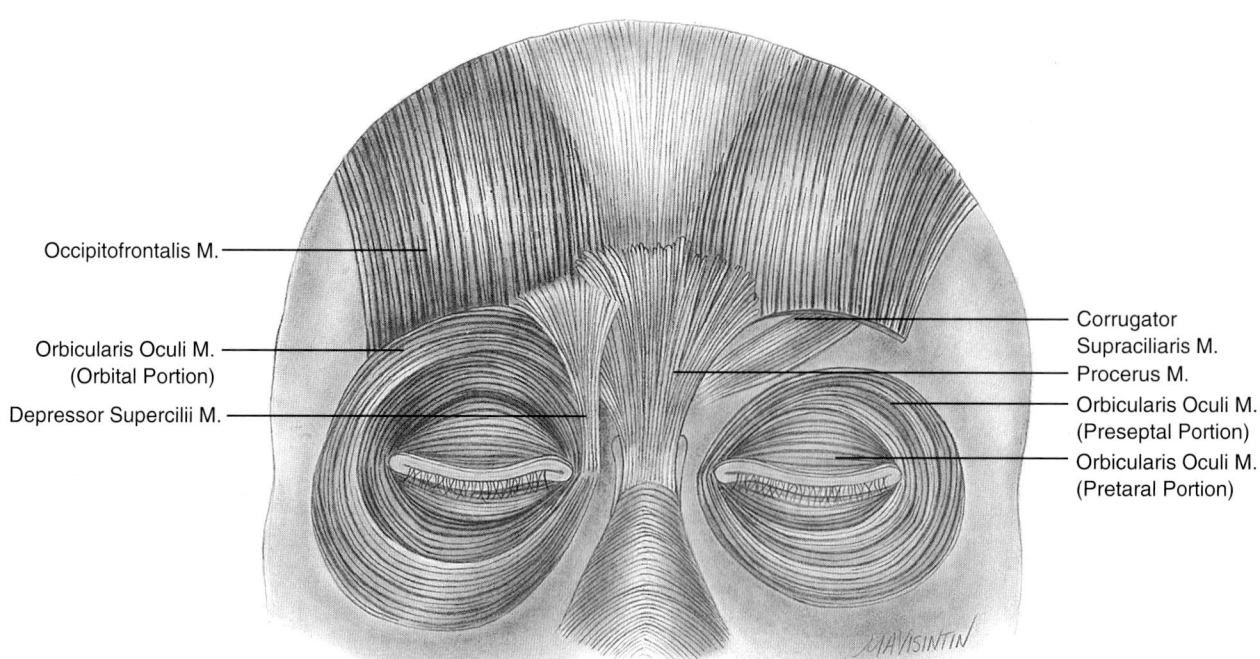

Figure 2.2. Muscles of the periorbital region and forehead.

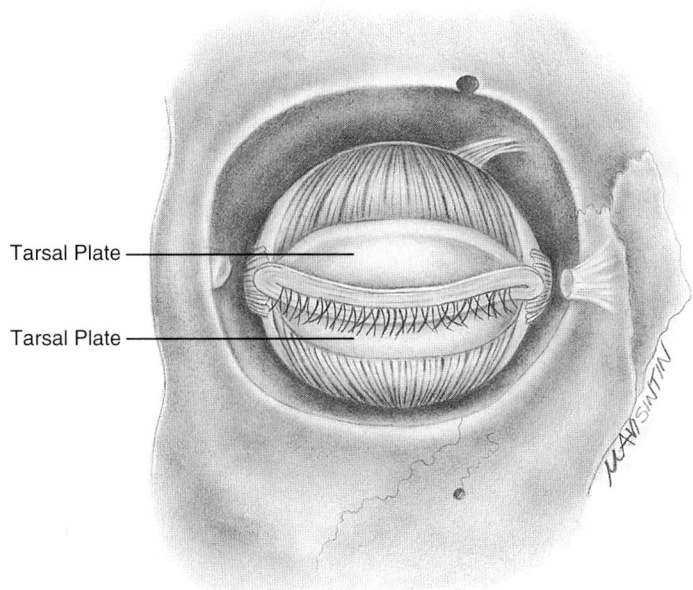

Tarsal Plate

Tarsal Plate

Figure 2.3. The tarsal plates. The upper eyelid tarsus is approximately 2.5 times the height of its lower eyelid counterpart.

limeters above the superior tarsal border: in the Oriental lid it occurs anterior to the tarsal plate. In the lower eyelid, the orbital septum fuses with the lower lid analog of the levator aponeurosis (the capsulopalpebral fascia) prior to inserting on the tarsal plate (7) (Figure 2.4).

Orbital fat is found posterior to the orbital septum. The anterior portion of the orbital fat is usually removed as part of upper and lower blepharoplasty surgery and it is thus important for the aesthetic surgeon to understand the distribution of this fat so as to avoid incomplete fat resection. There are three anterior fat pads in the inferior orbit, but only two in the superior orbit as the lacrimal gland occupies the space corresponding to the lateral fat pad of the lower eyelid (Figure 2.5). In the superior orbit, the central fat pad is always found posterior to the orbital septum and anterior to the levator aponeurosis (8). This fat pad is an extremely useful landmark in eyelid surgery, but care must be taken not to confuse this preaponeurotic fat pad with fatty degeneration of the levator aponeurosis itself, a condition commonly seen in older patients. Failure to make this distinction has led to inadvertent excision of the levator aponeurosis during blepharoplasty surgery. The medial fat pad in the upper and lower eyelids may be separated by fibrous septae into two portions, each of which must be identified (9). The three fat pads of the lower eyelids are found in the medial, central and lateral portions of the lid, respectively.

Asking patients to direct their eyes superiorly during the preoperative evaluation before lower blepharoplasty surgery is important, as lower eyelid fat pads become more apparent in upgaze. The central fat pad is seen most easily in a straight-up gaze, while the medial fat pad is best seen in a superior and lateral gaze, and the lateral fat pad is best seen in a superior and medial gaze. The medial and central fat pads are separated by the inferior oblique muscle, which is often encountered during transconjunctival blepharoplasty (10, 11). Manipulation of this muscle and its fibrous sheath should be avoided during blepharoplasty surgery (12–14). The central and lateral fat pockets are separated by a fibrous structure extending from the inferior oblique muscle to the lateral orbital wall, which is known as the *arcuate expanse of the inferior oblique* (Figure 2.6). As opposed to the inferior oblique muscle, the arcuate expanse may be divided without complications. Although considered a single fat pad by anatomists, clinically the lateral fat compartment is usually separated into two portions: one located more posterior and lateral to the other. The more posterior portion of the lateral fat pad is often missed by inexperienced blepharoplasty surgeons (15–17).

Sensory Innervation

The fifth cranial nerve supplies the sensory innervation of the eyelids, forehead, and midface. It arises from several subnuclei within the brain stem and spinal cord and has three major branches: the ophthalmic, maxillary, and mandibular. The ophthalmic division (V1) travels within the cavernous sinus where it branches into the lacrimal, frontal, and nasociliary nerves. The lacrimal nerve enters the orbit through the superior orbital fissure above the annulus of Zinn and courses along the lateral orbital wall where it is joined by fibers from the zygomatic nerve carrying parasympathetic innervation to the lacrimal gland. The lacrimal nerve then exits the orbit and provides sensory innervation to the skin of the lateral upper eyelid. The frontal nerve, the largest of V1's three branches, also enters the orbit through the superior orbital fissure, traveling along the orbital roof between the levator and the periorbita before dividing into its two terminal branches: the supraorbital and supratrochlear nerves. These nerves exit the orbit to provide innervation to the remainder of the upper eyelid, the brow, and the forehead. The supraorbital and supratrochlear nerves may be anesthetized with a single injection placed in the region of the supraorbital notch to provide excellent anesthesia for brow

LASERS IN FACIAL AESTHETIC AND RECONSTRUCTIVE SURGERY

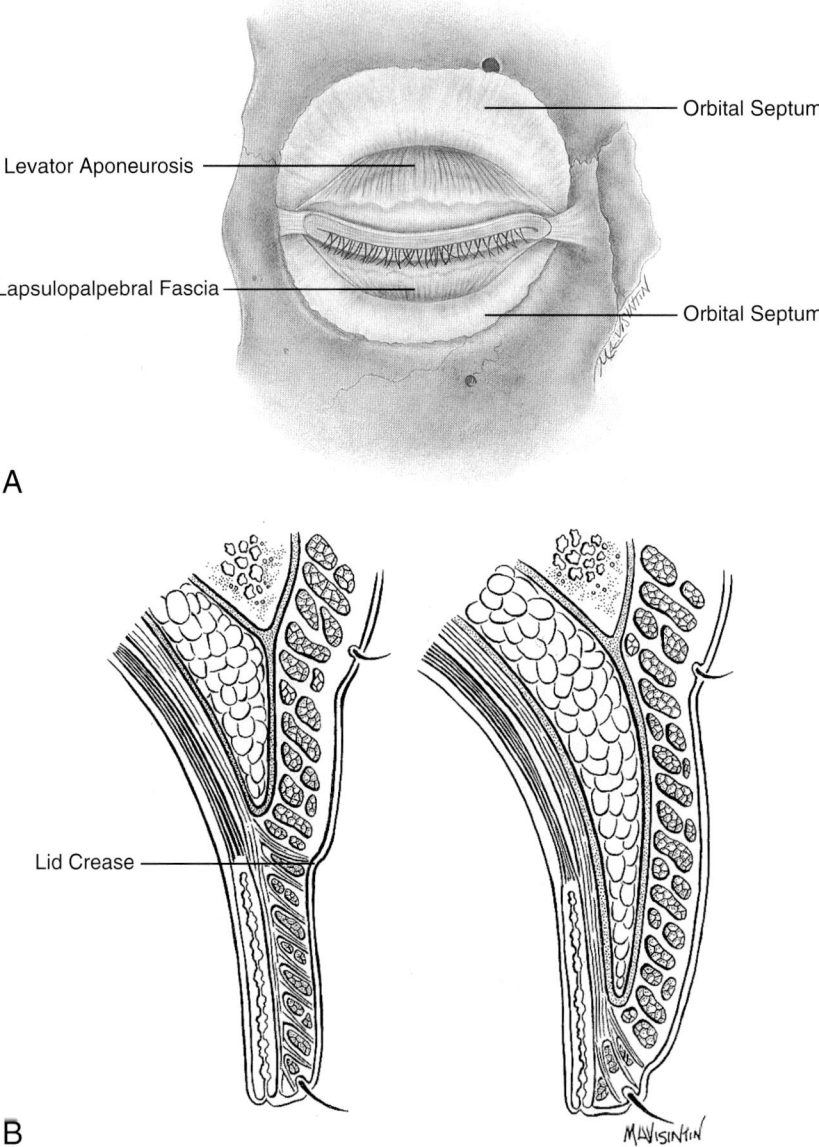

Figure 2.4. A. The orbital septum as observed in the occidental eyelid. **B.** Sagittal view comparing occidental eyelid (left) to Asian eyelid (right). The orbital septum and preaponeurotic fat extend further inferiorly in the Asian eyelid than the occidental eyelid. The eyelid crease is located just above the superior tarsal border in the occidental lid and is absent in the Asian lid.

lifting or skin resurfacing. The third division of V1 is the nasociliary nerve. It also enters the orbit through the superior orbital fissure and then travels along the medial orbital wall where it produces the anterior and posterior ethmoidal nerves before terminating as the infratrochlear nerve. The infratrochlear nerve exits the orbit to supply sensory innervation to the lacrimal sac, conjunctiva, and skin of the medial canthal region (Figure 2.7).

The maxillary division of the trigeminal nerve (V2), provides sensory innervation to the cheek and side of the face, lower eyelid, lateral aspect of the nose, upper lip, and upper teeth via the infraorbital, zygomaticotemporal, and zygomaticofacial, nerves. The infraorbital nerve exits the maxilla through the infraorbital foramen, approximately 7-10 mm inferior to the zygomaticomaxillary suture, nearly directly below the supraorbital notch (foramen), where it divides into four branches: the inferior palpebral, external and internal nasal, and superior labial. A bony prominence overlies the superior portion of the infraorbital foramen, protecting the nerve from trauma. When

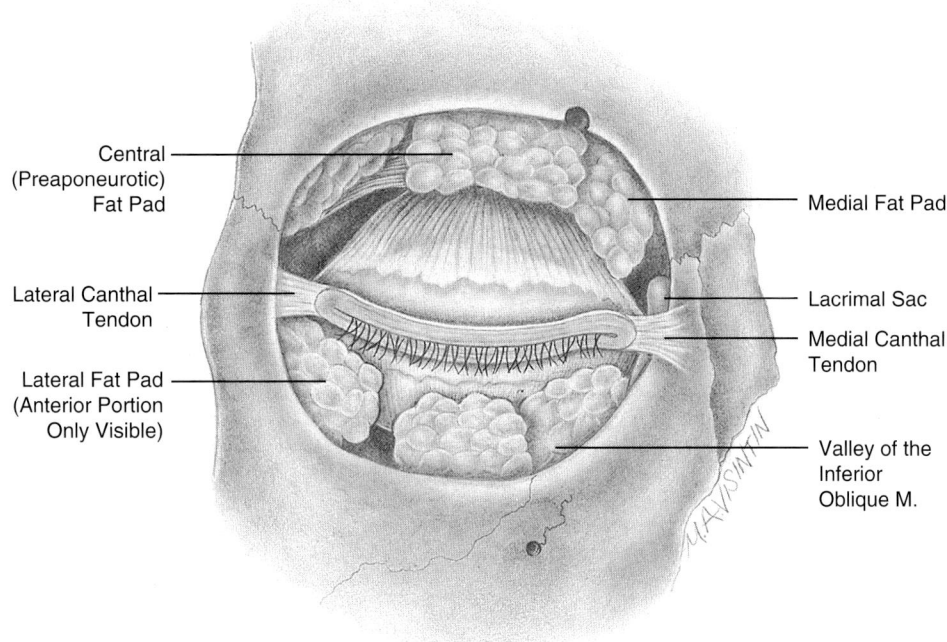

Central
(Preaponeurotic)
Fat Pad

Lateral Canthal
Tendon

Lateral Fat Pad
(Anterior Portion
Only Visible)

Medial Fat Pad

Lacrimal Sac

Medial Canthal
Tendon

Valley of the
Inferior
Oblique M.

Figure 2.5. Schematic representation of the anterior orbital fat pads. The fat pads in the upper lid have been displaced superiorly to demonstrate their relationship to underlying structures.

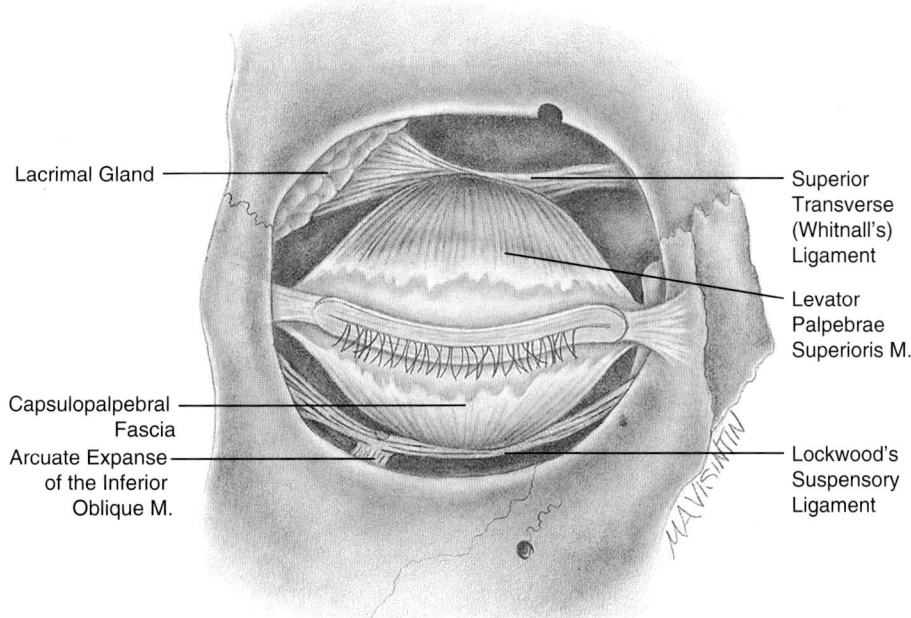

Lacrimal Gland

Capsulopalpebral
Fascia
Arcuate Expanse
of the Inferior
Oblique M.

Superior
Transverse
(Whitnall's)
Ligament

Levator
Palpebrae
Superioris M.

Lockwood's
Suspensory
Ligament

Figure 2.6. The upper and lower eyelid retractors and their respective suspensory ligaments.

administering an infraorbital nerve block, anesthesia is most complete when the nerve is approached inferiorly via the gingival buccal mucosa. This approach allows the anesthetic access to all branches of the nerve, including those protected by the bony prominence (18). Anesthesia of the zygomaticotemporal and zygomaticofacial divisions of V2 does not provide suitable anesthesia of the skin due to crossover innervation with branches of V3.

The third division of the trigeminal nerve (V3) has both motor and sensory components. The motor branch of V3 supplies the muscles of mastication; a more detailed discussion of these branches is beyond the scope of this text. There are four clinically important sensory branches to the mandibular nerve: the auriculotemporal, buccal, lingual, and inferior alveolar nerves. Sensory innervation of the lateral cheek skin is provided by the auriculotempo-

ral and buccal nerves. However, regional blockade of these nerves does not provide adequate sensory anesthesia to permit skin resurfacing due to coinnervation by branches of the greater auricular and anterior cutaneous nerves arising from cervical nerves C2 and C3. Direct infiltration remains the most reliable means of achieving adequate anesthesia of the lateral cheek. The mental nerve, a terminal branch of the inferior alveolar, supplies sensory innervation to the skin of the lower lip and chin. A regional blockade of the mental nerve is an easily accomplished, effective means of anesthetizing these areas for skin resurfacing. The lingual nerve innervates only intraoral structures and will not be discussed in detail (19) (Figure 2.8).

While a complete discussion of the autonomic nerve supply of the face is beyond the scope of this chapter, at

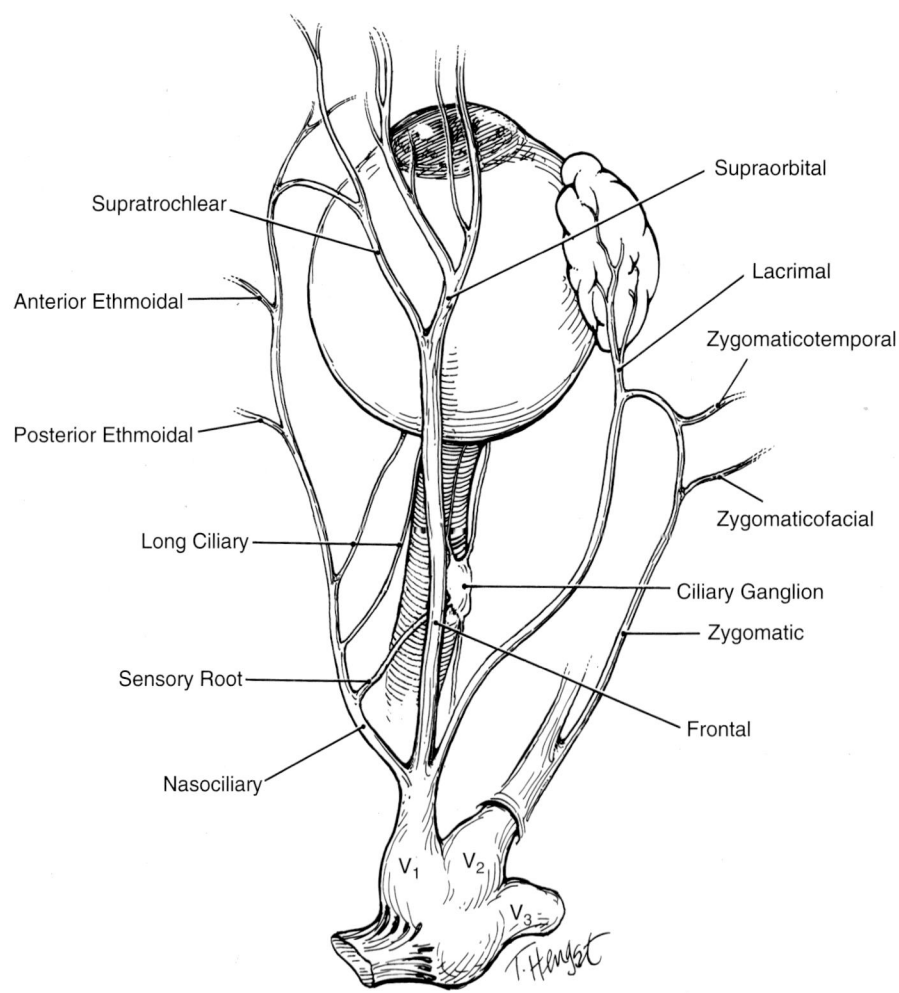

Figure 2.7. The proximal course of the first two divisions of the trigeminal nerve. These divisions supply the forehead, periorbital region, and midface. (Reprinted with permission from Dr. M.T. Doxanas. Appeared originally in Doxanas and Anderson clinical orbital anatomy. Baltimore: Williams & Wilkins, 1984.)

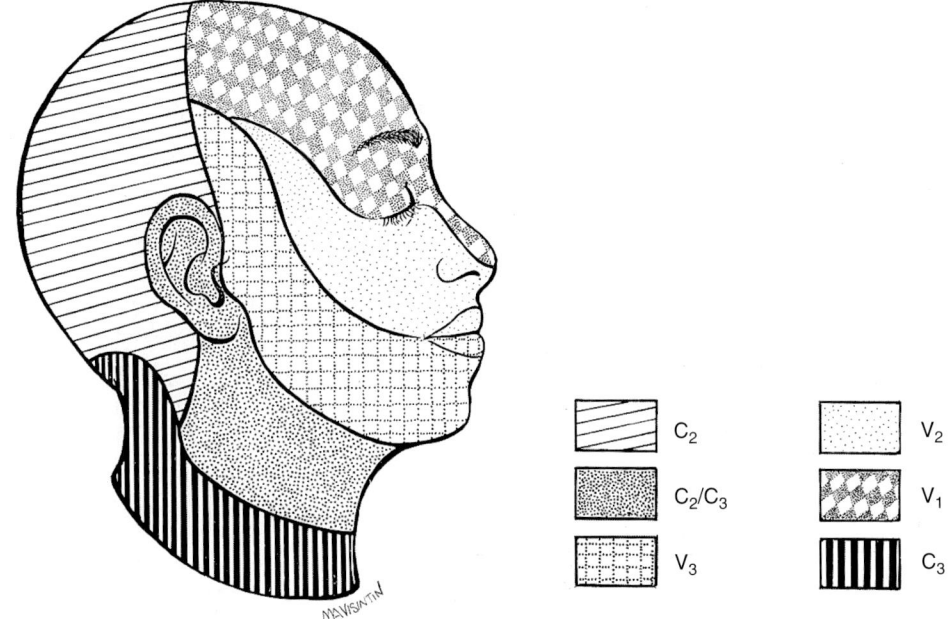

Figure 2.8. Sensory innervation of the face and forehead. C= cervical nerves, V= trigeminal nerves.

least two important clinical correlates of interest to the aesthetic surgeon should be noted. First, the parasympathetic nerve fibers, which control pupillary constriction, are carried to the globe with the nerve to the inferior oblique muscle. When administering local anesthesia through the conjunctiva (as for transconjunctival blepharoplasty), if the needle is directed too far posteriorly pupillary dilation may occur. This is a harmless condition that resolves as the anesthetic effect wears off, but can be the cause of great anxiety to surgeons unfamiliar with it. To understand the second important clinical situation in which the autonomic nervous system is involved requires recognition that sympathetic fibers supplying the orbit innervate the iris dilator muscle and Müller's muscle, a retractor of the upper and lower lids. Interruption of ocular sympathetics results in blepharoptosis (drooping of the eyelid) from lack of innervation of Müller's muscle, miosis (small pupil) from loss of innervation to the iris dilator, and sometimes anhydrosis (loss of sweating). This constellation of symptoms is known as Horner's syndrome and patients with this condition may present primarily to the aesthetic surgeon for the evaluation of ptosis (20).

EYELID RETRACTORS

The levator palpebrae superioris originates from the lesser wing of the sphenoid and passes anteriorly above the superior rectus muscle until it becomes tendinous approxi-

mately 10 mm posterior to the orbital septum. The tendon then passes anteriorly and inferiorly to insert on the anterior, superior third of the tarsus and on the skin, thus forming the eyelid crease. Prior to its insertion on the tarsus, the levator tendon fuses with the orbital septum. The levator receives support from the insertion of its medial and lateral extensions (known as horns) that insert on the posterior lacrimal crest and lateral orbital tubercle, respectively. The lateral horn of the levator muscle divides the lacrimal gland into its orbital and palpebral lobes. Whitnall's ligament is a special modification of the levator muscle. This fibrous structure acts as a check/suspensory ligament preventing excessive posterior movement of, and providing mechanical support for, the levator. The orientation of the muscle fibers changes in the region of Whitnall's ligament from anterior-posterior to superior-inferior. It is an important landmark in eyelid surgery and in repairing severely traumatized lids (21). The lower eyelid analog of Whitnall's ligament is Lockwood's suspensory ligament. Lockwood's ligament is a fibrous structure formed by fascial contributions from Tenon's capsule, the intermuscular septum, and the capsulopalpebral fascia. It inserts laterally at the lateral retinaculum, a structure consisting of the LCT, lateral horn of the levator aponeurosis, Lockwood's ligament, and the check ligament of the lateral rectus muscle (22) (Figure 2.6).

Müller's superior tarsal muscle is the only orbital muscle that is not formed by striated muscle; it is formed by smooth muscle. It arises from the posterior aspect of the levator muscle near Whitnall's ligament and is found

Figure 2.9. Bilateral lacrimal gland enlargement producing fullness in the lateral portion of the upper eyelids.

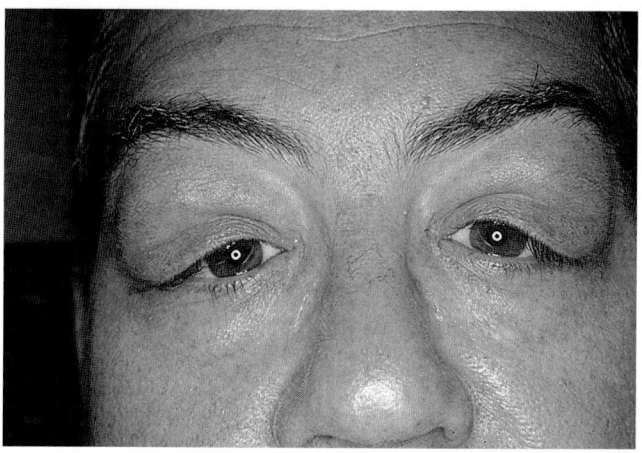

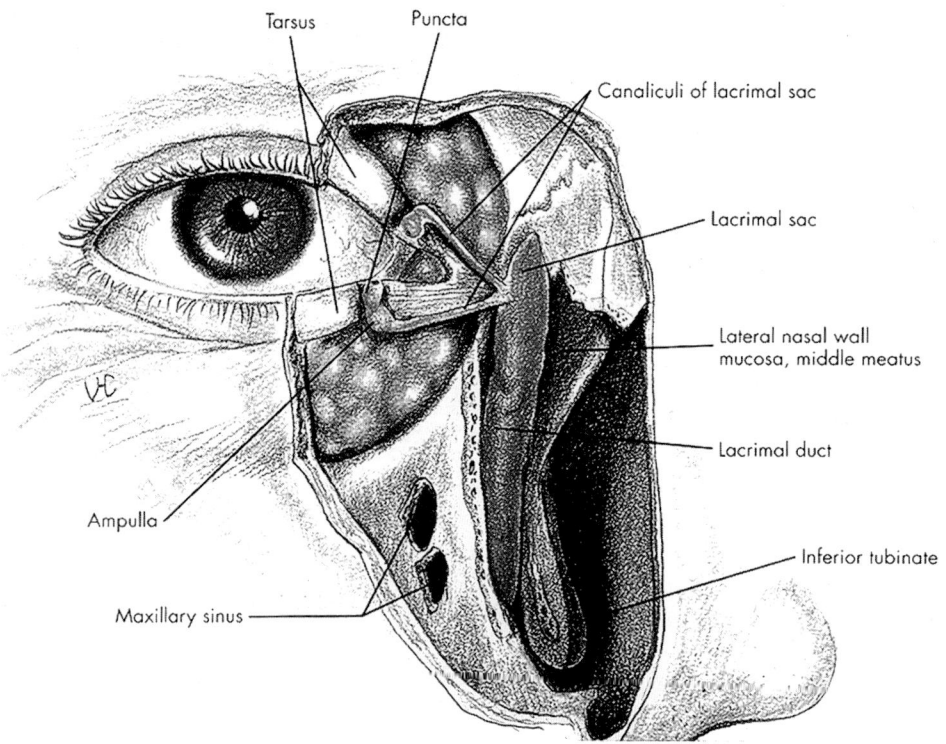

Figure 2.10. Lacrimal excretory system. (Reprinted with permission from Nesi FA, Lisman RD, Levine MR, eds. Smith's ophthalmic plastic and reconstructive surgery, 2nd ed. St. Louis: Mosby, 1998.)

between the conjunctiva and levator aponeurosis. It inserts onto the superior tarsal border and acts as a protractor of the lid. It has a lower lid counterpart that is often less well defined. In both upper and lower lids, Müller's muscle is sympathetically innervated (23).

The primary retractor of the lower eyelid is known as the capsulopalpebral fascia (CPF). The CPF arises from fascia surrounding the inferior rectus muscle, continues an-

teriorly where it splits to surround the inferior oblique muscle, and then fuses again to form Lockwood's suspensory ligament, the lower eyelid analog of Whitnall's superior transverse ligament found in the upper eyelid. Anterior to Lockwood's ligament, the CPF continues superiorly where it has three insertions: the deepest layer inserts into Tenon's layer of connective tissue surrounding the globe, the central, main layer inserts onto the inferior tarsal border, and the most superficial layer fuses with the orbital septum approximately 5 mm below the inferior tarsal border. The external most portion of the CPF is the lower lid analog to the levator aponeurosis. In contrast to the levator, because of the relative lack of movement of the lower eyelid, the CPF may be divided without adverse sequelae (24). This fact is used to the surgeon's advantage when performing transconjunctival blepharoplasty.

THE LACRIMAL SYSTEM

The lacrimal system can be divided, for the purpose of description, into secretory and excretory components. Together these components produce a tear film that adequately moisturizes and maintains the external ocular surface.

The lacrimal secretory system is composed primarily of the accessory and main lacrimal glands. The accessory lacrimal glands are found within the conjunctiva: Krause's glands are found in the fornices, and Wolfring's glands near the tarsal border. A greater number of accessory lacrimal glands are found in the superior than the inferior fornix. The accessory lacrimal glands are believed to be responsible for baseline tear production (25).

The main lacrimal gland lies within the lacrimal fossa in the superolateral orbit. It is divided into a larger superior (orbital) and a smaller inferior (palpebral) lobe by the lateral horn of the levator aponeurosis. The orbital lobe may prolapse into the central portion of the upper eyelid where it may be confused with preaponeurotic fat and excised by the unsuspecting surgeon (Figure 2.9).

The lacrimal excretory system drains tears from the eye in a regulated way so that the ocular surface is kept moist while preventing spillovers onto the eyelids and cheeks. Along the upper and lower eyelid margin, approximately 5 mm from the medial canthal angle, are elevated nipple-like lacrimal papillae. Each papilla represents the opening into the lacrimal canaliculus, an epithelial-lined structure that serves as a conduit for tears from the external surface of the eye to the lacrimal sac. The lacrimal canaliculi have a vertical component measuring about 2 mm and a horizontal component measuring about 8 mm (25, 26). In a normally functioning system, tears flow from the canaliculi into the lacrimal sac and then through the nasolacrimal duct, before exiting beneath the inferior turbinate (Figure 2.10). The punctae and canaliculi may be damaged during eyelid surgery. Upper blepharoplasty incisions generally should not ex-

tend below a point 4-5 mm above the superior punctum, or medial to a line drawn vertically through the superior lacrimal punctum to avoid a medial canthal band or "web" formation. Conjunctival incisions must be made at least 3 mm below the lid margin in the medial portion of the eyelid to avoid damage to the lacrimal canaliculus.

ANATOMY OF THE FOREHEAD AND TEMPORAL REGION

Understanding the anatomy of the forehead and temporal region is particularly important to the aesthetic surgeon as actinic damage and rhytids of the skin, eyebrow ptosis, and deep horizontal forehead furrows are common patient complaints. These problems are best treated when the surgeon has complete knowledge of their etiology and anatomic basis.

The scalp is generally considered to have five layers, the outer three functioning as a unit. These layers may easily be remembered with the mnemonic SCALP. From superficial to deep the layers are as follows: skin, subcutaneous tissue, aponeurosis (galea), loose areolar tissue, and periosteum. The skin of the forehead and temporal region is usually relatively thick, rich in sebaceous glands, and may be treated aggressively during laser skin resurfacing. However, in some elderly patients the skin of the temporal forehead, lateral to the frontalis muscle, may be quite thin and consequently requires a greater degree of care during resurfacing. The muscles of the forehead and scalp are covered by a layer of subcutaneous fascia. This fascia supports superficial nerves and vessels and is thinner on the forehead than the scalp. Laterally, this fascia has a deep layer known as the temporalis fascia. Above the temporal lines on each side of the skull from the superior nuchal line to the supraorbital ridges the deep fascial layer is absent, creating a space containing only loose areolar tissue. The aponeurotic layer consists of the epicranial aponeurosis, which is a tendinous sheet extending from the medial supraorbital ridge to the medial two thirds of the superior nuchal line. It is attached laterally to the superficial temporal fascia. The galea aponeurotica is continuous with the occipitofrontalis muscle at its anterior and posterolateral borders. The periosteal layer of the scalp represents the pericranium covering the outer surface of the skull bones. The pericranium is elevated quite easily in most areas but is tightly adherent to the superior orbital rim where it must be released completely to achieve adequate forehead and eyebrow elevation (27-29).

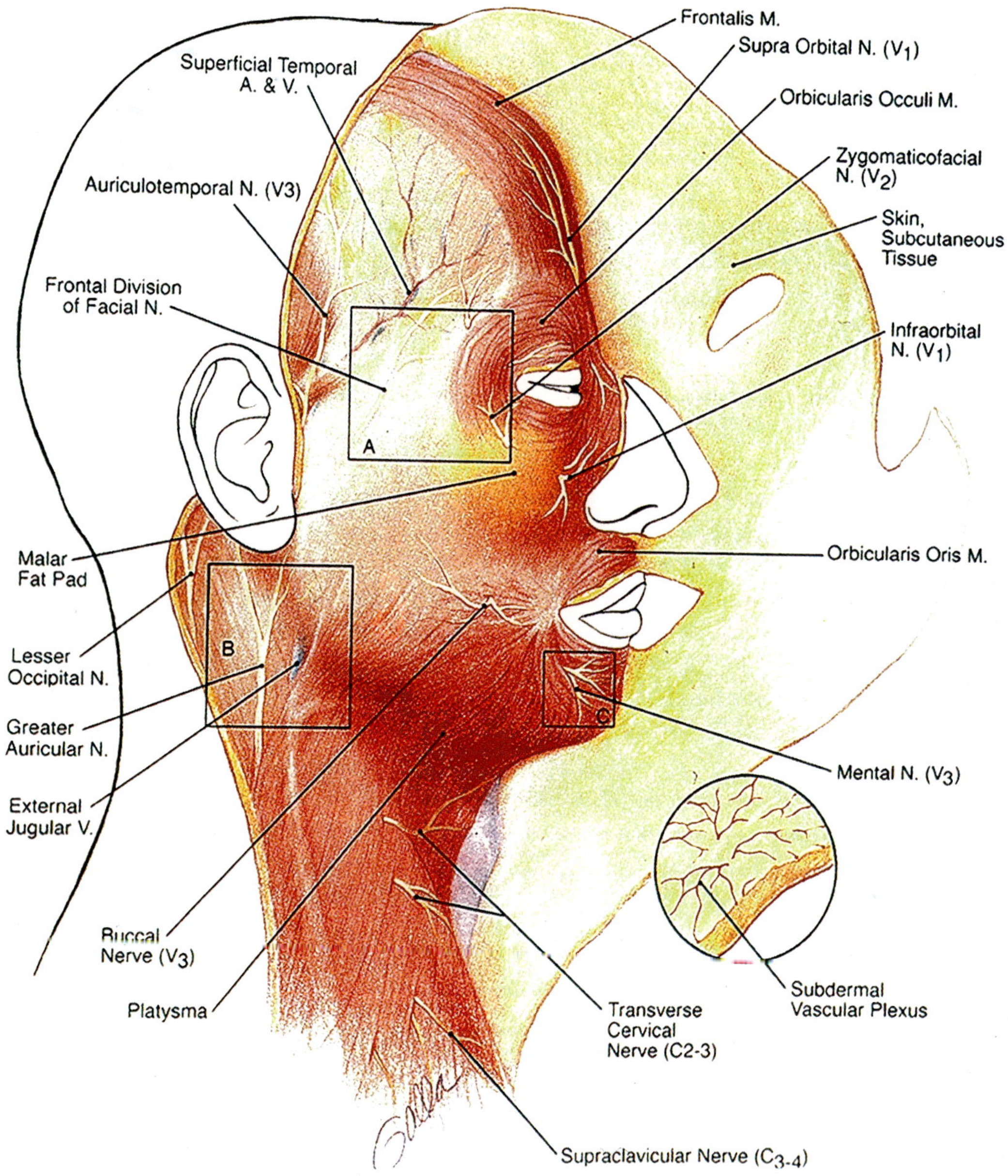

Figure 2.11. Superficial anatomy of the face highlighting structures pertinent to the aesthetic surgeon. (Reprinted with permission from Cheney ML. Facial surgery. Plastic and reconstructive. Baltimore: Williams & Wilkins, 1997.)

MUSCLES OF THE FOREHEAD

The primary elevator of the forehead is the occipitofrontalis muscle, a fibrous muscular sheet composed of two muscle bellies joined through an aponeurotic tissue. It arises posteriorly at the superior nuchal line of the occipital bone and extends anteriorly to insert deeply into the forehead skin. The occipitofrontalis muscle fuses laterally with the orbicularis oculi muscle and superficial temporal fascia, medially with the procerus muscle (and occasionally the frontal belly of the contralateral occipitofrontalis muscle), and inferiorly with the corrugator, depressor supercilii, and orbicularis oculi muscles. Contraction of the occipitofrontalis muscle as a whole results in elevation of the eyebrows with the development of horizontal creases in the forehead. The occipital belly contracts to allow movement of the galea over the periosteum. The frontal belly of the occipitofrontalis muscle is innervated by the temporal branch of the facial nerve and the occipital belly is innervated by the largest branch of the posterior auricular nerve (Figure 2.11).

The depressors of the forehead include the procerus, corrugator, and orbicularis oculi muscles. The procerus muscle is a pyramid-shaped muscle that travels in the same plane as the frontal belly of the occipitofrontalis, but is innervated by buccal branches of the facial nerve. It arises from tendinous fibers and fascia overlying the inferior portion of the nasal bone and the superior lateral portion of the nasal cartilage, and inserts into the skin and subcutaneous tissue between the eyebrows. Contraction of the procerus muscle results in pulling down of the medial eyebrow and wrinkling of the nasal skin in a transverse fashion. The corrugator supercilii muscle arises from the medial orbital rim and may be pyramidal or linear in shape. It inserts into the skin of the medial portion of the eyebrow and its contraction produces a vertical wrinkling of the forehead. The supraorbital neurovascular bundle often travels through the corrugator muscle. Motor innervation to the corrugator supercilii is carried by the temporal and zygomatic branches of the facial nerve. Contraction of the corrugator muscle draws the head of the eyebrow medially and downward. The orbicularis oculi muscle has been described above. It is innervated by the temporal and zygomatic branches of the facial nerve and acts in conjunction with the corrugator supercilii and procerus muscles to counteract the action of the occipitofrontalis muscle (30).

The supraorbital notch is found lateral to the corrugator muscle, at approximately the junction of the medial and middle thirds of the superior orbital rim. In some patients, the "notch" will actually be a foramen completely surrounded by bone. The notch transmits the supraorbital nerve and the supraorbital artery and vein. The supraorbital nerve courses on the undersurface of the frontalis muscle and galea, and supplies sensation to the central and lateral forehead. The supratrochlear nerve also emerges from the medial orbit in the region of the orbital rim. This nerve passes within the corrugator muscle and may be damaged if the corrugator is resected or ablated. Care should be taken to avoid injury to the supraorbital and supratrochlear nerves as the numbness and dysesthesias that may result are quite bothersome to patients.

ANATOMY OF THE TEMPORAL REGION

The temporal region is also considered to have five layers: the skin, superficial temporal or temporoparietal fascia, loose areolar tissue, deep temporal or temporalis muscle fascia, and temporalis. Lateral to the occipitofrontalis muscle, the galea aponeurotica is continuous with the superficial temporal or temporoparietal fascia, an extension of the SMAS. This fascial plane is fixed firmly to the skin and subcutaneous tissue above the level of the zygoma, and contains the superficial temporal artery and vein as well as the temporal branch of the facial nerve. Inferiorly as the zygoma is approached, the superficial temporal fat pad will be encountered. This fat pad often contains branches of the facial nerve and should be elevated from the underlying temporalis fascia if necessary. The temporoparietal fascia inserts on the zygomatic arch. The temporalis fascia is separated from the temporoparietal fascia by a layer of loose areolar tissue, which may be separated easily with blunt dissection. The temporalis fascia splits into superficial and deep layers, which are separated by the superficial temporal fat pad. When performing endoscopic brow elevation, dissection in this region may be accomplished either just above or just below the superficial layer of temporalis fascia, but should not extend into the superficial temporalis fascia. The deep fat pad is found deep to the deep layer of temporalis fascia. In the temporal crest region, the deep temporal fascia is adherent to periosteum and the galea fuses with the superficial temporal fascia. Dissection in this region should always be performed in a temporal-to-central direction to avoid injury to the frontal branch of the facial nerve (29, 31) (Figures 2.12, 2.13).

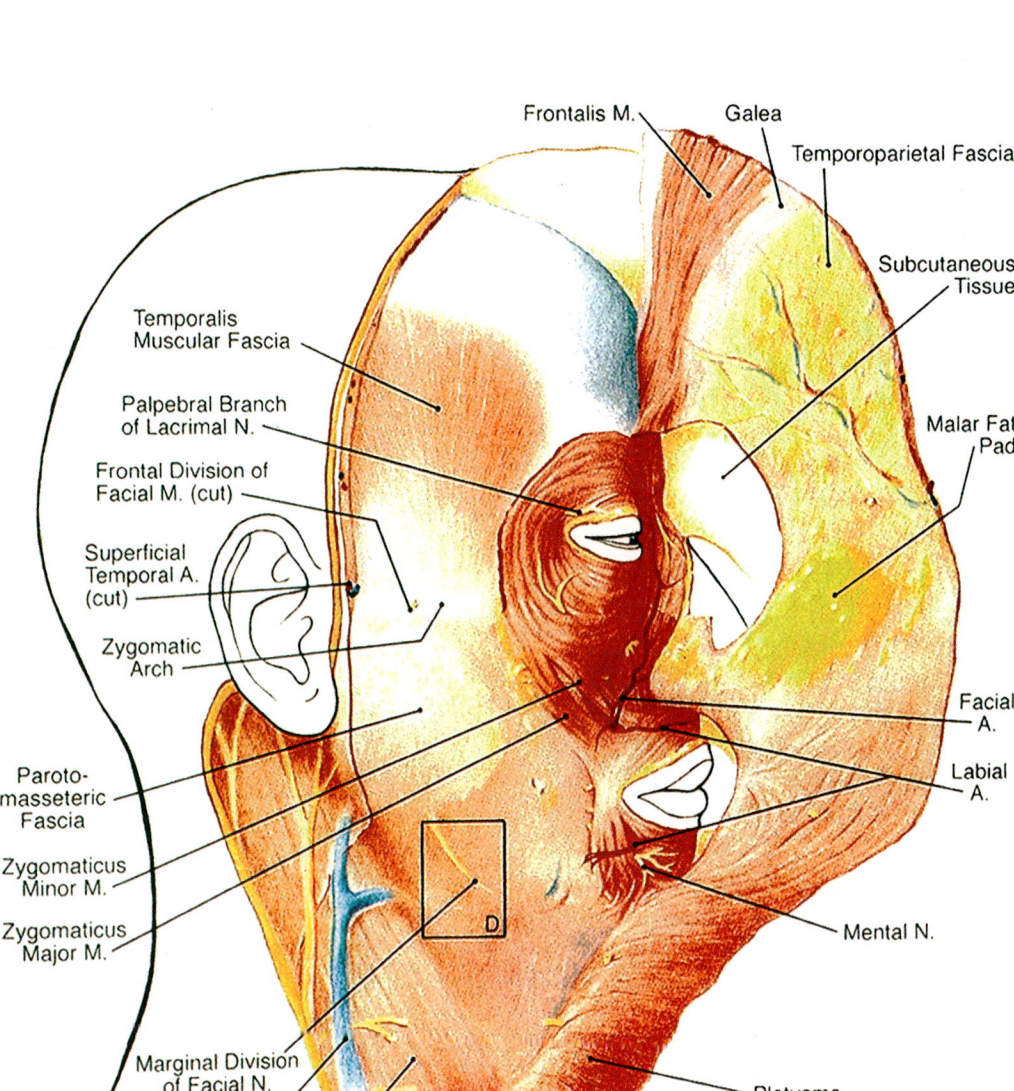

Figure 2.12. Deep anatomy of the temporal region. The superficial layer has been elevated. Note the position of the malar fat pad. (Reprinted with permission from Cheney ML. Facial surgery. Plastic and reconstructive. Baltimore: Williams & Wilkins, 1997.)

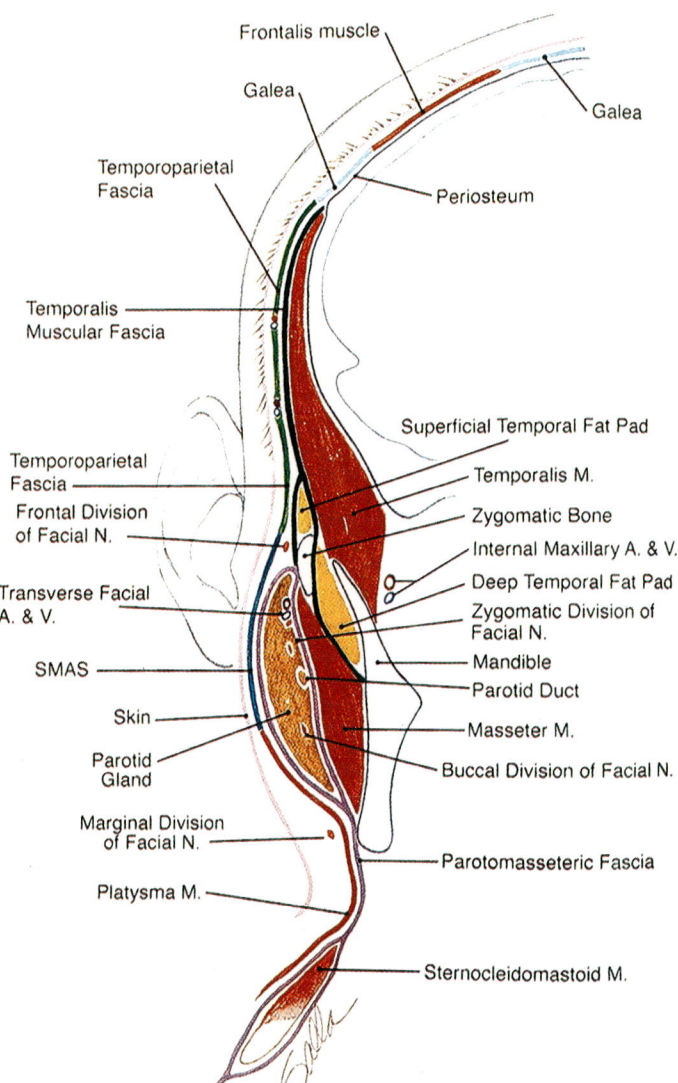

Figure 2.13. Coronal view of temporal region demonstrating important structures and their spatial relationships. (Reprinted with permission from Cheney ML. Facial surgery. Plastic and reconstructive. Baltimore: Williams & Wilkins, 1997.)

Frontalis muscle

Galea

Galea

Temporoparietal Fascia

Periosteum

Temporalis Muscular Fascia

Superficial Temporal Fat Pad

Temporoparietal Fascia

Temporalis M.

Frontal Division of Facial N.

Zygomatic Bone

Internal Maxillary A. & V.

Transverse Facial A. & V.

Deep Temporal Fat Pad

Zygomatic Division of Facial N.

SMAS

Mandible

Parotid Duct

Skin

Masseter M.

Parotid Gland

Buccal Division of Facial N.

Marginal Division of Facial N.

Parotomasseteric Fascia

Platysma M.

Sternocleidomastoid M.

REFERENCES

1. Anderson RL, Beard C. The levator aponeurosis attachments and their clinical significance. Arch Ophthalmol 1997;95:1437.
2. Aguilar GL, Nelson C. Eyelid and anterior orbital anatomy. In: Hornblass AH, ed. Oculoplastic orbital and reconstructive surgery. Baltimore: Williams & Wilkins, 1988;1:4.
3. Callahan M, Beard C, eds. Beard's ptosis, 4th ed. Birmingham, AL: Aesculapius Publishing, 1990.
4. Sires BS, Lemke BN, Kincaid MC. Orbital and ocular anatomy. In: Wright KW, ed. Textbook of ophthalmology. Baltimore: Williams & Wilkins, 1997:10–11.
5. Wesley RE, McCord CD, Jones NA. Height of the tarsus of the lower eyelid. Am J Ophthalmol 1980;90:102.
6. Doxanas MT, Anderson RL. Clinical orbital anatomy. Baltimore: William & Wilkins, 1984.
7. Putterman AM, Urist MJ. Surgical anatomy of the orbital septum. Ann Ophthalmol 1974;8:339.
8. Clemente CD. Anatomy: a regional atlas of the human body. Baltimore: Urban & Schwarzenberg, 1981: Fig. 591.
9. Ullmann Y, Levi Y, Ben-Izhak O, et al. The surgical anatomy of the fat in the upper eyelid medial compartment. Plast Reconstr Surg 1997;99:658–61.
10. Lemke BN, Lucarelli MJ. Anatomy of the ocular adnexa, orbit and related facial structures. In: Nesi FA, Lisman RD, Levine MR, eds. Smith's ophthalmic plastic and reconstructive surgery, 2nd ed. St. Louis: Mosby, 1997: 18–19.

11. Zarem HA, Resnick JL. Expanded applications for trans-conjunctival lower lid blepharoplasty. Plast Reconstr Surg 1991;88:215-220.

12. Hayworth RS, Lisman RD, Muchnick RS, et al. Diplopia following blepharoplasty. Ann Ophthalmol 1984;16:448-451.

13. Harley RD, Nelson LB, Flanagan JC, Calhoun JH. Ocular motility disturbances following cosmetic blepharo-plasty. Arch Ophthalmol 1986;104:542-544.

14. Jameson NA, Good WV, Hoyt CS. Fat adherence simulating inferior oblique palsy following blepharoplasty. Arch Ophthalmol 1992;110:1369.

15. Doxanas MT. Minimally invasive lower eyelid blepharo-plasty. Ophthalmology 1994;101:1327-1332.

16. Putterman AM. The mysterious second temporal fat pad. Ophthal Plast Reconstr Surg 1985;1:83-86.

17. Palmer FR III, Rice DH, Churukian MM. Transconjuncti-val blepharoplasty. Complications and their avoidance: a retrospective analysis and review of the literature. Arch Otol-Head & Neck Surg 1993;119:993-999.

18. Rosenberg M, Yagiela J. Maxillary anesthesia: increasing the success of injection techniques. Westborough, MA: Astra USA, 1997 (video).

19. Miller NR, ed. Walsh and Hoyt's clinical neuro ophthal-mology, 4th ed. Baltimore: Williams & Wilkins, 1983;2.

20. Thompson HS, Mensher JH. Horner's syndrome. Am J Ophthalmol 1974;78:739.

21. Anderson RL, Beard C. The levator aponeurosis attach-ments and their clinical significance. Arch Ophthalmol 1977;95:1437.

22. Hawes MJ, Dortzbach RK. The microscopic anatomy of the lower eyelid retractors. Arch Ophthalmol 1982;100:1313.

23. Beard C. Mullers superior tarsal muscle: anatomy, physi-ology, and clinical significance. Ann Plast Surg 1985;14:324.

24. Hawes MJ, Dortzbach RK. The microscopic anatomy of the lower eyelid retractors. Arch Ophthalmol 1982;100:1313.

25. Jones LT. The lacrimal secretory sytem and its treat-ment. Am J Ophthalmol 1966;62:47.

26. Iwamoto T, Jakobiec FA. Lacrimal glands. In: Duane TD, Jaeger EA, eds. Biomedical foundations of ophthalmol-ogy. Philadelphia: Harper & Row, 1988;1.

27. Hollingshead WH, ed. The head and neck. Anatomy for surgeons. Hagerstown, MD: Harper & Row, 1968;3.

28. Larrabee WF Jr, Makielski KH. Surgical anatomy of the face. New York: Raven Press, 1993.

29. Cheney ML. Facial surgery. Plastic and reconstructive. Baltimore: Williams & Wilkins, 1997.

30. Abramo AC. Anatomy of the forehead muscles: the basis for the videoendoscopic approach in forehead rhytidoplasty. Plast Reconst Surg 1995:7:1170-1177.

31. Owsley JQ. Aesthetic facial surgery. Philadelphia: WB Saunders, 1994.

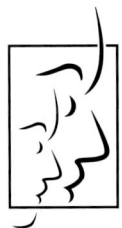

Chapter Three

Anatomy and Physiology of the Skin

Christine M. Hayes

The skin is the largest organ system of the body. It provides many functions: temperature regulation, immunologic surveillance, sensory reception, and serves as a barrier between a person and the environment. The skin consists of the outer keratinocytic layer, the epidermis, and the connective tissue layer, the dermis. The subcutaneous tissue is often directly below the dermis, however, in some areas, such as the periorbital skin, the dermis overlies muscle. The skin also contains appendiceal structures such as hair, sebaceous glands, eccrine glands, apocrine glands, and nails.

EPIDERMIS

The epidermis is the outermost layer of the skin. The thickness of the epidermis is 0.04–1.5 mm in thickness as compared with the total thickness of skin, which is 1.5–4.0 mm (1). The epidermis is a stratified, squamous epithelium, largely made up of continually replicating keratinocytes. The squamous epithelium also produces the skin appendages: hair, nails, sweat, and sebaceous glands.

The epidermis is primarily composed of ectodermally-derived keratinocytes that produce filamentous proteins called keratins. These proteins are of low molecular weight in the basal and germinative layers, and a higher weight in the stratum spinosum and granular layers. The cells in the stratum corneum, the outermost layer of the epidermis, are dead and continually sloughed and re-placed. Other cells present in the epidermis are melanocytes, Merkel cells and Langerhans cells, which migrate into the epidermis during development.

The epidermis is organized into layers, which have different functional activities and represent various levels of differentiation. As the cells differentiate, proteins involved in keratinization are synthesized: coordinated degradation of cellular organelles occurs. This leads to the final stage of the keratinocytes, programmed cell death. The terminally differentiated keratinocyte is composed of proteins and lipids, and is nonviable. Differentiation is a highly controlled sequence of events, which is susceptible to change. Disorders of keratinization can lead to a disease state and regulation of this process is critically important.

The epidermis rests on the basement membrane, a structure that provides support and acts as a semi-permeable interface between the epidermis and dermis. Its components are from the basal keratinocytes and the dermal fibroblasts. The basal keratinocytes contribute hemidesmosomes, anchoring filaments, lamina densa, and the lamina lucida. The dermal fibroblasts contribute the anchoring fibrils. The hemidesmosome is a specialized junction between the basal keratinocytes and the lamina densa, from which the anchoring filaments extend. The lamina densa is primarily made up of Type IV collagen and functions as a barrier and filter to macromolecules. The lamina lucida is a clear zone that contains many glycoproteins including laminin, bullous pemphigoid antigen, and fibronectin, all of which are important in promoting adhesion between the epidermal cells and the lamina densa. Separation of the epidermis and dermis is seen in bullous pemphigoid when autoantibodies to the bullous pemphigoid antigen result in cleavage at the lamina lucida (2). Anchoring fibrils are short, broad fibers which begin at the lamina densa and extend into the papillary dermis with its collagen fibrils.

The epidermal layers from the basement membrane to the outermost layer consist of the stratum germinativum, the stratum spinosum, the stratum granulosum and the stratum corneum (Figure 3.1A, B).

The stratum germinativum is also called the basal layer. It is composed of basal cells, which are situated on the basement membrane, are mitotically active, and are arranged perpendicular to the stratum corneum. The basal cells divide and produce the cells of the other layers. Transit time to the layer of the stratum corneum is roughly 14 days and through the stratum corneum and desquamation requires another 14 days. The basal cells are connected to the basement membrane via hemidesmosomes and to other keratinocytes via desmosomes. The keratin filaments in basal cells are lower-weight, intermediate filaments arranged in bundles around the nucleus, and in hemidesmosomes and desmosomes. The keratin filaments provide structural support to the cells. They also contain microtubules and microfilaments (actin, myosin and α-actinin), which assist in upward cell migration. The large nucleus has a prominent nucleolus, and the cytoplasm contains organelles including rough endoplasmic reticulum, Golgi bodies, mitochondria, lysosomes, ribosomes, and melanosomes, which have been transferred from melanocytes.

The stratum spinosum gets its name from the spiny-like processes apparent on routinely stained tissue. The spines represent desmosomes, which provide cell-to-cell attachment (3). Cell-to-cell adhesion is accomplished by desmosomes, tight junctions, and gap junctions. None are permanent structures but develop and disappear to allow keratinocyte movement. Desmosomes are present in all layers but are more apparent in this layer. Spinous cells contain keratin filaments of a higher molecular weight in addition to the low molecular weight keratins. The keratins are present around the rounded nucleus and the desmosomes. The cells in the upper spinous layers are larger and flatter and contain organelles including rough endoplasmic reticulum, Golgi bodies, mitochondria, lysosomes, and ribosomes. New organelles, lamellar granules, begin to appear in the upper spinous layer, which contain sugars conjugated to protein and lipid, other lipids, and hydrolases including acid phosphatase. The function of the lamellar granule is unclear. Involucrin, a cystine-rich protein, is produced in the spinous layer.

The stratum granulosum is named for the obvious granules noted on routine histologic examination. These basophilic granules, called keratohyalin granules, are composed of a precursor form of the histidine-rich protein, filaggrin. Conversion of profilaggrin to filaggrin is thought to occur during the transition of the granular cells to the cornified cells. Filaggrin is felt to function as a protein that embeds and may promote the aggregation of keratin filaments. Involucrin is concentrated and cross-linked in the granular layer. Keratin filaments of the granular layer have a higher molecular weight subunit as compared with the lower weight keratins present in the lower layers.

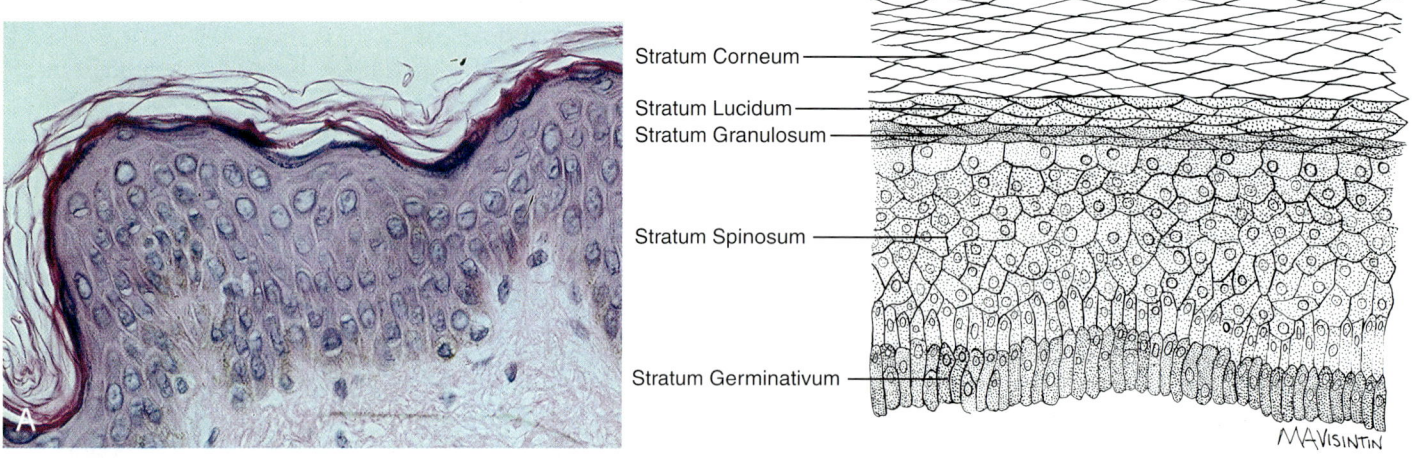

Figure 3.1. A, B. Photomicrograph and diagram demonstrating normal epidermis with the stratum germinativum, stratum spinosum, stratum granulosum and stratum corneum.

Transition from the granular layer to cornified layers involves a few steps. The lamellar granules aggregate in groups, fuse with the plasma membrane and, by exocytosis, release their contents into the intercellular space. The nucleus, organelles, and most cellular contents are lost, resulting in flat, dead keratinocytes, which make up the stratum corneum. The stratum corneum provides the major barrier of the skin. These large, cornified cells are flat and overlapping at the lateral margins. They primarily consist of high-molecular-weight keratins, filaggrin, and organelle remnants. The cells, joined by modified desmosomes, appear to align in columns (stacking). Stacking has been shown to correlate with trans-epidermal water loss.

Keratinocytes have remarkable endocytic and phagocytic capacities. During wound healing after injury, keratinocytes can engulf cellular debris, fibrin, and other materials. Nondigestible materials are carried into the stratum corneum where they are eventually desquamated. The extracellular compartment of the epidermis contains the surface coats of the apposing membranes of adjacent keratinocytes, which provide intercellular stability and cohesion and binds water to allow passage of water-soluble substances.

Complex and varied factors exist that may play a role in the regulation of epidermal growth and differentiation: multiple extrinsic factors can affect the proliferation, growth and differentiation of the keratinocytes. These include epidermal growth factor (EGF), transforming growth factors -α and -β (TGF-α, TGF-β), keratinocyte growth factor (KGF), keratinocyte-derived cytokines (IL-1α, IL-6, IL-8, GM-CSF), and hormones: estrogen, progesterone, and adrenalin, and vitamin A and other retinoids (1). The dermis also has regulatory effects on epidermal thickness and organization. Intrinsic factors, which can have effects on proliferation, include chalones and cyclic nucleotides such as prostaglandins. Chalones are hormone-like and produced by the cells on which they act.

The regulation of keratinization is important, and when altered may result in a disease state. Known disorders of keratinization include psoriasis and the ichthyoses.

RESIDENT EPIDERMAL CELLS

The vast majority of cells in the epidermis are keratinocytes, which are ectodermally derived and discussed in detail above. Other cells found in the epidermis include melanocytes, Merkel cells, and Langerhans cells. These cells arrive either during embryonic development or postnatally and interact with the keratinocytes.

Melanocytes are derived from neural crest tissue and are confined to the basal layer. Approximately one for every nine keratinocytes, they have an oval nucleus, pale cytoplasm, and an organelle, the melanosome, which contains pigment called melanin. The size of the melanosome is genetically determined and larger in black skin. Melanosomes transfer pigment to the keratinocytes, where it is distributed primarily through the basal layer. Within the keratinocyte, the melanosomes exist individually or in aggregates.

Merkel cells are from either neural crest tissue or ectoderm. They have pale cytoplasm with a lobulated nucleus and are present in the basal layer in various regions of the body including the digits, lips, regions of the oral cavity, and in touch domes, specialized structures involved in touch. They contain an organelle, a granule, with metenkephalin-like contents. Merkel cells are slow-adapting, type I mechanoreceptors.

Langerhans cells are derived from precursor cells in the bone marrow, migrate into the epidermis from the circulation early in development, and continue to repopulate the epidermis throughout life. Dendritic cells found in the basal, spinous and granular layers of the epidermis, they account for approximately 4% of the total number of epidermal cells. They are pale staining with a convoluted nucleus and contain a characteristic, tennis racket shaped Birbeck granules, which may be seen on the ultrastructural level. Langerhans cells are responsible for the recognition, uptake, processing and presentation of specific antigens to resident cutaneous T-cell lymphocytes. They are involved in the production of cytokines and other cellular mediators, express on the cell surface receptors for the Fc portion of IgG and C3b component of complement, and synthesize and express Ia antigen. Langerhans cell activity is decreased by ultraviolet radiation therefore decreasing immune surveillance. Langerhans cells are important in immunosurveillance and play an important role in contact dermatitis and skin graft rejection.

Indeterminate cells are a cell population that resemble Langerhans cells but lack Birbeck granules. Their function is unclear but are felt to be related to Langerhans cells.

DERMIS

The dermis is the connective tissue layer of the skin. It lies immediately below the epidermis and contains the skin appendages: hair follicles, sebaceous glands, eccrine glands, apocrine glands, smooth muscle fibers and nails, also the blood vessels, lymph channels and nerve bundles. The dermis consists of connective tissues such as collagen and elastin in a ground substance milieu.

Connective Tissue of the Dermis

Collagen and elastin account for most of the fibrous connective tissue of the dermis. Nonfibrous components of the connective tissue include the glycosaminoglycans and glycoproteins. Collagen makes up about three quarters of the dry weight of skin and provides both tensile strength and elasticity to the dermis. Collagen is made of fibrous proteins organized into bundles. There are various types of collagen (Table 3.1). Type I collagen makes up 80–85% of collagen in adult skin and Type III collagen 15–20%. Type I collagen provides tensile strength and extensibility while Type III collagen provides support and compliance. Blood vessels, the basement membrane zone, nerves, and smooth muscle are surrounded by a basal lamina made of Type IV collagen.

The assembly of collagen is highly organized. Three collagen chains make up a collagen molecule. The collagen molecules are then processed first intra- and then extra-cellularly before being cross-linked in the extracellular space and then assembled into collagen fibrils. The fibrils then organize into larger fiber bundles, which then organize into interwoven layers. Abnormalities in collagen biosynthesis have been described in a few types of Ehlers-Danlos syndrome. These patients have soft, thin, hyperextensible skin as well as hyperextensible joints, vascular fragility, and delayed wound healing with poor scars.

Elastic fibers form a network in the dermis and provide elasticity to the skin. Elastic fibers are also found in:

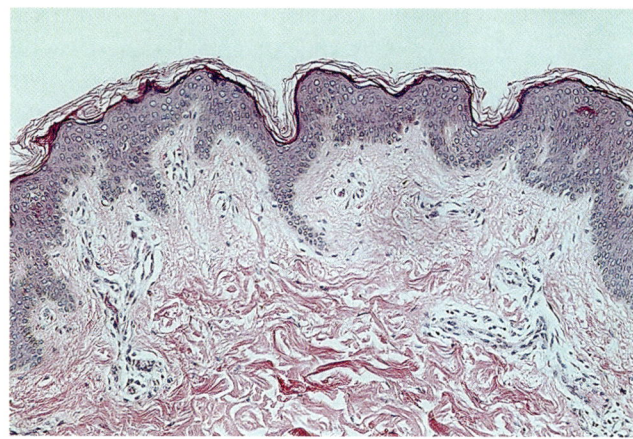

Figure 3.2. Photomicrograph demonstrating the thin, fibrillar papillary dermis immediately below the epidermis with the reticular dermis below.

blood vessel walls, lymphatic walls, hair follicle sheaths, eccrine and apocrine sweat glands. Elastic fibers account for about 1–2% of the dry weight of the dermal proteins. Elastic fiber assembly begins with the synthesis of microfibrils, which are laid in a pattern and fastened together with an elastin matrix. Fully formed elastic fibers are 90% elastin. Elastic fiber bundles border the collagen bundles. Abnormal elastic fibers are seen in patients with pseudoxanthoma elasticum, a disease that affects the skin, eyes and blood vessels. On the skin, yellow, chicken-skin like patches are seen on the neck, antecubital fossae and axillary folds.

Other molecules in the dermis include glycosaminoglycans and glycoproteins, which make up the ground substance. In adult skin, the major glycosaminoglycans are hyaluronic acid and dermatan sulfate; the minor glycosaminoglycans are chondroitin 4-sulfate and chondroitin 6-sulfate. The glycoprotein fibronectin ensheathes collagen bundles and the elastic network, among other roles.

Dermal Organization

The dermis has two components, the papillary dermis and the reticular dermis. The papillary dermis is immediately below the epidermis and basement membrane zone and is roughly the same thickness as the epidermis. The reticular dermis is below this, and extends to the subcutis, making up the bulk of the dermis (Figure 3.2). The dividing line between the papillary dermis and the reticular dermis is identified by a horizontal subpapillary plexus of arterioles and postcapillary venules.

TABLE 3.1 Collagen types

Collagen Type	Tissue Distribution
I	Skin, bone, tendon
II	Cartilage, vitreous
III	Fetal skin, blood vessels, intestine
IV	Basement membranes
V	Ubiquitous
VI	Aortic intima, placenta
VII	Amnion
VIII	Cell cultures of endothelial cells

The papillary dermis is primarily made of Type III collagen with a small amount of Type I collagen and fibronectin. Active fibroblasts are present along with microfibrillar elastic fibers and many capillaries, which supply both the papillary dermis and the epidermis.

The reticular dermis is primarily made of Type I collagen organized into large bundles. Type III collagen and fibronectin are part of a network that integrates the collagen bundles. The elastic fibers and collagen bundles get increasingly larger in size as they extend down toward the subcutaneous tissue.

RESIDENT DERMAL CELLS

Many cells exist in the dermis including fibroblasts, macrophages and mast cells. They are found in higher density in the papillary dermis, but are present in the reticular dermis.

The fibroblast is mesenchymal in origin and is responsible for the synthesis of collagen and elastic fibers in normal skin and healing wounds. Fibroblasts migrate to a wound site in response to cytokines. Fibroblasts also synthesize and secrete collagenase and gelatinase, which break down collagen fibrils.

Macrophages arise from precursor cells in the bone marrow, which differentiate into monocytes in the blood, and then terminally differentiate into macrophages in the tissue. Macrophages have cell surface receptors for the Fc portion of IgG and C3b component of complement and can process and present specific antigens to immunocompetent lymphoid cells. They are involved in the production of enzymes, cytokines and other cellular mediators and contain lysosomal enzymes. They are important in healing wounds to phagocytize bacteria and injured tissue and promote angiogenesis (4).

Mast cells are bone-marrow-derived cells present in the dermis, but especially around the blood vessels. They are recognized by their dark staining intracytoplasmic granules, which are both secretory and lysosomal. The secretory granules contain various vasoactive and chemotactic mediators, while the lysosomal granules contain degradative enzymes. They are perceived to be necessary for normal wound healing.

APPENDICEAL STRUCTURES

Hair Follicles

The hair follicle and its associated structures are complex in their organization and development. In early develop-

ment, three bulges are present on the surface of the hair follicle: the lowest bulge becomes the attachment of the arrector pilorum, the next bulge becomes the sebaceous gland, and the third bulge develops into an apocrine gland or involutes. Anatomically, the hair follicle is divided into three parts: the deepest portion starts at the base of the follicle and ends at the insertion of the arrector pilorum, the second portion, or isthmus, extends from the insertion of the arrector pili muscle to the duct of the sebaceous gland, the third, or infundibulum, begins at the sebaceous gland and ends at the skin surface. The hair follicle and sebaceous gland develop together and function as a unit. The hair follicle consists of an inner and outer root sheath, which are vital to the regrowth of epidermal skin after wounding (Figure 3.3).

The appearance of the hair follicle changes as the hair cycles through the anagen, catagen and telogen stages. The anagen stage is the stage of active hair growth and lasts three years, catagen, the phase of regression, lasts three weeks, and telogen, the resting period, lasts

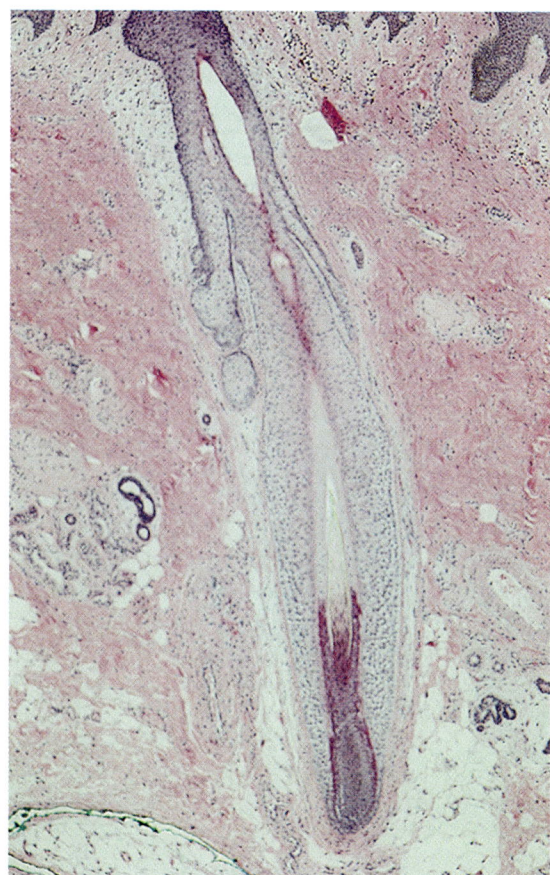

Figure 3.3. Photomicrograph demonstrating a hair follicle with the inner and outer root sheaths evident along with sebaceous glands.

about three months (4). Melanocytes are present in the basal layer of the hair matrix and produce melanosomes, which are responsible for hair color. Three types of melanosomes are possible, resulting in the various hair colors. In gray or white hair the melanocytes are absent or decreased in number.

The hair follicle is a critical structure in the regrowth of the epidermis after wounding as keratinocytes migrate from the follicle to repopulate the epidermis.

Sebaceous Glands

Sebaceous glands are present on all skin except on the palms and soles. The meibomian gland of the eyelid is a specialized sebaceous gland. Sebaceous glands may have one or more lobules and are found in association with hair follicles or, occasionally, may occur freely (Figure 3.3). They are well developed at birth, atrophy at a few months, and increase in size at puberty in response to androgens. They are considered to be holocrine glands as the secretion is composed of cell decomposition. The cellular fragments are lipid-rich and are composed of triglycerides, phospholipids, esterified cholesterol, and waxes (4). They secrete the contents (sebum) via a duct into the follicular structure at the junction of the isthmus and infundibulum. Obstruction of sebum secretion results in acneiform lesions (acne).

Eccrine Sweat Glands

Eccrine glands are secretory sweat glands found everywhere on the skin except the lips, nail beds, labia minora and glans penis. More prevalent on the palms, soles and axillae, they are important in thermoregulation. The eccrine glands are made of the secretory portion, a coiled tubule in the deep reticular dermis or subcutis (Figure 3.4A, B). From this the intradermal duct, a straight tubule, ascends and conducts the secreted sweat toward the skin surface. The epidermal duct, called the acrosyringium, then enters the epidermis, and reassumes a spiral pattern to end in a sweat pore at the skin surface. Eccrine sweat is composed of sweat, sialomucin, and glycogen. Obstruction of eccrine sweat secretion results in miliaria or heat rash.

Apocrine Sweat Glands

Apocrine sweat glands are scent glands and are only present in the axillae, anogenital region, and mammary glands. Specialized apocrine sweat glands exist in the eyelid (Moll's glands) and in the external ear canal (ceruminous glands). Apocrine glands, as compared with eccrine glands, are fewer, larger, and found deeper in the dermis or subcutis. Their organization is similar to eccrine glands. Apocrine secretion consists of protein, carbohydrate, am-

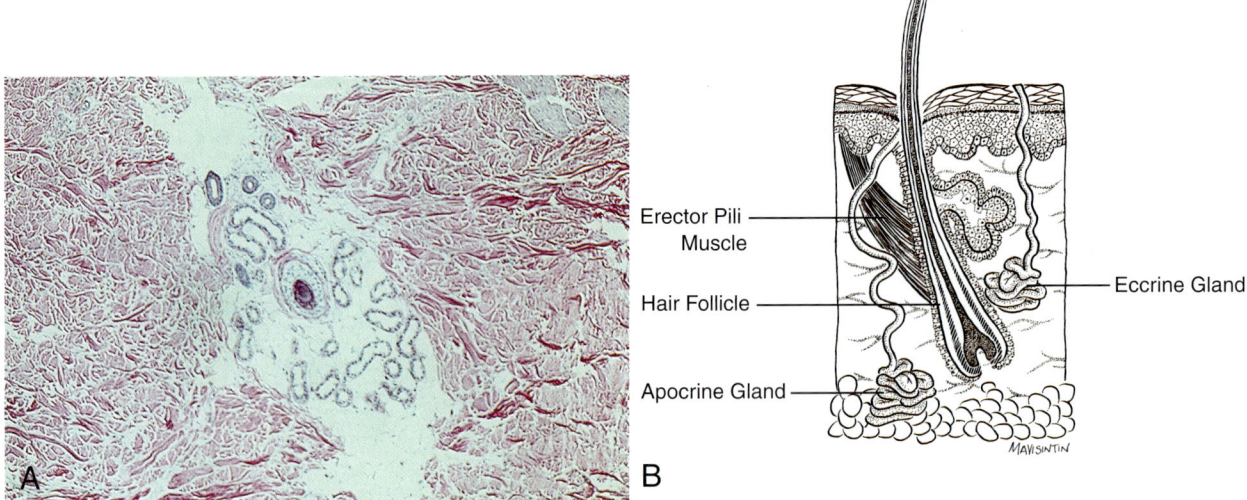

A   B

Erector Pili Muscle

Hair Follicle

Apocrine Gland

Eccrine Gland

Figure 3.4. A, B. Photomicrograph and diagram demonstrating eccrine ducts and glands surrounding a hair follicle.

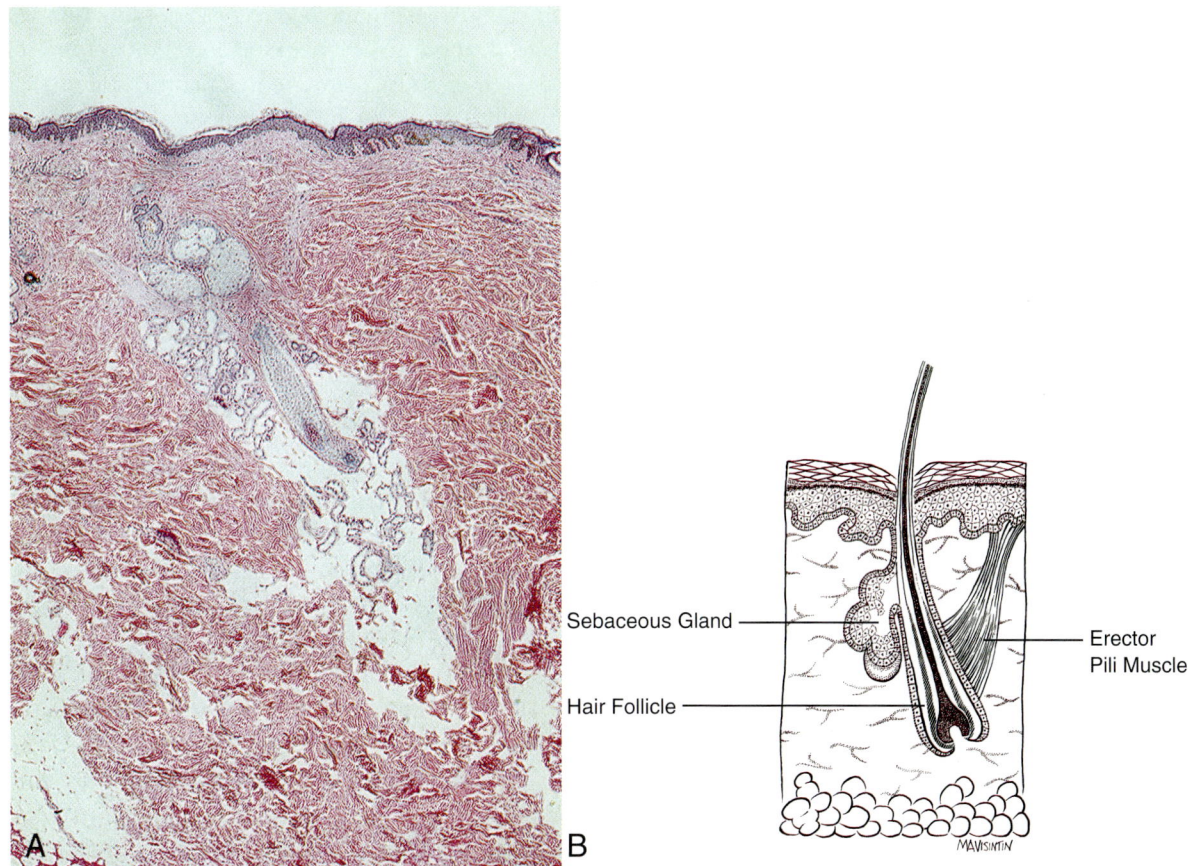

Figure 3.5. A, B. Photomicrograph and diagram of full skin including epidermis and dermis. A hair follicle with sebaceous glands, arrector pilorum muscle, and eccrine glands in the reticular dermis is displayed. Note the orientation of the hair follicle is at an angle with the epidermis.

monia and lipids. The duct of the apocrine gland enters the infundibular portion of the hair follicle above the entrance of the sebaceous glands: the apocrine secretion is mixed with the secretion from sebaceous glands. Apocrine secretion may be associated with a scent or odor.

Smooth Muscles

Smooth muscles are present in the skin of the areolae, the scrotum as the tunica dartos muscle, and the arrector pilorum muscles. The arrector pilorum arise in the connective tissue of the dermis and are attached to hair follicle below the sebaceous glands (Figure 3.5A, B). Contraction of the arrector pilorum cause the hair, which at rest is at a slant, to become perpendicular to the skin surface, clinically evident as goose bumps.

Nails

The nail is a hard, keratin structure, which is the end product of dead matrix cells. The nail is formed from the thick nail matrix that lies at the proximal portion of the nail unit immediately below the proximal nail fold and joins distally with the nail bed at the lunula or moon. The nail plate lies on the nail bed, which is composed of epidermis and dermis and has a rich vascular network. The nail plate is tightly adherent to the nail bed and is surrounded by the proximal and lateral nail folds.

Dermal Vessels

A rich vascular network exists in the dermis. The dermal vessels are branches from the musculocutaneous arteries that enter the subcutaneous fat, and then traverse the deep reticular dermis in a vertical fashion, perpendicular to the epidermis. These arterioles give off branches at various levels, which form horizontal vascular plexuses, one of which, the subepidermal plexus, is present at the level of the junction of the papillary and reticular dermis (Figure 3.6). A plexus begins with a muscular walled arteriole that gives off thin-walled capillaries, both of which have a continuous endothelium. Capillary loops come off the arterioles of the subpapillary plexus to feed the dermal papillae at a rate of one capillary per papillae. The descending limb of the capillary drains into a postcapillary venule. The venous system lies in a plane parallel to, and above and below, the arteriolar plexus. The walls of postcapillary venules are sensitive to mediators, such as histamine, which induce the development of gaps between endothelial cells, resulting in the loss of cells and fluid from the vessel. This can be seen as a result of urticaria or hives. Fluid loss or edema is also seen after skin wounding with laser or chemical peels.

Lymphatic channels are present in the skin and function to clear the tissue of extravasated fluid, cells, and protein, and regulate interstitial fluid pressure (1). The lymphatic capillaries are found in the papillary dermis in a random pattern and drain into larger channels in the subpapillary plexus.

Nerves

The skin has an extensive nervous supply consisting of somatic sensory and sympathetic autonomic fibers. Free nerve endings function alone, or in conjunction with specialized nerve structures as sensory receptors of touch, pain, temperature, itch, and mechanical stimuli. The density and type of receptors vary based on location. Sympathetic nerve fibers travel with sensory nerves in the dermis and innervate the sweat glands, vascular smooth muscles, and arrector pilorum.

Cutaneous nerves are large, myelinated branches of musculocutaneous nerves from spinal nerves. Branches from these nerves ascend to the level of the deep dermis and then branch, further forming a deep and more superficial subpapillary plexus. Cutaneous branches of the trigeminal nerve provide sensory innervation to the face. The sensory nerves supply individual dermatomes, but there is overlapping innervation to these areas.

Free nerve endings are common in the papillary dermis. Those present on nonhair-bearing skin, such as the palms and soles, function in fine discrimination and supply greater than half the papillae there. Free nerve endings are also associated with hair follicles and thought to be slow-adapting receptors that respond to the bending of hairs.

In hair-bearing skin, penicillate fibers are the major nerves present. They are rapidly adapting receptors that function in touch, temperature, pain and itch. The innervation from penicillate fibers is indiscriminate and overlapping. Two specialized mechanoreceptors are the Meissner's and Pacinian corpuscle. Meissner's corpuscle is present in the dermal papillae of digital skin, oriented vertically to the epidermal surface. Pacinian corpuscles are located in the deep dermis and hypodermis and respond to vibrational stimuli.

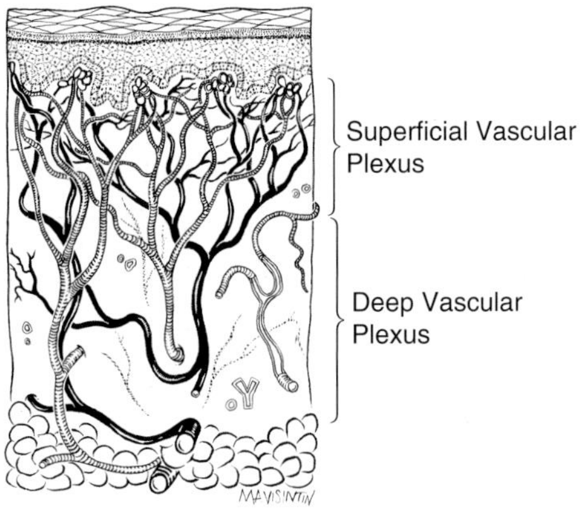

HYPODERMIS/SUBCUTIS

The subcutis rests immediately below the reticular dermis and there is a sudden transition. The tissue consists of groups or lobules of fat cells or adipocytes, surrounded by fibrous septa. Hair follicles and apocrine glands may be present in the lobules. The arteriolar and venous channels, lymphatic channels and nerve bundles course through the septa. The subcutis provides insulation for the body, acts as a cushion for trauma, allows for mobility of skin over underlying structures, and provides contour for cosmesis. The absence of fat in lipodystrophy, where there is a decreased number of fat cells and the cells are smaller than normal, the affected area appears abnormal and cachectic. Lipodystrophy can be partial or generalized.

Figure 3.6. Diagram of the horizontal arterial and venous plexuses of the skin.

Superficial Vascular Plexus

Deep Vascular Plexus

TABLE 3.2 Factors affecting wound healing

Causes of Delayed Wound Healing

Vascular diseases

Venous
　Impaired venous return
　Compromised lymphatic function

Arterial
　Arteriosclerosis
　Drug use, e.g., nicotine, alcohol

Nutritional deficiency
　Vitamins, e.g., A, B_6, B_{12}, C, folate
　Minerals, e.g., zinc, iron, calcium
　Protein (kwashiorkor)
　Protein/calories (marasmus)

Compromised immune system
　Immunosuppressive drug
　HIV/AIDS
　Radiation therapy history

Metabolic disorders
　Diabetes

Infections (local or systemic)
　Bacterial (e.g., *S. aureus*)
　Viral (e.g., herpes)

Advanced Age

WOUND HEALING

Wound healing is complex and can be affected by variables including overall health, nutritional status, age, predisposing conditions such as diabetes mellitus, and agents such as ionizing radiation and retinoids (Table 3.2). After a wound occurs, various steps take place. Following the initial fibrin clot formation, monocytes and granulocytes migrate into the injured area. Angiogenesis, the formation of new vascular growth from preexisting vessels, and fibroblast proliferation are important components of granulation tissue development.

Hemostasis begins with the deposition of fibrin and glycosaminoglycans including hyaluronic acid. The initial matrix upon which cell migration and proliferation occurs in wounded skin may begin with a complex of fibrin and hyaluronic acid. Fibronectin, a glycoprotein that promotes wound healing, is deposited by circulating plasma and resident fibroblasts and functions as a binding site for fibroblasts and migrating cells and as a scaffold for the deposition of collagen fibers. The matrix is replaced first by Type III collagen, followed by Type I collagen. The colla-

gen continues to be remodeled and strengthened by cross-links during the healing process.

While the dermal healing is on-going, the epidermal basal keratinocytes migrate from the wound edges and appendiceal structures. Keratinocyte migration is promoted by fibronectin, Type I collagen, and Type IV collagen.

Monocyte macrophages secrete many cytokines that affect wound healing: interleukin I (IL-1), tumor necrosis factor-α (TNF-α), epidermal growth factor (EGF), platelet derived growth factor (PDGF), and transforming growth factor-β (TGF-β). Promoters of inflammation include IL-1 and TNF-α while EGF, PDGF, and TGF-β are growth factors.

AGING SKIN

Numerous changes in the skin occur with age. There is an overall thinning of the dermis and epidermis with flattening of the dermal-epidermal junction (Figures 3.7, 3.8). The adhesion between the dermis and epidermis is

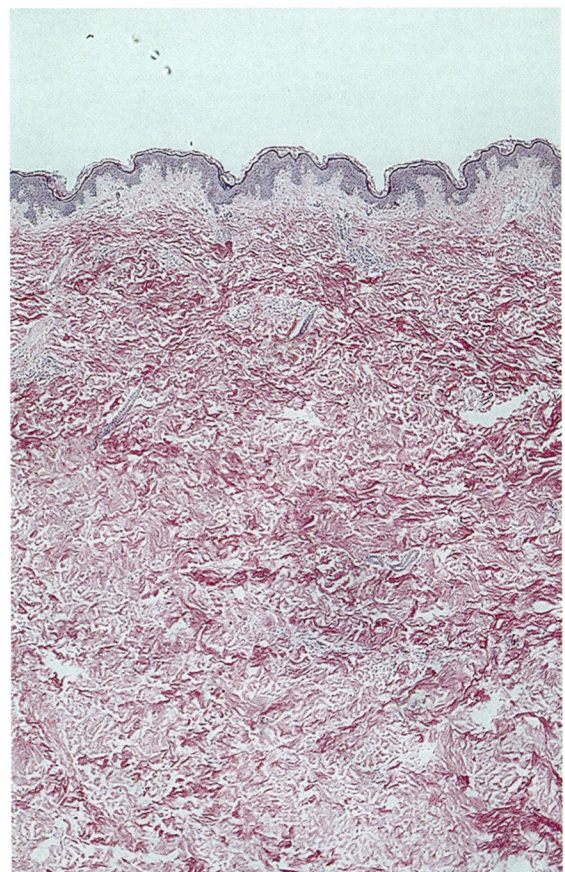

Figure 3.7. Photomicrograph demonstrating the relative thickness of the epidermis and dermis in young skin.

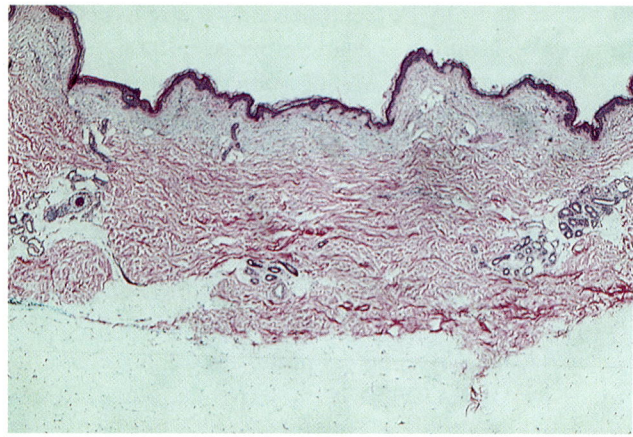

Figure 3.8. Photomicrograph demonstrating the relative atrophy of the epidermis and dermis in aged, sun-damaged skin.

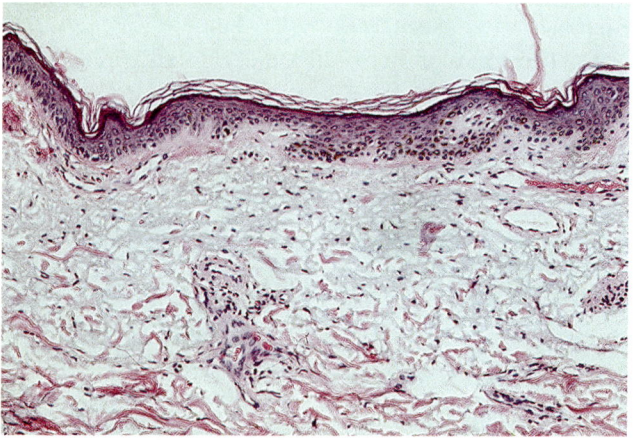

Figure 3.9. Photomicrograph demonstrating aged, sun-damaged skin. The epidermis is thinner, with loss of the rete ridges and solar elastosis. Dilated blood vessels (telangicctasias) are evident in the papillary dermis. The collagen bundles in the reticular dermis are fragmented and fewer in number.

diminished, resulting in an increased tendency to torn skin and abrasions. A decrease in epidermal turnover rate and repair rate occurs (5). Blood vessels fewer and less responsive. Appendiceal structures are also altered as hairs are fewer, finer and grow slower, and eccrine glands are decreased in number and output. Elastic fibers are fewer, thicker, and less elastic. Collagen fibers show an increase in incomplete cross-linking. Overall, with age, the dermis becomes more stiff, inelastic and inflexible (Figure 3.9).

Clinical signs of photoaging include rhytides, lentigines, keratoses, telangiectasias, and sallow skin. A classification of photoaged skin has been devised (6). Type I skin has no keratoses and little wrinkling. Type II skin displays few actinic keratoses and wrinkles in motion only. Type III skin has a moderate amount of actinic keratoses, sallow skin, telangiectasias and wrinkles at rest. Type IV skin displays a significant amount of actinic keratoses and notable wrinkling.

SUMMARY

The skin is a vast and complex organ that has many functions: temperature regulation, immunologic surveillance, sensory reception, and environmental barrier. It is a complex system composed of many specialized components and has extraordinary regenerative capacities. The interrelationship of the epidermis, dermis, subcutis and appendiceal structures, and also resident cell types, is important to keep in mind when performing procedures on the skin.

REFERENCES

1. Holbrook KA, Wolff K. The structure and development of skin. In: Fitzpatrick R, Eisen AZ, Wolff K, Freedberg IM, Austen KF, eds. Dermatology in general medicine. New York: McGraw Hill, 1993:99–145.
2. Wolff K, Kibbi AG, Mihm MC. Basic pathologic reactions of the skin. In: Fitzpatrick R, Eisen AZ, Wolff K, Freedberg IM, Austen KF, eds. Dermatology in general medicine. New York: McGraw Hill, 1993:66–87.
3. Holbrook KA. Structure and development of the skin. In: Soter NA, Baden HP, eds. Pathophysiology of dermatologic diseases. New York: McGraw Hill, 1984:3–43.
4. Bernstein EF, Mauviel A, McGrath JA, Bolton L. Wound healing. In: Lask GP, Moy RL, eds. Principles and techniques of cutaneous surgery. New York: McGraw Hill, 1996:1–22.
5. Gilbhrest BA. Aging of skin. In: Fitzpatrick R, Eisen AZ, Wolff K, Freedberg IM, Austen KF, eds. Dermatology in general medicine. New York: McGraw Hill, 1993: 150–157.
6. Glogau RG. Aesthetic and anatomic analysis of the aging skin. Seminars in Cutaneous Medicine & Surgery 1996;15:134–138.

Chapter Four

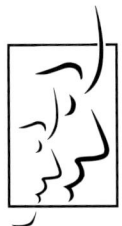

Anesthesia for Facial Aesthetic Surgery

Brian S. Biesman and Daniel E. Buerger

The goal of any aesthetic surgical procedure is to accomplish the desired result with as little anxiety and disruption of the patient's life as possible. Preoperatively, each individual has a unique set of fears, preconceptions, and misgivings, which must be explored if this goal is to be realized.

Commonly expressed surgery concerns: preprocedure anxiety, fear of discomfort before, during, or after surgery, amount of postoperative swelling and bruising, length of time away from work or social activities (which may be related to postoperative swelling and bruising), requirements for postoperative care, discomfort associated with suture removal, and, of course, postoperative results. While surgeons may focus on the latter, some patients may be equally concerned, or perhaps even more so, with these other issues. A knowledge of current techniques in anesthesia can help the surgeon plan the ideal procedure for each patient. This chapter addresses the anesthetic agents commonly used in facial aesthetic surgery, their intended application, methods of administration, and major risks and complications associated with their use.

ANATOMY

The anatomy of the sensory innervation of the face is described in Chapter 2.

GENERAL MEDICAL CONSIDERATIONS

A careful and complete medical history must be taken before performing any surgical procedure. Specific questions regarding cardiopulmonary symptoms must be asked as patients may be unable or unwilling to freely volunteer this information. Systemic problems, including hypertension, diabetes mellitus, thyroid dysfunction, renal insufficiency, and systemic inflammatory diseases, should be stable. Other general medical considerations may affect the administration of anesthesia: patient age, ability to lie flat for the duration of the operation, arthritis that may affect the cervical spine, airway abnormalities such as acute rhinitis, nasal tumors or deformity, acute respiratory disease, psychiatric disorders, and pregnancy. Patients should be encouraged to continue taking as many of their usual medications as possible on the day of surgery. Medications may be taken at home with a sip of water, and nonessential products (e.g. vitamins) may be withheld. Vitamin E should be discontinued 2 weeks before incisional surgical procedures. Despite occasional patient pressure to proceed with surgery as soon as possible, elective procedures should be postponed until other medical conditions have been thoroughly assessed and determined to be stable. Communication with the patient's primary care physician is important as even "minor" procedures may evoke enough anxiety in an unstable patient to cause serious cardiovascular events.

TABLE 4.1 American Society of Anesthesiology Patient Classification

ASA Patient Classification

1. A normal, healthy patient

2. A patient with mild systemic disease

3. A patient with severe systemic disease that limits activity but is not incapacitating

4. A patient with an incapacitating systemic disease that is a threat to life.

5. A moribund patient not expected to survive over 24 hours with or without surgery

The American Society of Anesthesiology (ASA) has developed a uniform system classifying each patient into one of five categories based on their overall health. The ASA class should be determined for each patient as part of the routine preoperative evaluation to assess the *relative* risk of the proposed procedure (1) (Table 4.1). While no *direct* correlation exists between ASA class and operative morbidity, overall morbidity is 4–5 times greater in Class 3 and 4 patients than in Class 1 patients. Aesthetic surgery should never be performed if the anesthesiologist or primary care physician feels that additional medical evaluation is necessary to properly assess a patient's medical status (2, 3).

LOCAL ANESTHETIC AGENTS

Local anesthetic agents are used extensively in facial aesthetic surgery. There are two major categories of local anesthetics: those that are applied topically and those that require injection. The injectable agents may produce either a regional nerve block, in which the entire distribution of a nerve is anesthetized, or a local effect in the immediate area of injection. Although these agents are generally safe and well tolerated, it is important to recognize their potential complications and side effects.

All local anesthetic agents currently available are tertiary amines classified as esters or amides based on the nature of the linkage between the aromatic lipophilic component with the hydrophilic amine. Commonly used esters include procaine (Novocaine, Sanofi Winthrop, NY, NY), cocaine, tetracaine, proparacaine, and benoxinate (used topically on the eye). Some of the frequently used amide local anesthetics include lidocaine (Xylocaine, Abbott Laboratories, N. Chicago, IL), bupivacaine (Marcaine, Astra Pharmaceuticals, Westboro, MA), mepivi-

caine (Carbocaine, Sanofi Winthrop, NY, NY), and etidocaine (Duranest, Sanofi Winthrop, NY, NY). The ester group of local anesthetics are broken down rapidly in the bloodstream by plasma cholinesterase, and more slowly in tissue by tissue cholinesterase. A byproduct of the degradation of the ester anesthetics, with the exception of proparacaine, is paraaminobenzoic acid, a highly allergenic compound. This accounts for the greater incidence of allergic reaction to the ester anesthetics and severely limits their use in local injection. The amide group, in contrast, is not degraded in tissue or the bloodstream, but in the liver, and has largely replaced the esters because of their stability and the decreased incidence of allergic reactions (4, 5).

Both the amide and the ester groups of drugs are available commercially as organic salts (they are unstable in their base amine form). The injectable agents are supplied in an isotonic saline solution and are most potent over a pH range of 3.0–6.5, and begin to precipitate with increasing alkalinization. The addition of sodium bicarbonate to stock solutions of local anesthetics has been suggested for raising the pH and thus improving the comfort level of injection. However, caution is required as the pH of each stock solution may vary, and addition of a standard amount of bicarbonate without pH control can result in the development of a precipitate. If this occurs, upon injection the precipitate will be deposited in the tissue and appear as a tattoo (6).

The injectable local anesthetic agents used most often in facial aesthetic surgery are bupivacaine and lidocaine. While lidocaine is often used independently of bupivacaine, the latter is not usually used alone because of the prolonged delay in the onset of its analgesic effects (30–45 minutes) as compared to lidocaine's nearly instantaneous onset of action. Conversely, lidocaine is metabolized relatively rapidly (1.5–2 hours half-life), while bupivacaine produces a more lasting analgesia (about 3.5 hours half-life). For this reason, lidocaine and bupivacaine are sometimes administered as a mixture to either maintain analgesia for a lengthy case or to provide several hours of postoperative pain relief following a shorter procedure.

Local anesthetics often are supplied in a solution containing epinephrine added in a ratio of 1:100,000 or 1:200,000. Epinephrine prolongs the duration of anesthetic effect and decreases systemic toxicity by causing local vasoconstriction. The same vasoconstrictive effect that increases the safety margin from a dosing standpoint may be used to the surgeon's benefit by reducing the amount of intraoperative hemorrhage (7, 8). To take maximum advantage of this effect, a full 15 minutes should be allowed to pass before making an incision. If proper monitoring is available, the local anesthetic may be injected while the patient is in the holding area to save time and expense in the operating room.

Bupivacaine hydrochloride is available in concentrations of 0.25%, 0.5%. and 0.75%. The highest concentration is not recommended for use as a single agent because of an unacceptably high incidence of serious complications. It may be administered as a mixture with other agents for periorbital surgery. All three concentrations are available with epinephrine added at a ratio of 1:200,000 (8).

Lidocaine for injection is also supplied as a hydrochloride salt and is available in concentrations of 0.5%, 1.0%, 1.5%, and 2.0%. All of the concentrations are available plain or with epinephrine added at a 1:200,000 dilution; the 1% and 2% solutions are available with epinephrine diluted at 1:100,000 (8). Solutions containing epinephrine should not be autoclaved and should be protected from sunlight. Lidocaine is also available as a 4% solution and indicated for topical use only. As a result of solubility problems, the 4% solutions are prepared in sterile water and are extremely painful when injected.

The maximum recommended total dose of bupivacaine administered to a healthy adult is approximately 2 mg/kg (or a total dose of 175 mg): lidocaine should not exceed 4.5 mg/kg (300 mg). If the anesthetic preparations contain epinephrine as an additive, the total dose of bupivacaine may be increased to approximately 2.5 mg/kg (225 mg total), and the total dose of lidocaine is increased to about 7.5 mg/kg (500 mg total). Dosages should be reduced for children, elderly patients, and those with liver disease. While these dosages may appear to offer a large safety zone given the usual requirements for a typical facial procedure, the surgeon is reminded that 1 ml of 1% solution of anesthetic contains 10 mg of drug, and that 1 ml of a 2% solution contains 20 mg of drug.

Topically applied anesthetic agents such as EMLA cream (Astra Pharmaceuticals, Westboro, MA) (lidocaine 2.5% and prilocaine 2.5%), 30% lidocaine/Velvachol cream, and others, have been used prior to laser skin resurfacing (9). The topical agents are usually delivered in a cream base applied to the intact skin surface under an occlusive dressing such as Tegaderm (3M Health Care, St. Paul, MN). The onset, depth, and duration of analgesia from topical creams are primarily dependent upon the duration of application. A minimum of 1 hour is required to achieve anesthesia sufficient for superficial cutaneous laser or surgical procedures. Two-to-three hours of application are required to realize a maximal effect. Analgesia persists for 1-2 hours after removal of the cream (8). Superficial Er:YAG resurfacing may be performed after application of topical anesthetic in some patients. Deeper Er:YAG or CO_2 laser resurfacing is difficult to perform with topical anesthesia alone.

Systemic absorption of topical anesthetic agents correlates to the area of application, the duration of application, and the integrity of the skin (broken or inflamed skin increases absorption). Systemic toxicity arising from the use of topical anesthetic agents is uncommon. It is unknown if lidocaine or prilocaine are metabolized by the skin. As they are not indicated for use on mucous membranes or the eye, caution must be exercised with their use on periocular skin. Chemical burns of the cornea following periocular use have been reported (10). Adverse reactions to topical anesthetic preparations are mainly local or regional: pallor with blanching, erythema, edema, itch, and rash. These symptoms usually resolve spontaneously within 1-2 hours of discontinuation of the agent.

LOCAL AND REGIONAL ANESTHESIA FOR FACIAL AESTHETIC SURGERY AND FULL FACE LASER SKIN RESURFACING

Most facial aesthetic surgery may be performed under local or regional anesthesia, with or without supplemental intravenous sedation (11). When performing relatively short procedures, which require a limited volume of agent and are expected to produce minimal postoperative discomfort, 1-2% lidocaine with epinephrine 1:100,000 is effective. For longer procedures, or those which may produce more postoperative discomfort (e.g., brow and forehead lifting, full face skin resurfacing), a 1:1 or 1:2 mixture of 0.5-0.75% bupivacaine and 1-2% lidocaine containing epinephrine 1:100,000 is recommended.

Local anesthesia for most eyelid and periorbital procedures is administered via direct subcutaneous injection. The volume of agent injected is usually not of critical importance, but in preparation for adult ptosis surgery, only a minimal volume (approximately 1 ml) is administered so as to avoid partial or complete akinesia of the levator muscle. See chapter 10 for further discussion. A 27- or 30-gauge needle is used to decrease patient discomfort and to minimize trauma to the eyelid tissues. Adequate ocular protection should be in place and the needle should be directed away from the globe so that unanticipated patient movement will not jeopardize the eye when injecting the eyelids.

The forehead may be readily anesthetized with regional blockade of the supraorbital and supratrochlear nerves. Together these nerves supply the majority of the

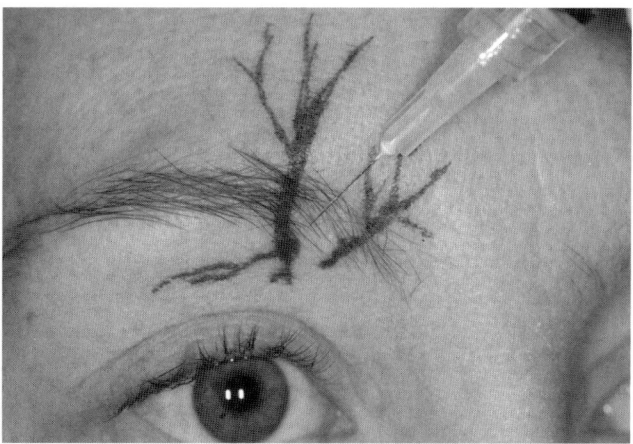

Figure 4.1. Location of the supraorbital and supratrochlear nerves. Local anesthesia is injected in the area of the supraorbital notch to block both of these nerves.

sensory innervation to the forehead and anterior scalp, with the exception of a small area above the lateral brow supplied by the lacrimal nerve. The supraorbital and supratrochlear nerves may be anesthetized with a single injection of local anesthetic given in the region of supraorbital notch (Figure 4.1). A 27- or 30-gauge needle is passed through the skin to the periosteum where approximately 1 cc of agent is injected. Care must be taken to withdraw the plunger before injection to avoid an inadvertent intravascular injection.

Anesthesia of the eyelids is usually best achieved via direct subcutaneous infiltration. Alternatively, some surgeons prefer a regional blockade of the frontal nerve to minimize distortion of eyelid tissues. A 30-gauge long or 25-gauge retrobulbar needle is advanced along the roof of the orbit, in line with the supraorbital notch, and approximately 0.5 cc of anesthetic is injected. If surgery is to be performed in the medial or lateral aspects of the upper lid as well, a supplemental blockade of the infratrochlear or lacrimal nerves, respectively, may be required. The infratrochlear nerve is anesthetized by injecting about 0.5–1.0 cc of agent medial to the supraorbital notch, while the lacrimal nerve is blocked by injecting 0.5–1.0 cc of anesthetic along the roof of the anterior lateral orbit (Figure 4.2). To avoid akinesia of the extraocular muscles or the levator palpebrae superioris, the injection should be given external to the intermuscular septum.

The lower eyelid may be anesthetized via direct subcutaneous infiltration or with an infraorbital nerve block. The course and distribution of the infraorbital nerve is described in the anatomy of the eyelids in chapter 2. The infraorbital nerve may be approached transconjunctivally,

percutaneously, or via the gingival buccal mucosa. The transconjunctival infraorbital nerve block is given by pulling the lower lid inferiorly, thus exposing the inferior fornix. A 30-gauge needle is introduced through the fornix, until it lies anterior to the inferior orbital rim. It is then advanced down the anterior surface of the maxilla along a vertical line drawn inferiorly from the supraorbital notch, a structure that can be easily palpated along the superior orbital rim. The infraorbital nerve block may be administered percutaneously by placing the needle adjacent and just above the lateral alae of the nose along the same line drawn vertically through the supraorbital notch. To approach the infraorbital nerve through the gingival buccal mucosa, advance a 27- or 30-gauge needle just lateral to the canine tooth along the anterior surface of the maxilla, directing the needle toward the infraorbital foramen (which may be readily palpated). The transconjunctival and transoral approaches avoid bleeding that may occur when passing a needle through the facial musculature in a percutaneous approach.

The lateral portion of the upper and lower face is best anesthetized by direct infiltration of anesthetic agent, as opposed to regional blocks. A fair amount of overlap to the innervation in this area makes regional blocks ineffective. Injections are administered with a 27-gauge needle bent at a 60–75° angle, with the syringe so that the needle remains in the subcutaneous plane. At least 10 cc of anes-

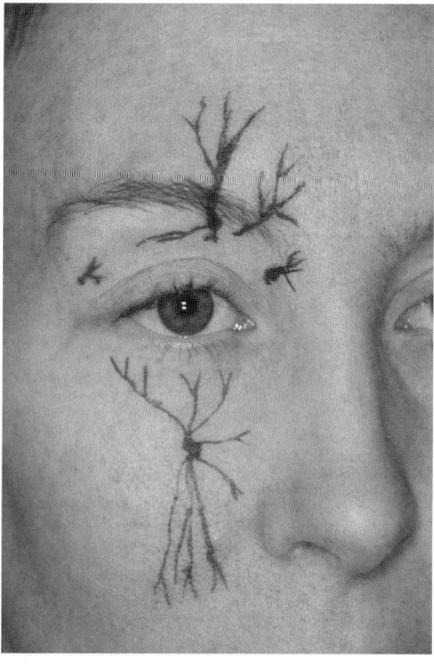

Figure 4.2. Distribution of the lacrimal, supratrochlear, infratrochlear, and infraorbital nerves.

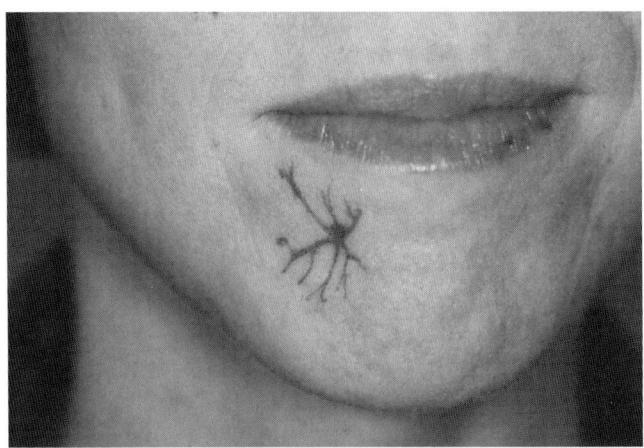

Figure 4.3. Distribution of the mental nerve.

thetic are generally required to produce adequate anesthesia of the lateral portions of the face.

The perioral region is satisfactorily anesthetized with a combination of regional blocks and local infiltration. The upper lip is effectively anesthetized with an infraorbital nerve block as described above. The lower lip and chin may be anesthetized with a regional block of the mental nerve, the terminal branch of the mandibular nerve. The mental nerve exits the mandible through the mental foramen, a bony opening in the mandible, which lies approximately in the midpupillary line (Figure 4.3). The mental nerve may be anesthetized via an intraoral approach by injecting 0.5–1.0 cc of agent through a 27- or 30-gauge needle against the mandible along a line drawn vertically through the pupil. If a 30-gauge, short (⅝″) needle is used, it is advanced to its hub. Once the infraorbital and mental nerve blocks have been administered bilaterally, the lateral aspect of the oral commissure must be directly infiltrated as this area is not well anesthetized by either regional nerve block.

COMPLICATIONS OF LOCAL ANESTHETIC AGENTS

Careful consideration must be given to the toxicity of local anesthetics, an often overlooked topic in surgical texts. Toxic reactions may be related to overdosage, inadvertent intravenous injection, hypersensitivity reaction, or an idiosyncratic reaction, and may be serious or fatal. An overdose of local anesthetic may affect the central nervous system, the cardiovascular system, or both. The central nervous system (CNS) may become stimulated or de-

pressed at a much lower dose of lidocaine (8–10 μg/ml) than that associated with cardiovascular effects (20 μg/ml). Bupivacaine toxicity occurs in the CNS and cardiovascular system at the same serum concentration (3–5 μg/ml). Central nervous system stimulation may manifest as restlessness, tremors, lightheadedness, nervousness, apprehension, euphoria, confusion, tinnitus, diplopia, twitching, or shivering and may progress to seizures. Coma and respiratory arrest may follow CNS stimulation or may present as the first sign of local anesthetic overdose. Cardiovascular effects may include depressed conduction leading to heart block and severe bradycardia, ventricular arrhythmias, hypotension, and cardiovascular collapse. The management of systemic toxic reactions to local anesthetic agents begins with the establishment and maintenance of an airway and effective ventilation with 100% oxygen. If seizure activity occurs, the development of hypoxia, hypercarbia, and acidosis will be rapid. Seizure activity may be controlled with intravenous benzodiazepines or antiseizure agents. Succinylcholine may be administered to induce paralysis if necessary. The cardiovascular system must be addressed and supported with intravenous fluids or pressors as necessary. Hemodialysis is generally of little benefit in the management of local anesthetic overdose (12, 13). Inadvertent intravenous injection of epinephrine-containing solutions can induce severe hypertension and tachycardia. Alpha and beta adrenergic blockers should be available whenever these agents are administered in the region of a blood vessel large enough to receive an intraluminal injection. Intravenous injection of bupivacaine can result in profound cardiac depression with asystole unresponsive to resuscitation efforts because of avid binding of this agent to nonspecific cardiac protein-binding sites (5).

Complications of local anesthetic injections in the eyelids are rare. A hematoma may form if the injection is given intramuscularly rather than subcutaneously. Patients should be warned before introduction of the needle to avoid inadvertent head movements that may endanger the eye itself. To help prevent accidental intraocular injection, the tip of the needle should always be directed away from the globe and, if necessary, the patient's head and hands may be stabilized.

Allergic reactions to local anesthetics are rare and may occur as a result of sensitivity to the drug itself or to antimicrobial preservatives (such as methylparaben), which are added to most multidose vials. Most local anesthetic agents are available in methylparaben-free preparations. The symptoms and signs of a true hypersensitivity reaction to a local anesthetic agent are any Type IV reaction: urticaria, pruritus, erythema, angioneurotic edema, tachycardia, sneezing, nausea, vomiting, dizziness, sweating, fever, and even hypotension. Treatment of an allergic reaction to a local anesthetic does not differ from the management of any other Type IV reaction.

Care should always be taken to confirm the contents of a syringe before administering an injection. Injection of the wrong agent has been performed with devastating consequences. All syringes and solutions on the sterile field must be clearly and properly marked. If there is any doubt as to the proper identification of a solution, it should be discarded.

SEDATION

Before administration of a general or a local anesthetic, pharmacologic agents are often given to promote relaxation and relieve anxiety before surgery. Sometimes, they are given to induce sedation and amnesia for a short period while a noxious stimulus, such as injection of a local anesthetic, is applied. Sedative agents may be given orally, sublingually, or intravenously.

The benzodiazepines are anxiolytics whose effect is believed to be related to action on the limbic system, the thalamus, and the hypothalamus. The benzodiazepines commonly used by the facial aesthetic surgeon include diazepam (Valium, Roche Products, Manati, Puerto Rico), lorazepam (Ativan, Wyeth-Ayerst, Philadelphia, PA), and midazolam (Versed, Roche Laboratories, Nutley, NJ). These drugs differ primarily in their half-lives and time to onset of action. They may be administered orally (diazepam, lorazepam), intravenously, intramuscularly, sublingually, or by inhalation (midazolam). Midazolam has the shortest half-life (1.2-12.3 hours) as compared with lorazepam (16 hours) and diazepam (2-3 days). The clinical effects of midazolam generally last 2-6 hours. Because of its short half-life and duration of effect, midazolam is the benzodiazepine used most often as an adjunct to aesthetic facial surgical procedures (14).

Besides their anxiolytic effects, benzodiazepines are also skeletal muscle relaxants and amnesia-producing sedatives. Following intravenous administration of midazolam, sedation occurs within 3-5 minutes and peak sedation occurs in about 30 minutes and lasts for 2 hours. The sedative effect of benzodiazepines is accentuated by premedication with narcotics, and the dosages should be decreased by at least one third when narcotics are used (8).

All benzodiazepines must be administered in a careful, patient-specific manner. As the respiratory depressant effects may not become manifest immediately, midazolam must be administered intravenously in small doses of 1-2 mg. Diazepam is less potent than midazolam and is usually given in doses of 2.5-5 mg intravenously. Great care must be taken not to use *diazepam* dosing when administering *midazolam*. This mistake was made frequently when midazolam was first introduced, leading to unexpected respiratory depression (7). Some discomfort occurs with the intravenous administration of diazepam as it is supplied for injection in a solution of propylene, ethanol, and water.

The major adverse effects of the benzodiazepines include CNS and respiratory depression. Respiratory arrest and cardiovascular collapse can occur. Thus, careful monitoring of respiration, pulse, and blood pressure is required when these drugs are administered. Excessive dosages are manifest clinically by snoring, followed by airway obstruction that usually responds to jaw-lift maneuvers to maintain the airway. As opposed to narcotic overdosage, the patient overdosed with benzodiazepines will often make a respiratory effort. Ventilation is not usually required. When severe respiratory depression does occur, a benzodiazepine antagonist, flumazenil (Romazicon, Hoffman-LaRoche, Nutley, NJ), may be administered intravenously in doses of 0.4 mg. As flumenazil has been associated with seizures, it should only be used when necessary. While the sedative and psychomotor effects of benzodiazepines may be reversed, the half-life of flumazenil is short and resedation may occur. Airway and cardiovascular support must be maintained even if flumazenil is used (8).

A more minor adverse effect found in approximately 4% of patients receiving midazolam is hiccoughs (8). This is insignificant unless it should occur intraoperatively when delicate maneuvers are being performed.

Recently, two new ultra-short acting medications, diprivan (Propofol, Glaxo Wellcome, Research Triangle Park, NC) and remifentanil (Ultiva, Zeneca, Wilmington, DE), have become available and have proven to be extremely useful to the aesthetic surgeon. Propofol is a sedative hypnotic with minimal water solubility supplied in a white oil-in-water emulsion for intravenous administration. Following injection, hypnosis is usually induced with one circulation through the CNS. Following a single injection, peak hypnosis usually occurs within 2 minutes. Hypnosis is usually profound, and this drug is extremely useful before injection of local anesthetics. Patients will be fully awake several minutes after a single bolus. Apnea may occur, and may be profound, although it usually resolves within one minute. Propofol may also be administered as a continuous drip to maintain sedation throughout a procedure. This is particularly useful when operating on extremely anxious patients or when doing lengthy procedures under local anesthesia. Following a 1-hour continuous infusion of propofol, serum levels are nearly zero 20 minutes after discontinuation of the drug. This makes propofol ideal for use in an outpatient surgery setting (15, 16).

The usual dosage of propofol for induction of general anesthesia is 2.0-2.5 mg/kg in healthy adults and 1.0-2.0 mg/kg in elderly or debilitated adults, given over 10 seconds until induction onset occurs. Alternatively, to initiate monitored sedation and to avoid hypotension and apnea, slow infusion of 0.5 mg/kg may be given over 3-5 minutes. This may be followed immediately by an infusion of 30-50 mcg/kg/min. Bolus dosing should be avoided in ASA class 3 or 4 patients. Failure to observe careful aseptic technique during the preparation of propofol for injection has resulted in iatrogenic infection (17), including infectious endophthalmitis (18). Rapid growth of microorganisms can occur in the propofol solution (19). Because of the content of the emulsion in which propofol is supplied, patients with allergies to eggs should receive this medication slowly.

The major adverse effects of propofol are related to cardiovascular and respiratory depression. Arterial hypotension is common and this drug should be used with extreme caution in ASA 3 and 4 patients. Respiratory depression may result in apnea, airway obstruction, and oxygen desaturation. Propofol should be given only by persons trained in the administration of general anesthesia and should not be given by the surgeon performing the operation or procedure (19). Continuous monitoring of the airway, respiratory status, and cardiovascular status is not only critical, but is considered standard of care. Ventilatory and circulatory support, including oxygen artificial respiration, and airway management including endotracheal intubation, should be immediately available (19-22).

Remifentanil is an opioid agonist with rapid onset and short duration of action that reaches its peak effect quickly. Unlike other opioids, remifentanil is metabolized by nonspecific blood and tissue esterases, and therefore, the pharmacodynamics are not changed in patients with renal or hepatic impairments (23). After a single injection, its analgesic effect is gone within minutes. Even following continuous infusion there is no residual opioid activity 5-10 minutes after discontinuing the drug (24, 25). It is supplied as a lyophilized powder that may be reconstituted in either sterile water or saline. It should not be admixed with lactated Ringer's solution.

Remifentanil is an analgesic that blunts the pain caused by a noxious stimulus. It is recommended for use at dosages that produce minimal loss of consciousness and amnesia. When used alone, remifentanil may be ad-

ministered: as a single intravenous dose of 1 μg/kg 90 seconds before administering a local anesthetic injection, or as a continuous infusion at a dose of 0.1 μg/kg/min started 5 minutes before a local injection, and then 0.05 μg/kg/min to maintain analgesia during a procedure. Bolus dosing is not recommended simultaneously with a continuous infusion as hypoventilation may occur. Remifentanil potentiates the sedative effect of benzodiazepines and propofol and is often used in conjunction with one of these agents. In these situations, the dosing of both agents is substantially decreased: remifentanil by 50% and sedative hypnotics by up to 75% (25, 26). At these dosages, the amnestic and analgesic effects are realized while the sedative effect is minimized, allowing patients to respond to verbal commands. Thus, the risk of hypoventilation is decreased while maintaining patient comfort.

The major adverse effects of remifentanil are similar to fentanyl and related to respiratory depression, bradycardia, hypotension, and skeletal muscle rigidity (19). These effects dissipate within minutes of stopping the infusion. Like propofol, continuous monitoring of the airway, respiratory status, and cardiovascular status is not only critical but is considered standard of care. Ventilatory and circulatory support, including oxygen artificial respiration, and airway management including endotracheal intubation should be immediately available. Other side effects noted more commonly include nausea, vomiting, pruritus, headache, shivering, and dizziness. These are fairly uncommon, especially with the lower dose of remifentanil when used with midazolam. Remifentanil should be given only by persons trained in the administration of general anesthesia and should not be given by the surgeon performing the operation or procedure.

GENERAL ANESTHESIA

While most patients undergoing aesthetic facial surgery prefer local or regional anesthesia in combination with intravenous sedation, some will request general anesthesia. The general anesthetic state is characterized by an induced state of unconsciousness, during which surgical stimulation elicits only autonomic reflex responses. The patient should not exhibit any voluntary movements, but changes in vital signs may be monitored. This definition differs from that of the analgesic state, in which there is no sensibility to pain. The analgesic state may be produced by narcotics in much smaller doses than are required to produce unconsciousness.

Inhalation general anesthetic agents are traditionally administered via an endotracheal or nasotracheal tube.

More recently, the laryngeal-mask airway has been introduced to provide airway control while eliminating the need for laryngoscopy and tracheal intubation. The main shortcoming of this device relative to an endotracheal tube is its inability to protect the respiratory tree from aspiration of gastric contents. However, for patients without gastroesophageal reflux, hiatal hernia, severe obesity, or other similar conditions, the laryngeal-mask provides an attractive alternative for airway support during anesthesia. It may also be used during deep intravenous sedation without the use of inhaled agents.

The inhalation anesthetic agents commonly used include enflurane (Ethrane), isoflurane, desflurane, sevoflurane and nitrous oxide. Halothane is the primary inhalation agent used in children, but should not be used in adults because of concern about hepatotoxicity (27, 28). Isoflurane has been the mainstay of inhalation anesthesia for many years (29). It is not associated with renal or hepatotoxicity, but may adversely affect myocardial perfusion in patients with underlying coronary artery disease. Desflurane and sevoflurane are newer agents (30). Desflurane has low solubility, leading to rapid onset of anesthesia and rapid elimination of agent upon its discontinuation. Widespread use of this agent has been limited in part by its expense and the requirement of a heated vaporizer for delivery. Sevoflurane has been used in a large number of patients without apparent toxic effects. It has a more pleasant odor than other agents and may be useful in children. It is metabolized into potentially toxic byproducts, which has caused severe renal problems in animal models (31, 32) but not in humans. Nitrous oxide is one of the earliest inhalation anesthetics, and is still widely used. Care must be taken to avoid the use of nitrous oxide in patients who may have had intraocular gas injections following repair of a retinal break or detachment. In such cases, the nitrous oxide will fill the eye and may raise the intraocular pressure high enough to cause a central retinal artery occlusion. Nitrous oxide has been implicated as a cause of bone marrow depression, severe neurologic defects, and suppression of important enzymatic reactions (19).

General anesthesia may be supplemented with injections of epinephrine-containing local anesthetic agents to improve intraoperative hemostasis and to help control postoperative pain. If postoperative pain control is not likely to be a major source of concern, 1% lidocaine with epinephrine 1:100,000 is used for local infiltration. For longer postoperative pain relief, a 1:1 mixture of 1–2% lidocaine with epinephrine 1:100,000 and 0.25–0.75% bupivacaine mixture is recommended.

The decision as to which anesthetic agents to use, and under which conditions surgery should be performed, should be made with the best interests of the patient and surgeon in mind. A surgeon will be most comfortable with a relaxed, cooperative patient. The patient's wishes must also be considered. While most patients will trust a surgeon's judgement, some will have had adverse experiences that will affect their approach to their care. A relaxed, informative preoperative office visit allows the surgeon to explore these issues and to choose the best anesthetic for each individual patient.

REFERENCES

1. Menke H, Klein A, John KD, Junginger T. Predictive value of ASA classification for the assessment of the perioperative risk. Intl Surg 1993;78:266–270.
2. Fagraeus L. Anesthesia. In: Sabiston DC, ed. Essentials of surgery. Philadelphia: WB Saunders, 1987.
3. Jackson D, Chen AH, Bennett CA. Identifying true lidocaine allergy. J Am Dent Assoc 1994;25:1362–1366.
4. Gills JP, Hustead RF, Sanders DR. Ophthalmic anesthesia. New York: McGraw-Hill, 1993:75–77.
5. Wiklund RA, Rosenbaum SH. Anesthesiology: second of two parts. New Engl J Med 1997;337:1215–1219.
6. Hinshaw KD, Fiscella R, Sugar J. Preparation of pH adjusted local anesthetics. Ophthalmic Surgery 1995; 26:194–199.
7. Epstein GA. Anesthesia in ophthalmic plastic surgery. In: Hornblass A, ed. Oculoplastic, orbital and reconstructive surgery. Vol 1. Baltimore: Williams & Wilkins, 1988.
8. Physicians desk reference. 49th ed. New Jersey: Medical Economics, 1995.
9. Lener EV, Bucalo BD, Kist DA, Moy RL. Topical anesthetic agents in dermatologic surgery. A review. Dermatol Surg 1997;23:673–683.
10. Brahma AK, Inkster C. Alkaline chemical ocular injury from Emla cream (Letter). Eye 1995;9:658–659.
11. Khan J, Wegner P. Extensive orbital bone and soft tissue surgery under IV sedation with local anesthesia: a dynamic approach to intraoperative pain. Presented at the 25th annual meeting of the American Society of Ophthalmic Plastic and Reconstructive Surgery, Atlanta, Georgia. November, 1995.
12. Baker TJ, Gordon HL, Stuzin JM. Surgical rejuvenation of the face. St. Louis: Mosby, 1996.
13. Gilman AG, Rall TW, Nies AS, et al. The pharmacological basis of therapeutics, 8th ed. New York: Pergamon Press, 1990.
14. White PF, Vasconez LO, Mathes SA, Way WL. Comparison of midazolam and diazepam for sedation during plastic surgery. Plast Reconstr Surg 1988;81:703.

15. Sebel PS, Lowdon JD. Propofol: a new intravenous anesthetic. Anesthesiology 1989;71:260–277.
16. Smith I, White PF, Nathanson M, Gouldson R. Propofol: an update on its clinical use. Anesthesiology 1994;81:1005–1043.
17. Bennett SN, McNeil MM, Bland LA, Arduino MJ. Postoperative infections traced to contamination of an intravenous anesthetic, propofol. N Engl J Med 1995;333:184–185.
18. Daily MJ, Dickey JB, Packo KH. Endogenous Candida endophthalmitis after intravenous anesthesia with propofol. Arch Ophthalmol 1991;109:1081–1084.
19. Wiklund RA, Rosenbaum SH. Anesthesiology: first of two parts. New Engl J Med 1997;337:1132–1140.
20. Davies BW, Pennington GA, Guyuron B. Clinical office anesthesia: the use of propofol for induction and maintenance of general anesthesia. Aesth Plast Surg 1993;17:125–128.
21. Friedberg BL. Propofol-ketamine technique. Aesth Plast Surg 1993;17:297–300.
22. Hustead RF, Hamilton RC. Pharmacology. In: Gills JP, Hustead RF, Sanders DR, eds. Ophthalmic anesthesia. New York: McGraw-Hill, 1993.
23. Burkle H, Dunbar S, Van Aken H. Remifentanil: a novel, short-acting, opioid. Anesth Analg 1996;83:646–651.
24. Michelsen LG, Hug CC Jr. The pharmacokinetics of remifentanil. (Review). J Clin Anesthesia 1996;8:679–682.
25. Patel SS, Spencer CM. Remifentanil (Review). Drugs 1996;52:417–427.
26. Avramov MN, Smith I, White PF. Interactions between midazolam and remifentanil during monitored anesthesia care. Anesthesiology 1996;85:1283–1289.
27. Kenna JG, Jones RM. The organ toxicity of inhaled anesthetics. Anesth Analg 1995;81(suppl):S51–S66.
28. Summary of the National Halothane Study. Possible association between halothane anesthesia and postoperative hepatic necrosis. JAMA 1966;197:775–788.
29. Stevens WC, Cromwell TH, Halsey MJ, Eger EI II. The cardiovascular effects of a new inhalation anesthetic, Forane, in human volunteers at constant arterial carbon dioxide tension. Anesthesiology 1971;35:8–16.
30. Eger EI II. New inhaled anesthetics. Anesthesiology 1994;80:906–922.
31. Gonsowski CT, Laster MJ, Eger EI II, Ferrell LD. Toxicity of compound A in rats: effect of a 3-hour administration. Anesthesiology 1994;80:556–565.
32. Gonsowski CT, Laster MJ, Eger EI II, Ferrell LD. Toxicity of compound A in rats: effect of increasing duration of administration. Anesthesiology 1994;80:566–573.

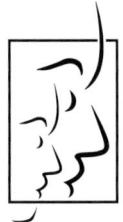

Chapter Five

A Comparison Between Laser Skin Resurfacing and Chemical Peeling

Kenneth D. Steinsapir

The field of cosmetic surgery is concerned with the structural improvements that are possible with incisional surgery, and skin quality improvements that result following skin rejuvenation through the application of mechanical, chemical or photic injury. Despite the injury method, the subject of skin resurfacing represents a discipline unto itself. Understanding the limitations of this technology, and comparing the injury it creates with the alternative methods of chemical peeling and dermabrasion, is essential for the cosmetic surgeon offering laser resurfacing. Control and finesse is what distinguishes the master chemical peeler. As more experience is gained with laser resurfacing, our understanding of the limitations and capabilities of laser resurfacing has become more sophisticated, creating the opportunity for finesse with laser resurfacing.

This chapter compares the wounding results obtained with resurfacing lasers and chemical agents. This discussion will help place laser resurfacing into the larger context of skin rejuvenation procedures. Chemical peelers think in terms of light, medium, and deep chemical peels. Many clinicians are new to the subject of skin resurfacing. For reasons that will be discussed below, laser resurfacing is an excellent modality for safely performing skin rejuvenation. Consequently, many cosmetic surgeons performing laser resurfacing are not fully familiar with chemical peels. Lacking this perspective, appreciating that the field of laser resurfacing is evolving is difficult. Laser resurfacing must be thought of as light, medium,

and deep treatments, and need to be selected based on the cosmetic defect to be treated. This chapter will also highlight the limits and advantages of laser resurfacing.

A BRIEF HISTORY OF CHEMICAL PEELING AND LASER RESURFACING

The desire to rejuvenate the face and restore a youthful look is not unique to modern history. In the Edwin Smith Papyrus, a description of an ointment was said to remove the signs of aging (1). However, the modern literature of chemical peeling dates to the nineteenth century. Ferdinand Hebra, a Viennese physician and a pioneer in dermatology, was one of the first to describe the use of caustic agents on the face for the removal of lentigines (2). The relationship between lay peelers and the progress of medical peelers is murky. Montgomery described a Fifth Avenue "beautifier" who was using phenol as a peeling agent as early as the 1880s (3). So this work was probably known to the physicians of the day. MacKee, a very prominent dermatologist of his time, experimented with phenol as a peeling agent as early as 1903, but did not publish his work until 1952 (4). In the interim, two other papers reported the use of phenol to address facial scarring (5, 6). In the early 1960s, two groups of physicians filed and obtained patents for phenol solutions for chemical peeling (7). The technique of phenol peeling of the face became popularized with the work of Litton (8), and

Baker (9). In particular, it was the elegant and simple formula of Baker that was widely adopted by cosmetic surgeons (Table 5.1). At the time when phenol peels were broadly accepted in the medical community, Ayres described the use of various strengths of trichloroacetic acid (10). The 1980s saw the evolution of chemical peeling with the enunciation of the concept of light, medium, and deep peels (Collins PS. The spectrum of chemical peeling. American Academy of Dermatology Annual Meeting, Las Vegas, December 1985). The field has further matured with the introduction of alpha-hydroxy acid peels (11, 12) and the understanding of the importance of skin preparation with retinoic acid (13, 14).

The principle of light amplification by stimulated emission of radiation (LASER) was first described by Albert Einstein in 1917. The first practical demonstration of this concept did not take place until 1954 when Charles Townes reported on stimulated emission with microwave (MASER). In 1960, Theodore Maiman, a scientist at Hughes Aircraft Research Laboratory, reported the development of a ruby laser, which produced a highly collimated, coherent beam of light at a wavelength of 0.69μ (15). The first clinical application of laser was in ophthalmology less than one year later. Lasers have now found application in all fields of medicine. However, the application of lasers to skin resurfacing has been a relatively recent development.

The concept of skin resurfacing with the laser was first described by Laurence David and coworkers (16, 17). Their technique used a continuous wave CO_2 laser that was manually swept over the skin surface to be treated. This technique was highly operator-dependent and resulted in an unacceptably high rate of postoperative scaring as a result of unwanted spread of thermal damage beyond the region of skin ablation. Study of the continuous wave laser used for incisional purposes demonstrate an area of devitalized tissue adjacent to the wound measuring 250 μ in width (18, 19). Further, the continuous wave lasers ablate tissue slowly and consequently char formation and unwanted thermal heating resulted. If the zone of thermal damage is too large, the skin stem cells present in the dermal appendages (upon which healing is dependent) will be lost, and, following laser injury scarring, instead of skin rejuvenation, will result.

Practical skin resurfacing only became possible with the introduction of laser technology that strictly limits the zone of thermal necrosis beyond the tissue ablated by the laser. Studies have shown the benefits of the pulsed laser over the continuous wave CO_2 laser in reducing the zone of thermal necrosis in the wound bed (20, 21). Coherent Medical (Palo Alto, CA) invented the UltraPulse laser in 1991. For the first time, a laser could produce an optimized injury to the skin with a clearly defined depth of clean tissue ablation and a limited zone of thermal damage. The UltraPulse™ laser was first used to treat actinically damaged skin in 1992, and entered wide clinical use in 1994. Sharplan Lasers Inc., (Allendale, NJ) introduced the Silktouch™ laser, a continuous wave CO_2 laser that is rapidly scanned over the skin with an optomechanical device. This technology controls the dwell time of the laser beam at any given point, and thus permits controlled tissue ablation with limited thermal necrosis. The UltraPulse™ and the Silktouch™ CO_2 lasers are considered to be first generation resurfacing lasers. Several other companies have also introduced lasers that can successfully resurface the skin. Some of these systems result in a much more superficial skin injury and have created a second generation of instruments for resurfacing. The recently introduced Erbium:YAG laser represents the latest generation of skin resurfacing instruments and will be discussed briefly in this chapter.

SKIN HISTOLOGY AND SKIN DAMAGE

The skin is a remarkable organ essential for homeostasis. It defends the body from environmental insult. The primary sense organ of touch, skin is also very important in social interaction. It is not surprising then that changes in the skin, which convey a loss of youthfulness, is a cause of great concern for many patients. Intrinsic aging, sun damage, and the chronic environmental insults account for the loss of skin elasticity, alterations in skin tone, development of lentigines, and benign lesions that form the basis for facial skin changes that trouble patients.

Having an appreciation of the histologic anatomy of skin, the nature of its repair mechanisms, and how chronic sun damage affects the appearance of the skin is essential. Each of these areas will be briefly reviewed in this section. This information is the basis for understanding the nature of skin changes that affect appearance, how wounding

TABLE 5.1 Baker's Formula

Phenol	3 ml
Tap water	2 ml
Croton oil	3 drops
Septisol	8 drops

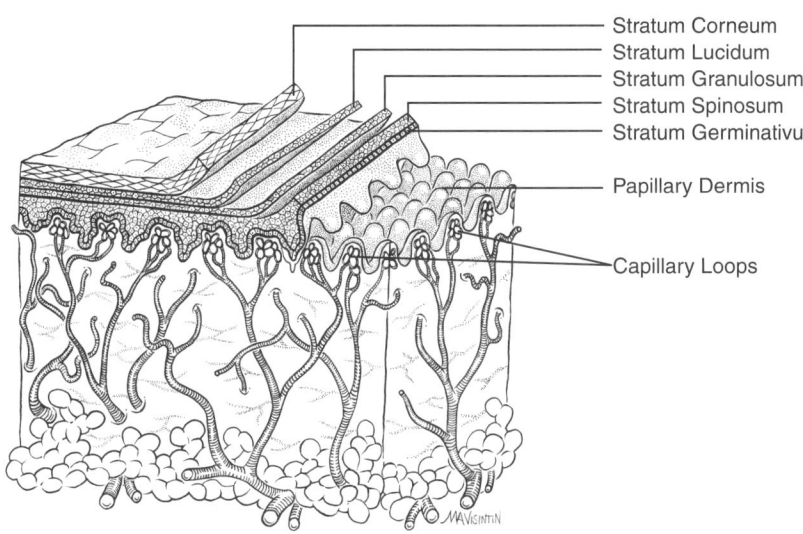

Stratum Corneum
Stratum Lucidum
Stratum Granulosum
Stratum Spinosum
Stratum Germinativum

Papillary Dermis

Capillary Loops

Figure 5.1. Histology of the normal skin. Note that the epidermis and the papillary dermis are of similar depth. In comparison, the reticular dermis is much thicker.

agents affect the skin and activate its reparative mechanisms, and how these mechanisms can and must be maximized to obtain optimal resurfacing results.

The skin is divided into an outer layer, known as the epidermis, and an underlying layer of connective tissue, the dermis. The epidermis is a stratified squamous keratinizing epithelium that also contains keratinocytes, Langerhans' cells, and melanocytes. Nutrients reach the epidermis by diffusion from capillaries in the dermis. Nerve fibers extend from the dermis into the epidermis. Keratinocytes are the main cells present in the epidermis. Keratinocytes mature from germinative cells in the basal layer, which rests on the basement membrane that separates the epidermis from the dermis. The keratinocytes mature into spinous cells and then granular cells before losing their nucleus to become cornified cells that compose the stratum corneum. Basal, spinous, and granular keratinocytes make up the malpigian layer of epidermis (Figure 5.1). The epidermis is continually renewed, with a typical turnover time of 28 days. Melanocytes are dendritic cells usually located in the basal cell layer that produce the melanin in skin. Melanin is distributed to the basal cells through the dendritic processes of the melanocytes. Langerhans' cells are the third cellular component of the epidermis. Also dendritic cells, which possess immunological surface markers consistent with monocytes and macrophages, they are thought to be involved in the initiation of the immune response.

The dermis is composed of a superficial layer, called the papillary dermis, and a deeper, thicker layer, the reticular dermis. The papillary layer is relatively thin and interfaces with the epidermis with irregular papillae. The papillae create finger-like projections that substantially in-

crease the surface area between the dermis and the epidermis relative to the skin surface area. Each dermal papillae contains collagen, elastin, and a small capillary venule to exchange nutrients with the epidermis. The reticular dermis lies below the papillary dermis (Figure 5.1). This is a thicker layer of connective tissue characterized by abundant collagen bundles, ground substance, and elastin. The dermis contains the skin appendages, blood supply, lymphatics, and nerves. Skin adnexa include hair follicles, sebaceous glands, apocrine glands, and eccrine glands. They are significant structures for chemical and laser resurfacing: the epidermal cells, which regenerate the epidermis following mechanical, pulse or flashscanned laser, or chemical injury to the skin, are thought to reside in the hair bulge and other skin appendages (22, 23).

Patients seeking cosmetic surgery for skin rejuvenation typically have one or more of the following concerns:

1. acne vulgaris with or without scarring
2. acquired hyperpigmentation
3. photoaging
4. intrinsic aging.

Importantly, chronic sun exposure accounts for many changes associated with aged skin including fine lines, creases and deep furrows; loss of skin elasticity; scaly, dry skin with irregular lentigines and premalignant or frankly malignant neoplasms; and an overall yellowish hue to the skin (24).

Histologically, with age and sun damage, the epidermis demonstrates loss of polarity or frank dysplasia, which is the loss of the normal uniform differentiation of the epithelium from the basal layer to the stratum corneum. Individual cells may exhibit atypia, dyskeratosis, and hyperkeratosis in the stratum corneum. The rete pegs flatten at the dermal-epidermal junction, the dermal matrix becomes disorganized, and elastin fibers show damage with thickening and curling. With sufficient actinic damage, loss of elastin fibers occurs (25), ultimately resulting in sagging skin that does not snap back to its original form when stretched. Loss of collagen also results in the dermis and a build up of ground substance, which is primarily composed of glycosaminoglycans (GAGs). In contrast, the changes associated with intrinsic aging represent bland atrophy with gradual thinning of the epidermis, and loss of collagen and elastin from the dermis (26).

The effect of a particular wounding modality is affected by its depth of penetration and, equally important, the depth of the skin to be wounded. Chemical peelers have long appreciated that the skin thickness in the face varies from the thinnest skin in the lower eyelids, temple area, and along the jaw line to the thickest skin around the mouth. Laser resurfacing has altered the clinical perspective. Laser ablation depth and zones of thermal necrosis have been studied to the micron, precision that has required a far more detailed knowledge of facial skin depth. By meshing skin depth with known laser ablation depths, the clinician can tailor the laser treatment appropriately. This information is helpful in clarifying the comparison between alternative laser modalities and chemical peeling, and can be readily obtained with high frequency ultrasound backscatter microscopy. Table 5.2 summarizes this information of the face. Data consistent with clinical impressions regarding the variation of skin depth, the thinnest areas in the chart correspond to the eyelid skin and the temple areas. Skin depth data will be referred to in comparing the effects of laser resurfacing and chemical peeling.

CHEMICAL REAGENTS

To have a basis of comparison between laser resurfacing and chemical peeling, the effects of the standard peeling reagents must be reviewed. Armed with this information, the effects of various lasers and laser parameters and the chemical peeling agents can then be compared. Commonly used peeling agents include the alpha hydroxy acids, Jessner's solution, trichloroacetic acid (with and without enhancement), phenol and Gordon Baker's phenol.

Alpha hydroxy acids (AHAs) are derived from fruit and dairy products. Glycolic acid is the most commonly used agent in this class, and it is available in a wide array of concentrations and formulations. Glycolic acid, like other AHAs, help reduce corneocyte adhesion and thin the stratum corneum resulting in a smoother skin. In addition, there is an increased turnover of the epithelium, which also facilitates the turnover of melanin. When these products are combined with skin bleachers, a synergistic effect lightens the skin. With chronic use of glycolic acid, new collagen and elastin are seen in the dermis. Glycolic acid also appears to help in the treatment of acne vulgaris, an effect that may be related to the desquamation of keratinous plugs, which are central to comedogenesis.

Glycolic acid products are available in a variety of strengths and formulations. Lower concentration products (2-15%) are available as over-the-counter skin rejuvenation products (27, 28). Higher strengths (8-30%) are distributed to estheticians for freshening facials, and 40-70% agents are available to the cosmetic surgeon for mild peeling. Stronger glycolic acid is effective in treating dyschromias such as pigmented lentigines, melasma, and berloque hyperpigmentation secondary to chronic perfume application (29). The effect of a glycolic acid peel is dependent on the concentration of the agent and on the length of time the acid acts on the skin before its pH is neutralized (30). Typically, a patient will require a series of peels to achieve a desired result. Stronger in-office peels can be combined with the use of mild, at-home products to create a very effective skin care program.

Histologically, applications of higher concentrations of alpha hydroxy acids (50-70%) penetrate through the epidermis to result in epidermal separations and focal

TABLE 5.2 Skin depth based on ultrasound biomicroscopy

Skin depth (microns)	Epidermis	Papillary dermis	Reticular Dermis
Forehead	75	100	2000
Nose	60	80	1800
Temple	50	100	1000
Cheek	60	100	2500
Eyelids	50	50	800

Ultrasound biomicroscopy is accurate to + 50 μ. Values are averaged from 5 subjects with no correction for age.

TABLE 5.3 Jessner's solution

Resorcinol	14 gm
Salicylic acid	14 gm
Lactic acid	14 ml
QS AD ethanol	100 ml

epidermolysis (31). Once healed, the treated skin demonstrates a thinner, smoother stratum corneum and thickening of the collagen in the papillary dermis (32). Collagen changes can be seen in the upper papillary dermis. Since the alpha hydroxy acids do not produce necrosis in the dermis, it has been suggested that the AHAs may serve as a co-factor in the synthesis of collagen (33).

Jessner's solution (Table 5.3) is a combination of resorcinol, salicylic acid, and lactic acid. It is a mild epithelial exfoliant and, as such, is considered a mild peeling agent. Histologically, skin treated with Jessner's solution demonstrates epidermal edema and no dermal changes (34). The ability of Jessner's solution to disrupt the barrier function of the epidermis can be exploited to enhance the penetration of Trichloroacetic acid (TCA) 35%. Trichloroacetic acid 35% is a mild-to-moderate peeling agent. However, it penetrates more deeply into the papillary dermis following the application of Jessner's solution, creating a peel of moderate depth with a good safety margin (35, 36).

Trichloroacetic acid is used in a variety of strengths depending on the desired effect. The higher the concentration of TCA, the deeper the peeling effect: the concentrations refer to weight to volume dilution (37, 38). Mild freshening peels can be obtained with a TCA 10% solution, which only penetrates into the stratum granulosum. This agent produces a mild burn and minimal frosting. The patient experiences redness and mild desequamation to reveal a fresher, smoother skin. This effect can be intensified with solutions consisting of up to 20% TCA. At concentrations of 25–35%, the peel is sufficiently uncomfortable; patients benefit from regional anesthesia and intravenous sedation. Wounding extends into the papillary dermis with necrosis of the epidermis. Trichloroacetic acid solutions in concentrations above 50% are unpredictable and can result in unexpected scarring (39). Brodland and coworkers measured the depth of necrosis caused by various strengths of TCA in a porcine model and showed a direct correlation between concentration

and depth of necrosis (Table 5.4) (40). When a 35% concentration is applied, patients will experience frosting of the skin following application. Over 24 hours, the skin initially reddens and then darkens. At 48–72 hours following the peel, the skin begins to shed to reveal a pink fresh epithelium, which may take several days before it is completely intact.

Phenol and Baker's phenol are powerful and highly effective agents for chemical peeling of the face. Phenol 89% is a supersaturated solution of phenol and is considered a medium-deep peeling agent. Phenol 89% is effective at addressing all but the deepest lines. Both phenol and Baker's phenol are capable, when used proficiently, of producing an overall tightening effect on the facial skin that can rival the results of a facelift. Both agents are able to significantly improve actinic sun damage, lentigines, actinic keratoses and frank in-situ squamous cell carcinomas. Baker's solution is capable of penetrating deeply in to the reticular dermis and thus effects a greater degree of change. Histologically, the effects of phenol on the skin are dose-dependent (41). Phenol causes tissue necrosis of the epithelium with varying degrees of edema and inflammation in the reticular dermis. The result is regeneration of the epithelium from skin appendages, dermal thickening, and new collagen and elastin deposition. Kligman showed that the improvement in the skin peeled with phenol could be seen in facelift skin specimens twenty years after the peel (42). A distinct band of new dermis was present overlying the old degenerated dermis (Figure 5.2). This band of expanded papillary dermis was referred to by Stegman as the Grenz zone (41). Stegman was also able to measure the effects of dermabrasion, phenol, and Baker's phenol, in sun damaged human skin 120 days after skin wounding. This study demonstrated that Baker's phenol and dermabrasion are associated with

TABLE 5.4 Wounding Depth of TCA

Concentration of TCA(%)	Necrosis Depth(mm)
20	0.044 ± 0.017
35	0.255 ± 0.023
50	0.500 ± 0.061
80	0.983 ± 0.172

Reprinted with permission from Brodland, et al. Depths of Chemexfoliation induced by various concentrations and application techniques of tricholoacetic acid in a porcine model. J Dermatol Surg Oncol 1989;15:967–971.

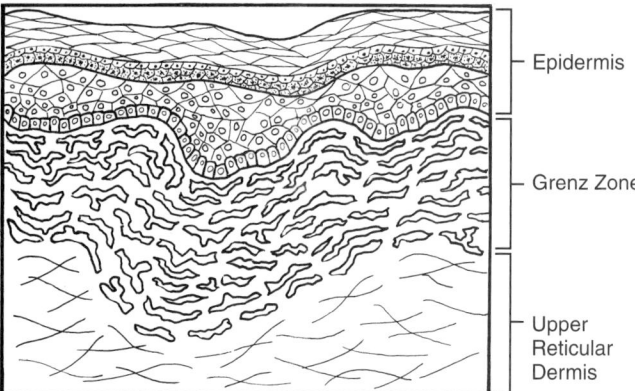

Figure 5.2. Skin postphenol peel. The peel results in the deposit of a new band of collagen referred to as the Grenz zone, which is the basis for long term skin tightening.

TABLE 5.5 Wounding Depth of Phenol: Measurements in Millimeters of Wound Depth, Epidermal Thickness, Grenz Zone Depth, and Dermal Scar in Sun Damaged Skin With Occlusion

	Phenol	Baker's Phenol	Dermabrasion
Wound depth (day 3)	0.4	0.85	0.85
Grenz zone (day 120)	0.08	0.18	0.09
Dermal scar (day 120)	0.35	0.45	0.55

Adapted from Stegman SJ. A comparative histologic study of the effects of three peeling agents and dermabrasion on normal and sun damaged skin. Aesth Plast Surg 1982;6:123–135.

wounds that extend deep into the dermis and account for the profound clinical improvements that occur following these treatments (Table 5.5).

The relative strength of these agents demands caution in their application. Overzealous application of Baker's phenol can result in disastrous facial scarring. Phenol is associated with cardiac arrhythmia (43–45). Consequently, patients require continuous cardiac monitoring. Since phenol is cleared by the liver and kidney, this type of peel is contraindicated in individuals with renal or hepatic impairment. Adequate intraoperative and postoperative hydration can expedite the excretion of the phenol (46). Postoperative pain management is a significant issue. Intraoperatively, patients require deep sedation or general anesthesia. Postoperatively, icing, long-acting nerve blocks, and narcotics may be needed. Patients who have had a Baker's phenol peel can take up to 21 days to

heal. During this period, the skin is gently debrided with dilute hydrogen peroxide if necessary, and dressed with a bland petrolatum. The skin can stay red up to 12 months, often requiring a cosmetic cover-up. Once the erythema subsides, permanent hypopigmentation becomes evident. Fair-skinned persons make excellent candidates, particularly older individuals who are committed to wearing cosmetics and sensible protection from damaging sun exposure.

LASER METHODOLOGIES

Laser resurfacing of the face is made possible by taking advantage of the short absorption length of the CO_2 laser, and more recently, the pulsed Erbium:YAG laser in skin. The CO_2 laser operates in the mid-infrared spectrum (10.6 μ) and has an absorption length of 20 μ in water, the predominant component of soft tissue. According to Beer's law, the absorption length is the thickness of tissue required to absorb 63% of the incident laser energy. Extinction length is another related concept, and represents the distance in tissue needed to absorb 90% of the incident laser energy. The extinction distance is about 2.3 times the absorption length. The laser energy absorbed in tissue is converted to heat, and is conducted to surrounding tissue in a process known as thermal relaxation. When intense laser energy is rapidly delivered into a small tissue volume, the tissue is heated to its boiling point in a process called ablation. In the case of the CO_2 laser, the critical energy density for tissue ablation with minimal thermal damage is a fluence of 5 J/cm² or greater. This energy must be delivered in less than a millisecond, the thermal relaxation time of skin. When the fluence is delivered in a longer period of time, significant conduction of energy takes place resulting in a greater zone of thermal injury. In contrast, when the energy density is above the critical value, and delivered in less time than the thermal relaxation time of the skin, tissue is ablated with minimal heat conduction to the surrounding tissues. Following CO_2 laser treatment, considerable desiccated material remains. Unless this devitalized tissue is debrided before a second laser pass, the desiccated tissue is heated as charred residue rather than ablated. This heat can then spread creating a deeper than anticipated thermal injury.

Two types of CO_2 laser technology are now available commercially to achieve optimal tissue ablation with minimal tissue char. The first of these are the short pulse duration CO_2 lasers like the UltraPulse™ laser (Coherent, Palo Alto, CA). Alternatively, critical fluence values for skin ablation have been achieved with a continuous wave laser delivered by an optomechanical scanning device (Sharplan lasers Inc., Allendale, NJ). A pulsed CO_2 laser with a fluence of 5 J/cm² has been found to vaporize 20–30 μ of tissue and leaves a 40- to120-micron zone of thermal damage (47). In a porcine model, a pulsed CO_2 laser with a fluence of 18J/cm² ablated the porcine skin to the mid-dermis and left a zone of thermal damage measuring 100μ (48) (Figure 5.3). Fitzpatrick and coworkers compared the effects of 1–3 passes of various pulsed laser fluences with the effects of TCAloroacetic acid, Baker-Gordon phenol, and dermabrasion. They found that 3 passes of 150 mJ (2.1 J/cm²) per pulse or 1-2 passes of 250 mJ (3.5 J/cm²) was histologically similar in effect to 35% TCAloroacetic acid peeling. Sites treated with 1-2 passes at 250 to 450 mJ (3.5 to 4.9 mJ) had histologic effects similar to dermabrasion. None of the laser treatments were comparable to treatment with Baker's phenol (49).

The flashscanner technology (Sharplan Lasers Inc., Allendale, NJ) uses a continuous wave CO_2 laser, to which a handpiece containing microprocessor- controlled rotating mirrors is attached. The rotating mirrors move the beam quickly over the skin resulting in a scanned beam that dwells on any one spot for less than the thermal relaxation time of the skin. This technology is associated with a slightly deeper zone of thermal damage for a given fluence (50). The Tru-pulse™ (Tissue Technologies Inc., Albuquerque, NM) is a pulsed CO_2 laser with a pulse duration that is short (60–90 microseconds) compared with the thermal relaxation time of the skin (1 millisecond). The result is an ablation profile much closer to that pre-

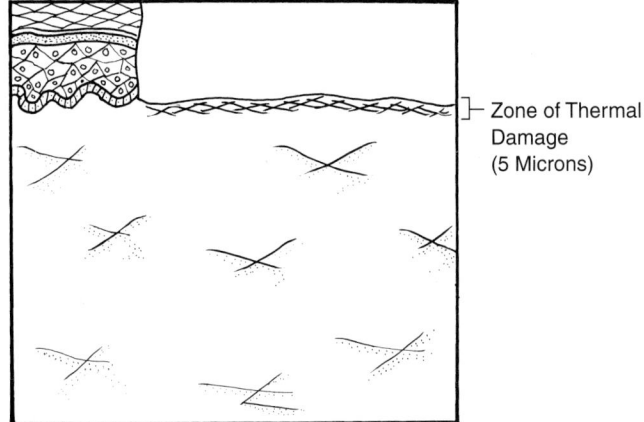

Figure 5.4. Erbium ablation. This illustrates the clean ablation effect of stacking three passes of a typical Erbium:YAG laser. Note that there is minimal thermal effect.

dicted by the absorption of the CO_2 laser in pure water. The average depth of ablation with a fluence of 6 J/cm² is 40μ so that two passes just removes the epithelium and leaves a zone of thermal damage measuring just 10 μ (51). This laser produces much less postoperative erythema, an observation that may be attributable to a thinner zone of thermal damage, or to the decreased depth of injury achieved.

The Erbium:YAG laser is also a mid-infrared laser with an emission wavelength of 2.94 μ. This coincides with the maximal absorption peak for water (52). Consequently, the absorption coefficient of water at 2.94 μ is 13,000 cm^{-1}, with an optical penetration depth of 1 μ. Clinically, the laser creates an ablation of 20–25 μ with a 5-micron zone of thermal damage (Figure 5.4). Ablated tissues are cleanly ejected from the ablation crater and must be collected by a smoke evacuator. Since the zone of thermal necrosis is so narrow, only a minimal coagulative effect to the laser is produced. Bleeding occurs when ablation reaches the papillary dermis. This is not an issue when the resurfacing procedure is intentionally limited to the epithelium. Because tissue is removed cleanly from the ablation site, very little thermal effect is seen and stacking of laser pulses causes only a slight increase in the zone of thermal damage (53). Interestingly, the predicted 1- to 2-micron zone of thermal damage is not realized because the laser-induced tissue stress is not confined to this narrow zone (53). With a moderate number of passes, this laser creates a superficial wound with a very narrow zone of underlying thermal damage. While these wounds usually heal rapidly and with minimal erythema, multiple passes are required to achieve a clinically

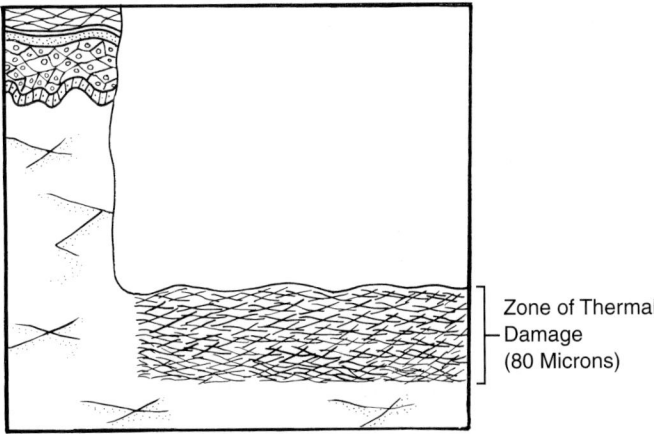

Figure 5.3. CO_2 laser ablation depth. The diagram demonstrates the effect of a CO_2 laser pass. Note that in addition to the significant removal of tissue, a residual zone of thermal injury is also left in the bed of the laser ablation.

Zone of Thermal Damage (80 Microns)

Zone of Thermal Damage (5 Microns)

desirable result. The underlying thermal effect becomes more significant and some perceived benefit of this modality is lost with enough successive passes.

Considerable controversy exists regarding the effect of laser resurfacing on collagen shrinkage. In the process of performing a laser resurfacing procedure, once the epithelium has been removed, subsequent passes of the laser produce dramatic tightening of the skin. This effect is thought to be related to the shrinkage of collagen. Studies show however, that clinical improvement following dermabrasion correlates with the synthesis of new collagen (54). This is also likely to be the case with laser resurfacing. The resultant skin tightening is well documented (55, 56). Collagen denatures near the temperatures produced by the laser. It is not clear whether skin tightening is because of the shrinkage of collagen from the direct effect of laser, or tissue remodeling as has been displayed with dermabrasion. However, histologically it is well established that a zone of dermal repair follows the laser resurfacing procedure (57). Shrinkage of collagen, from denaturation following laser resurfacing, results in the removal of the injured collagen and subsequent replacement as part of the repair process. Consequently, the depth of injury probably determines the nature of the rejuvenation that follows a particular resurfacing procedure, rather than a unique injury mechanism associated with laser resurfacing. It has been shown following laser resurfacing to the depth of the upper reticular dermis, that a new band of collagen forms analogous to the situation with medium and deep chemical peels (Figure 5.5).

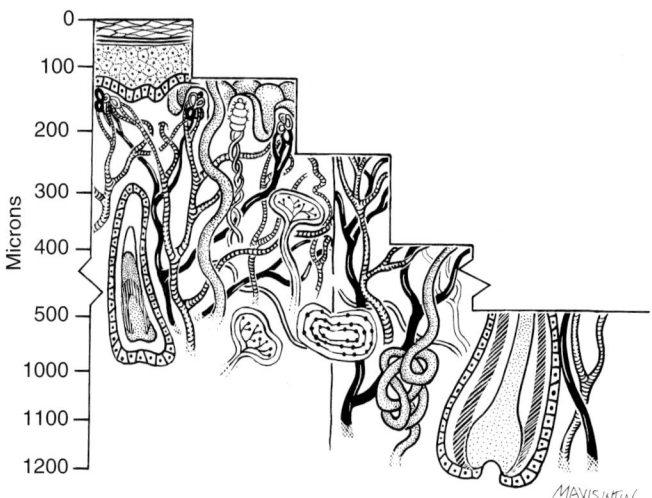

Figure 5.6. Comparing wounding agents. This diagram compares the effective depths of both chemical and laser resurfacing modalities.

LASER RESURFACING VERSUS CHEMICAL PEELING

To appreciate the differences between chemical peeling and laser resurfacing, one must consider the possible range of effects with the two techniques and also the factors required to obtain the desired results (Figure 5.6). These differences defy simplistic comparison. Clinically and histologically, chemical peels continue to have the widest range of effects. The lightest of clinical effects can be achieved with over-the-counter products that can safely be used at home without medical supervision. These are mild agents that, used consistently, produce subtle but satisfying results. Stronger glycolic peels in the 50–70% concentration, dilute TCA peels (10–15%), and Jessner's solution penetrate the epidermis, result in turnover of the epidermis, and mild dermal changes. These "minipeels" can temporarily improve the clarity of the skin, reduce hyperkeratosis, and temporarily benefit fine wrinkles. They are associated with minimal recovery and no down time for the patient. Comparable effects can now be achieved with the ultrashort duration CO_2 skin resurfacing lasers and the erbium lasers. Typically one or two passes of these lasers do not fully ablate the epithelium and are not associated with residual erythema or raw areas. Rapid recovery with an appreciable improvement in the smoothness of the skin, increased skin tone, clarity, and improvement in fine lines occurs. Consequently, skin rejuvenation at a superficial depth can be achieved with both chemical reagents and laser methods. There is a substantial cost difference in delivering the treatment with a laser, but this may be offset by patient demand for the procedure.

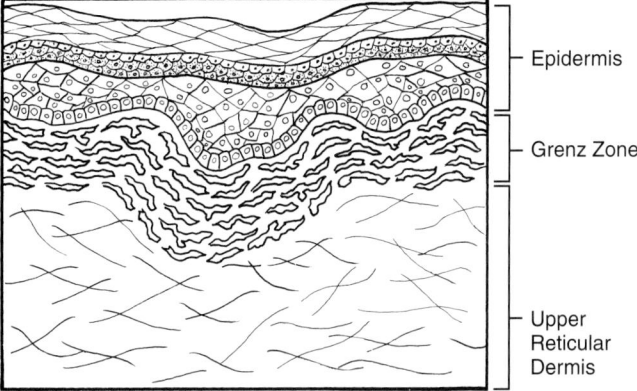

Figure 5.5. Late effects of CO_2 resurfacing. Note that a Grenz zone develops following laser resurfacing. The thickness of this zone may be related to the depth of laser resurfacing.

Higher-strength concentrations of TCA are associated with complete necrosis of the epithelium and a superficial injury to the papillary dermis. This effect can be enhanced with prior application of dry ice or Jessner's solution. Trichloroacetic acid 50% is unpredictable and has been associated with scarring. The Obagi solution is a modified 50% TCA that can be used to obtain a deeper peeling effect with more predictability and fewer complications. Phenol solution (89%) is an excellent medium-depth peeling agent that reliably penetrates to the upper reticular dermis. However, all of these methods require considerable experience to obtain optimum results. Additionally, there is tremendous intraoperator variation between chemical peelers. Therefore, chemical peeling is truly a clinical art. In contrast, laser resurfacing is very effective for performing skin wounding to the depth of the upper reticular dermis. The treatment effect is determined by the parameters of the laser system being used to perform the treatment, and the thickness of the skin being treated. The effect can be to a depth comparable to phenol solution or enhanced TCA peels. However, the laser resurfacing methods are not comparable to Baker's phenol peel, which penetrates almost 1 millimeter into the skin and results in the most significant of skin rejuvenations. However, it can take up to 3 weeks before the facial epithelium is intact following a Baker's phenol peel. Erythema may persist up to a year or longer and once it has resolved, the skin is left hypopigmented. Additionally, thinner skin may not tolerate Baker's phenol and significant scarring can result.

Laser resurfacing removes the outer protective layers of the skin at the time of the procedure. The skin must be dressed either with an occlusive membrane dressing such as Flexzan™ (Dow B. Hickam Pharmaceuticals, Sugar Land, TX) or N-terface™ (Winfield Laboratories, Inc., Dallas, TX), or occluded by bland petrolatum or vegetable shortening. In contrast, following a chemical peel, the necrotic skin requires several days before it sloughs off. It therefore acts as a natural dressing until the peeling necrotic skin reveals the raw, rejuvenating skin underneath. Patients are then instructed to use ointment to occlude the skin. It has been demonstrated that occluding the healing skin with ointment prevents drying of the skin surfacing and allows the epithelial cells to slide over the raw surface, significantly speeding the healing of the skin (58). Increasing the rate of healing can have a significant effect on the ultimate clinical outcome.

Perhaps the most important difference between chemical peeling and laser resurfacing is reproducibility. Consider the variables involved with a chemical peel:

1. How has the skin been prepared? Has the patient been using Retin A or other topical agents?

2. What is the skin degreasing protocol at the time of the peel and how vigorously is it applied?
3. What agent will be used?
4. How is the agent applied (wet, dry, scrubbed in, feathered)?
5. Will multiple peeling agents be used? Considerable variation in skin thickness exists: acne scarring, sebaceous activity, and adnexal density, which must be considered in applying a chemical peel.
6. What will constitute the post peel care?

Each of these factors is critical to the success of a peel. Even in controlling other factors, such as the force with which an agent is applied, perhaps the most individual element of the treatment can never be controlled. In contrast, with laser resurfacing, the laser does the work of skin wounding. The operator-dependent variables associated with laser resurfacing are reduced to a more manageable level compared with chemical peeling. This makes it possible to share treatment parameters with other surgeons. Where there is an infinite variation in how one applies say, a TCA 35% solution peel, the variation is finite with a particular laser technology. The operator must still learn, however, to titrate the laser treatment to skin variables such as skin depth and adnexal density.

Baker's phenol is a qualified gold standard for skin rejuvenation. It penetrates the deepest of any of the resurfacing agents: when used properly, it corrects the most severe of lines around the mouth. Yet it also has significant limitations. Used incorrectly, it can create devastating facial scars. Post treatment erythema can last for a year or longer. Patients must be prepared for this and use concealer makeup to hide the erythema. Once the erythema resolves, hypopigmentation becomes evident. In an individual with a fair complexion, the hypopigmentation may not be noticeable. In individuals with olive skin, the hypopigmentation can be disturbing. Phenol and deeper laser resurfacing procedures are also associated with hypopigmentation. Trichloroacetic acid (50%) and its modifications can be associated with splotchy hypopigmentation. It is not clear if the hypopigmentation is the result of toxicity or simply the result of altered melanocyte function.

Clinicians new to laser resurfacing are often surprised by the persistent postoperative erythema and usually so are their patients. Laser manufacturers are sensitive to this issue and have been touting new technology that produces less erythema. These systems are characterized by shorter pulse durations that produce less thermal injury and generally a shallower tissue ablation. They do produce less erythema, but they also do less clinical work. Significantly, there is great patient acceptance of these procedures, especially in younger patients who are more concerned with the overall clarity and quality of the facial skin and who are less troubled by deeper lines and acne scarring.

The clinical challenge remains meeting the needs of our patients with techniques possessing the smallest risk of morbidity. Nothing can substitute for knowing what the patient desires. The historic trend in chemical peeling has been the development of easily controlled and lighter treatments such as TCA and alpha hydroxy acids. This reflects a desire on the part of younger patients to have the benefit of skin rejuvenation without the downtime and adverse consequences of the stronger peeling agents. This pattern has been rapidly followed in the case of laser resurfacing. In just a few years, several generations of laser resurfacing instruments have been introduced with refinement in technology that also parallels an evolution in our understanding of laser resurfacing.

REFERENCES

1. Breasted JH. The Edwin Smith surgical papyrus. Vol 1. Chicago: University of Chicago Press, 1930:492-498.
2. Hebra F, Kaposi M. On diseases of the skin, including the exanthemata. Vol 3. London: New Sydenham Society, 1874:22-23.
3. Montgomery DW. Phenol. J Cutan Dis Syph 1917;35:157-162.
4. MacKee GM, Karp FL. The treatment of post-acne scars with phenol. Br J Dermatol 1952;64:456-459.
5. Eller JJ, Wolf S. Skin peeling and scarification in the treatment of pitted scars, pigmentation and certain facial blemishes. JAMA 1941;116:934-938.
6. Urkov JC. Surface defects of skin: treatment by controlled exfoliation. Ill Med J 1946;89:75-81.
7. Gross BG, Maschek F. Phenol chemosurgery for removal of deep facial wrinkles. Int J Dermatol 1980;19:159-164.
8. Litton C. Chemical face lifting. Plast Reconstr Surg 1962;29:371-380.
9. Baker TJ. The ablation of rhytides by chemical means. J Fla Med Assoc 1961;48:451-454.
10. Ayres S. Superficial chemosurgery in treating aging skin. Arch Dermatol 1962;85:385-393.
11. Coleman WP, Futrell JM. The glycolic acid trichloroacetic acid peel [Comments]. J Dermatol Surg Oncol 1994;20:76-80.
12. Moy LS, Murad H, Moy RL. Glycolic acid peels for the treatment of wrinkles and photoaging. J Dermatol Surg Oncol 1993;19:243-246.
13. Mandy SH. Tretinoin in the preoperative and postoperative management of dermabrasion. J Am Acad Dermatol 1986;15:878-879.
14. Hevia O, Nemeth AJ, Taylor JR. Tretinoin accelerates healing after trichloroacetic acid chemical peel. Arch Dermatol 1991;127:678-682.
15. Maiman TH. Stimulated optic radiation in ruby. Nature 1960;187:483-494.
16. David LM. Laser vermillion ablation for actinic cheilitis. J Dermatol Surg Oncol 1985;11:605-608.
17. David LM, et al. CO_2 laser abrasion for cosmetic and therapeutic treatment of facial actinic damage. Cutis 1989;43:583-587.
18. Cochrane JPS, et al. Wound healing after laser surgery: an experimental study. Br J Surg 1980;67:740-743.
19. Aronoff BL. Carbon dioxide laser in surgical oncology. Int Adv Surg Oncol 1978;1:243-263.
20. Baggish MS, Mohamed ME. Comparision of electronically superpulsed and continuous-wave CO_2 laser on the rate of uterine horn. Fertil Steril 1986;45:120-127.
21. Green HA, et al. Middermal wound healing: a comparison between dermatomal excision and pulsed carbon dioxide laser ablation. Arch Dermatol 1992;128:639-645.
22. Clark RAF. Cutaneous wound repair: molecular and cellular controls. Prog Dermatol 1988;22:1-12.
23. Mertz PM, Levin R, Bourguignon L. The expression of a transmembrane glycoprotein CD44 in keratinocytes during burn wound healing. J Invest Dermatol 1992;98:634.
24. Kligman LH, Kligman AM. The nature of photoaging, its prevention and repair. Photodermatology 1986;3:215.
25. Braverman IM, Fonferko E. Studies in cutaneous aging: the classic fiber network. J Invest Dermatol 1982;78:434.
26. Lavker RM. Structural alterations in exposed and unexposed aged skin. J Invest Dermatol 1979;73:59.
27. Dial WF. Preparations prescribed in anti-wrinkling therapy. Cosmet Dermatol 1990;3:6-7.
28. Jackson EM. AHA-containing products proliferate in 1993. Cosmet Dermatol 1993;6:22-26.
29. Garcia AJE, Fulton JE. The combination of glycolic acid and hydroquinone or kojic acid for the treatment of melasma and related conditions. Dermatol Surg 1996;22:443-447.
30. DiNardo JC, Grove GL, Moy LS. Clinical and histologic effects of glycolic acid at different concentrations and pH levels. Dermatol Surg 1996;22:421-424.
31. Moy LS, Peace S, Moy RL. Comparison of the effect of various chemical peeling agents in a mini-pig model. Dermatol Surg 1996;22:429-432.
32. Newman N, et al. Clinical improvement of photoaged skin with 50% glycolic acid. A double-blind vehicle-controlled study. Dermatol Surg 1996;22:455-460.

33. VanScott EJ, Yu RJ. Alpha hydroxyacids: procedures for use in clinical practice. Cutis 1989;43:222–229.

34. Brody HJ. Variations and comparisons in medium-depth chemical peeling. J Dermatol Surg Oncol 1989;15:953–963.

35. Monheit GD. The Jessner's + TCA peel: a medium-depth chemical peel. J Dermatol Surg Oncol 1989;15:945–950.

36. Monheit GD. The Jessner's-trichloroacetic acid peel. An enhanced medium-depth chemical peel. Dermatol Clin 1995;13:277–283.

37. Bridenstine JB, Dolezal JF. Standardizing chemical peel solution formulations to avoid mishaps. Great fluctuations in actual concentrations of trichloroacetic acid. J Dermatol Surg Oncol 1994;20:813–816.

38. Bridenstine JB. Errors in compounding acid chemical peel solutions [Letter; Comment]. Plast Reconstr Surg 1996;97:253–254.

39. Sperber PA. Chemexfoliation for aging skin and acne scarring. Arch Otolaryngol 1965;81:278–283.

40. Brodland DG, et al. Depths of chemexfoliation induced by various concentrations and application techniques of trichloroacetic acid in a porcine model. J Dermatol Surg Oncol 1989;15:967–971.

41. Stegman SJ. A comparative histologic study of the effects of three peeling agents and dermabrasion on normal and sun damaged skin. Aesthetic Plast Surg 1982;6:123–135.

42. Kligman AM, Baker TJ, Gordon HL. Long-term histologic follow-up of phenol face peels. Plast Reconstr Surg 1985;75:652–659.

43. Gross BG. Cardiac arrhythmias during phenol face peeling. Plast Reconstr Surg 1984;73:590–594.

44. Truppman ES, Ellenby JD. Major electrocardiographic changes during chemical face peeling. Plast Reconstr Surg 1979;63:44–48.

45. Beeson WH. The importance of cardiac monitoring in superficial and deep chemical peeling [Editorial]. J Dermatol Surg Oncol 1987;13:949–950.

46. Wexler MR, et al. The prevention of cardiac arrhythmias produced in an animal model by the topical application of a phenol preparation in common use for face peeling. Plast Reconstr Surg 1984;73:595–598.

47. Yang CC, Chai CY. Animal study of skin resurfacing using the Ultrapulse carbon dioxide laser. Ann Plast Surg 1995;35:154–158.

48. Green HA, et al. Middermal wound healing: A comparison between dermatomal excision and pulsed carbon dioxide laser ablation. Arch Dermatol 1992;128:639–645.

49. Fitzpatrick RE, et al. Pulsed carbon dioxide laser, trichloroacetic acid, Baker-Gordon phenol, and dermabrasion: a comparative clinical and histologic study of cutaneous resurfacing in a porcine model [letter] [see comments]. Arch Dermatol 1996;132:469–471.

50. Hruza GJ. Skin resurfacing with lasers. Fitzpatrick's Journal of Clinical Dermatology 1995;3:38–41.

51. Bass LS, SJ Aston. Shrinkage and thermal injury in human skin in vitro after resurfacing with carbon dioxide and erbium:YAG lasers. Lasers Surg Med 1997;9(suppl):30.

52. Hale GM, Querry MR. Optical constants of water in the 200-nm to 200-micron wavelength region. Appl Opt 1973;12:555–563.

53. Kaufmann RR. Hibst pulsed erbium:YAG laser ablation in cutaneous surgery. Lasers Med Surg 1996;19:324–330.

54. Nelson BR, et al. Clinical improvement following dermabrasion of photoaged skin correlates with synthesis of collagen. Archives of Dermatology 1994;130:1136–1142.

55. Weinstein C. Ultrapulse carbon dioxide laser rejuvenation of facial wrinkles and scars. American Journal of Cosmetic Surgery 1997;14:3–11.

56. Bass LS, Aston SJ. Shrinkage and thermal injury in human skin in vitro after resurfacing with carbon dioxide and erbium:YAG lasers. Lasers Surg Med 1997;9(Suppl):30.

57. Cotton J, et al. Histologic evaluation of preauricular and postauricular human skin after high-energy, short-pulse carbon dioxide laser [see comments]. Arch Dermatol 1996;132:425–428.

58. Fulton JE Jr. Dermabrasion, chemabrasion, and laserabrasion. Historical perspectives, modern dermabrasion techniques, and future trends. Dermatol Surg 1996;22:619–628.

Chapter Six

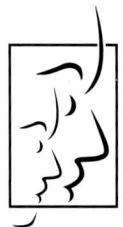

Laser Skin Resurfacing

Jeffrey S. Dover and George J. Hruza

Facial rejuvenation has always been of great interest. For thousands of years, topical agents, such as soured milk, vegetable extracts and mud packs, have been used with limited success. More recently, prepared concentrations of topical agents have been used, including vitamin A derivatives: retinoic acid and a group of hydroxy acids, most notably alphahydroxy acid. Public interest has been great, but the clinical effects only minimal.

A variety of chemical agents have been used to strip off a variable skin thickness to more effectively rejuvenate significantly photodamaged skin. The expectation is re-epithelialization resulting in a more youthful skin appearance. Mechanically removing varying layers of dermis with dermabrasion can also improve wrinkles.

In the 1980s and early 1990s, continuous wave CO_2 lasers were used to resurface photoaged skin (1). Although the results of this procedure (performed by a few) were quite impressive, the risk-benefit ratio of the procedure was very high. Dwelling too long on a specific area led to significant thermal diffusion and thermal damage, and resulted in scarring. The technique was never widely used for this specific reason. However, with the development of short pulse, high peak power, and rapidly scanned, focused-beam CO_2 lasers, and normal mode Er:YAG lasers, removing photodamaged skin precisely, layer by layer, while leaving behind a very narrow zone of thermal damage became possible (2-8). An explosion of interest in the use of this new technology to resurface

photoaged skin, as well as for the treatment of scars, has resulted.

LASER TISSUE INTERACTIONS FOR CO_2 AND Er:YAG LASERS

The use of lasers in dermatology is generally related to laser-induced heating. When this is accomplished with attention to the principles of selective photothermolysis, then very precise tissue effects can be achieved. The basic principles of this theory are that selective heating is achieved by preferential laser light absorption and heat production in the target chromophore, with heat being localized to the target by a pulse duration shorter than the tissue's thermal relaxation (cooling) time (9).

The tissue chromophore that absorbs the 10,600 nm wavelength of the CO_2 laser is water. The depth of penetration of this wavelength into tissue is dependent only on water content: pigmentation and vascularity are irrelevant. The extinction length, or thickness, of water that absorbs 90% of the radiant energy of the incident beam for the CO_2 laser is approximately 30 μm (10-12).

The vaporization or boiling temperature of water at 1 atmosphere pressure is 100°C. When the CO_2 laser is used in the continuous mode at modest powers for vaporization, the skin surface temperature fluctuates in cycles between 120-200°C during ablation. Charring occurs because of extreme heating of desiccated tissue, which carbonizes. The immediate tissue effects are dependent on spot size and power, and the speed with which the laser beam is moved across the tissue surface. When a very small beam diameter of 100–300 μm is used, very high irradiances may be achieved resulting in rapid tissue vaporization. However, unless the beam is moved rapidly across the tissue surface, desiccation, charring and heat diffusion occur. When a large beam size greater than 2 mm is used, nonvaporization heating occurs. The potential for deep thermal damage increases because of the need to apply the low irradiances for long tissue dwell times to achieve vaporization or visible thermal effects. In all of these situations, the time of laser-tissue interaction is the critical factor determining the depth of residual thermal damage (2).

Although the laser energy penetrates only 30 μm or so and is absorbed within that layer, thermal coagulation occurs to a depth of up to 1 mm because of heat diffusion. When visible tissue charring occurs, temperatures greater than 300°C are reached: when the laser is held stationary on this carbonized tissue until it glows red, as with burning coals, temperatures greater than 600°C may be achieved. This results in widespread thermal necrosis that interferes with wound healing and results in scarring.

The ability of the CO_2 laser to photocoagulate blood vessels less than 0.5 mm in diameter, and seal small lymphatics and nerve endings, has resulted in achieving virtually bloodless surgery with less postoperative edema and pain (13, 14). However, the risk of scarring and unpredictable levels of thermal damage with delayed healing have limited the clinical applications of the continuous CO_2 laser. The ability to achieve excellent clinical results has remained an art difficult to perfect.

To control the depth of thermal tissue damage, the continuous CO_2 laser beam must be scanned at a rate resulting in a tissue dwell time less than the thermal relaxation time: otherwise, the energy must be delivered in a pulse shorter than this time. The thermal relaxation time of the 30 μm tissue layer heated by the CO_2 laser has been calculated to be less than 1 msec (15).

Superpulsed CO_2 lasers were developed to deliver peak powers 2–10 times higher, and pulse durations 10–100 times shorter, than conventional CO_2 lasers with shuttered pulses. The basic principle of superpulsed CO_2 lasers is to use high peak powers with short pulse duration to vaporize tissue with minimal thermal injury (16–18).

Further calculations and experimental data reveal the necessary pulse fluence to achieve pulsed laser ablation of skin tissue to be approximately 5 J/cm^2 (10–12). When using a superpulsed laser, the pulse energy of a single pulse is in that 30–50 mJ range, so for single pulse vaporization to occur, the beam diameter must be less than 1 mm. A beam of such a small size cannot be used for resurfacing vaporization applications efficiently, as grooving of tissue occurs and the small beam size results in a slow and tedious procedure. In general, a beam size of at least 2.5 mm is desirable for these applications. In this situation, 6–10 pulses of 30–50 mJ are necessary to reach the tissue vaporization threshold. This can be accomplished by manually shuttering the beam to deliver these short bursts of pulses. However when the superpulse laser pulses are delivered in an uninterrupted stream of pulses, often at a rate of 200 Hz or more, this semicontinuous beam reacts no differently to tissue than a continuous beam. To prevent accumulation of heat between stacked pulses when the only mechanism for heat removal is conduction with no vaporization occurring, the maximum pulse rate should be less than 5 Hz (19). It is clear that the effects of multiple laser pulses impacting the same tissue points is deeper thermal damage.

High Peak Power Laser

Tissue needs to be vaporized in a single pulse to achieve maximal vaporization with minimal thermal damage. When using a beam diameter of 2.5 mm or greater, a pulse energy greater than 250 mJ is necessary, which delivers the required 5 or more J/cm^2. This laser energy will vaporize tissue to the 20–30 μm optical penetration depth of the laser and will leave 40–120 μm of residual thermal damage, which is 2–4 times the optical penetration depth (4, 5). This high energy pulsed laser has been developed by Coherent, Inc. and has been named the UltraPulse™ laser.

When the UltraPulse™ laser is used for single-pulse vaporization of the epidermis, intracellular water is vaporized leaving behind cellular proteinaceous debris. The depth of vaporization is directly proportional to the pulse energy. However, when the dermis is encountered, a large amount of extracellular matrix dominated by structural proteins exists: collagen and elastin. Elastin is very stable and may survive very high temperatures intact. Type I collagen has a sharp melting transition between 60–70°C. Energy densities much higher than 5 J/cm^2 are necessary to vaporize this proteinaceous matrix. Nonvaporization heating of the dermis will have little additive effect if the pulse duration is less than 1 msec and the pulses are delivered at a rate of 5 Hz or less (19). If the delivery rate is greater than this, heat accumulation in tissue will occur and thermal damage by diffusion may occur and may result in poor wound healing or scarring.

In a study conducted on pig skin, a resurfacing depth of 150–450 mJ per pulse delivered in 1–3 passes was compared to the depth achieved with 30% trichloroacetic acid (TCA) medium depth chemical peel, dermabrasion, and Baker's phenol deep chemical peel (4). Reepithelialization of all sites was complete at 7 days with the exception of the phenol-treated site, which required approximately 3 weeks to completely heal with a normally configured epidermis. Healing of the TCA-treated site, both clinically and histologically, was comparable to laser treatment sites receiving 150 mJ/pulse (3 passes) and 250 mJ/pulse (1 or 2 passes). Healing of the dermabrasion-treated site was comparable clinically and histologically to laser treatment sites receiving 250 mJ/pulse–450 mJ/pulse (2–3 passes). The phenol-treated site had not returned to normal at study's end (6 weeks), and represented a deeper and slower-healing wound than produced by any combination of laser pulse energy and numbers of passes studied. Overall, the severity of clinical wound healing parameters and time to resolution correlated with increased depth of tissue removal. Scarring was not observed in any of the treatment sites at study completion.

The precise depth of vaporization was difficult to measure: once the epidermis is removed, laser-tissue interaction with collagen results in heat-induced collagen contraction that alters visible dermal thickness as well. Instead, the total zone of vaporization/tissue contraction plus residual thermal damage was measured to determine the laser resurfacing depth. Since the thermally coagulated tissue sloughs within days, it is this combination of tissue effects that is relevant clinically. A single pass resulted in partial or complete epidermal loss with minimal dermal effects, regardless of the pulse energy, though higher energies resulted in more complete epidermal vaporization. Subsequent passes resulted in progressive tissue loss into the dermis. Dermal vaporization plus necrosis depth was directly proportional to pulse energy and the number of passes applied. The depth of residual thermal necrosis in the dermis after single laser passes of various energies was minimal (< 4 μm). However, with second and third passes, residual thermal damage ranged from 53–106 μm and increased with increasing pulse energy and increasing numbers of passes.

In rabbit skin, with its very thin epidermis, one laser pass with 250 mJ and 3 mm collimated spot size was found to vaporize the epidermis and portions of the papillary dermis and to leave behind approximately 70 μm of residual thermal damage (5).

On human skin, one pass with the UltraPulse™ laser leaves behind a 20-micrometer zone of thermal damage. A second pass increases that zone to 40 μm and a third pass increases it further to 70 μm (20).

Flashscanner

A focused CO_2 laser beam with a spot size of 0.1–0.25 mm can achieve complete vaporization of tissue water by delivering more than 5 J/cm^2 to the target tissue in less than 1 msec. A focused laser beam delivering such a high energy fluence would be very difficult to control freehand. A SilkLaser™ flashscanner (Sharplan SilkTouch™, FeatherTouch™) (with the help of rapidly oscillating mirrors in the handpiece), scans the focused laser beam in a spiral pattern across the tissue: the laser beam is kept at any given spot for less than 1 msec, which for the tissue is equivalent to a 1 msec laser pulse. This dwell time allows for complete target tissue vaporization of well-hydrated tissue, while being short enough to confine peripheral thermal damage to a 40–50 micrometer-zone around the impact site (6). The scanner is microprocessor-controlled and can be programmed to scan areas of various sizes from 0.6–15 mm in diameter depending on the handpiece lens focal length. Scan shapes can be circular, elliptical or even square. The SilkTouch™ flashscanner scans the shape twice with a tissue dwell time of less than 1 msec, while the FeatherTouch™ flashscanner scans the pattern just once at more than twice the speed resulting in a tissue dwell time in the range of 0.3 msec. In the FeatherTouch™ mode, the wattage used is doubled so that the energy fluence delivered to the tissue is above the 5 J/cm^2 vaporization threshold. The amount of tissue vaporized per pass and the zone of thermal damage are both greater per pass with the SilkTouch™ than the FeatherTouch™. A complete scan for skin resurfacing takes 0.03–0.52 sec depending on the scan size.

One pass with the SilkTouch™ flashscanner vaporizes the epidermis, leaving behind a 30 μm zone of thermally coagulated dermis. A second pass increases the zone of thermal damage to 80 μm and a third pass increases it to 150 μm (20). The additive depth of thermal damage observed is probably because of the desiccated thermally denatured collagen left behind from each previous pass. This material contains very little water, thus preventing significant additional vaporization after the initial pass. When less complete vaporization occurs, there is more energy left in the tissue to cause thermal coagulation. Histologic studies with the FeatherTouch™ have yet to be published but, based on the clinical tissue response, the thermal damage zone can be expected to be significantly smaller than with the SilkTouch™.

The SilkLaser™ has a "painting" mode in which the spiral scan is continuously repeated. The painting mode is useful when a large area of epidermis needs to be removed. In this mode, there may be added thermal damage as some overlap of scans is inevitable.

A new scanner system, called the SureTouch™ was introduced in 1997. This scanner can be used with most CO_2 lasers. Focusing the laser beam into a smaller spot size increases the irradiance, which allows the SureTouch™ scanner to generate more than 5 J/cm^2 with one half of the wattage required with the FeatherTouch™. The residual thermal damage zone with the FeatherTouch™ and SureTouch™ scanners are equivalent. Scans up to 17 mm are possible with 20 or 30 watt CO_2 laser systems. The scan pattern lays down rows rather than a spiral, and almost any geometric shape desired can be generated.

High Peak Power Laser vs. Flashscanner

With both laser systems, as tissue is vaporized, a noticeable shrinkage of the remaining dermis becomes evident. Collagen, as it is heated, will contract significantly. It is unclear, at this time, if this collagen shrinkage adds to the final clinical improvement, or if the collagen that has contracted is sloughed off with all the other necrotic material. Both lasers produce increased residual thermal injury with repeated passes to the same area, and eventually reach a limit where further passes do not produce further thermal injury. However, if pulses are stacked, i.e. successive passes are made over the same area without wiping the debris away first, the zone of residual thermal damage will continue to increase. Inadvertent pulse stacking substantially increases the risk of unwanted thermal injury and resultant scarring.

The different laser systems appear to achieve equivalent clinical results in properly trained hands. In clinical use, two passes with the SilkTouch™ are approximately equal to three passes with the UltraPulse™ and four passes with the FeatherTouch™ in terms of the amount of tissue removed and the depth of residual thermal damage left behind. The main differences are in the specific parameters used with each laser system (Table 6.1).

Contrary to many pulsed CO_2 resurfacing laser systems, increasing the wattage on the SilkLaser™ will increase the energy fluence delivered to the tissue: more tissue is vaporized per scan without an appreciable increase in the residual thermal damage zone. This makes the SilkLaser™ useful for the removal of bulk tissue such as rhinophyma or adnexal tumors or to rapidly resurface large areas with a lower number of laser passes required.

Erbium:YAG Laser

Among alternative lasers developed for skin resurfacing, the Er:YAG laser has been the most useful. Its emission wavelength of 2,940 nm is close to an absorption peak of water that is 16 times greater than that of CO_2 laser light (21). Shallower skin penetration of 1 μm, compared with 20 μm for CO_2 laser light, allows more precise ablation with less thermal damage (22).

Measurements on the Er:YAG laser predict an ablation threshold of 0.6–5 J/cm^2 (23–25). Although absorption takes place in the first 1–2 μm of tissue, fluencies of 80 J/cm^2 can ablate 400 μm of tissue, a finding that has not been satisfactorily explained. The Er:YAG laser has been tested in a pulsed (normal) mode with a pulse width of 200 μsec and in a Q-switched mode with a pulse width of 90 nsec. At fluencies below 25 J/cm^2, 2.5–30 μm of tissue was ablated and the zone of damage was limited to 10–40 μm with normal mode laser, and 5–10 μm with the Q-switched laser, when tested in guinea pig skin (23, 24). In the Q-switched mode, residual thermal damage is insufficient to coagulate blood vessels, leaving a bloody surgical field limiting its clinical utility. In the normal mode, skin vaporization leaves a relatively bloodless field after 2–3 passes. Bleeding becomes a greater problem with successive passes (26).

Whether the histological changes with the Er:YAG are similar remains to be determined. It appears that the depth of ablation increases with fluence up to 80 J/cm^2. Residual damage also rises with increasing fluence and with increasing pulse width (23, 24). There is insufficient thermal damage to produce immediate tissue contraction. Whether long-term wound healing is associated with contraction of collagen, which improves sagging skin, remains to be seen.

Other Lasers

Limitations of CO_2 laser resurfacing are oozing and crusting that lasts from 7 to 14 days after treatment, and ex-

TABLE 6.1 High Peak Power CO_2 Lasers vs. Flashscanner

	Coherent UltraPulse	Tissue technology TruPulse	Sharplan SilkLaser	Er:YAG Laser (various manufacturers)
Laser type	100 watt CO_2	6 watt CO_2	20 or more watt CO_2	Er:YAG
Wavelength	10.6 μm	10.6 μm	10.6 μm	2.94 μm
Delivery method	Individual Gaussian pulses	Individual square pulses	Spiral (SilkTouch, Feather-Touch) or rasterized (Sure-Touch) scan with focused beam	Individual pulses
Power	500 watts peak power, pulsed	10,000 watts peak power, pulsed	7–100 watts average power, continuous-wave beam	10–20 watts average power
Pulse duration	950 μsec	60–100 μsec	0.03–0.52 sec scan duration; 300–1000 μsec tissue dwell time	300 μsec
Energy	50–500 mJ/pulse Adjustable by changing pulse width	10–500 mJ/pulse Adjustable by changing peak power	N/A continuous wave laser	0.1–2 J/pulse adjustable
Energy fluence	5–7 J/cm²	5–7 J/cm²	5–15 J/cm² or more	1–50 J/cm²
Spot size	3 mm collimated; computer pattern generator (CPG)	1 and 3 mm	0.6–15 mm scan size with 0.1–0.25 mm focused beam	2–7 mm collimated or focused; pattern generator
Spot shape	Round spot; various with CPG	Square spot	Round, square or elliptical scan (SilkTouch, Feather-Touch); various (Sure-Touch)	Round; various with pattern generator
Effect of increasing power	Increases rate of pulsing	Increases rate of pulsing	Increases thickness of tissue removed with each scan	Increases rate of pulsing: 1–20 Hz

tensive erythema, which persists for at least 4–6 weeks, but sometimes more than 3 months (3, 8). Based on technology developed at the Los Alamos National Physics Laboratory, a high-peak power, short pulse but low average power, CO_2 laser has been developed by Tissue Technologies and approved for skin ablation by the FDA. This 6-watt laser, called the TruPulse™, produces high-peak power pulses that can achieve fluencies of over 5 J/cm², the ablation threshold of human skin, at variable pulse durations, from 30 μsec to 1 msec (Table 6.1). By using shorter pulse durations than the UltraPulse™ CO_2 laser, in the 60–100 μsec range, this device removes less tissue per pass (roughly 30 μm). The TruPulse™ laser requires more passes to ablate significantly photodamaged skin effectively, but also leaves less residual thermal damage (roughly 15 to 30 μm). In a bilateral comparison study with the UltraPulse CO_2 laser, when the endpoints of

treatment rather than the number of passes were fixed, there was no difference in healing time or outcomes, suggesting that the benefit of the shorter pulse duration was negated by the need for more passes to achieve clearing of rhytides (27).

PREOPERATIVE CONSIDERATIONS

Patient Selection (Table 6.2)

In evaluating the prospective patient and assessing the potential response to laser resurfacing, the two primary areas of attention are the perioral and periorbital regions. Wrinkling in these areas has been traditionally unresponsive to face-lifting procedures, as the laxity of skin removed and tightened by these techniques does not

TABLE 6.2 Indications for Resurfacing CO₂ and ER:YAG Lasers

Actinic cheilitis

Actinic keratoses

Adenoma sebaceum

Dermatosis papulosa nigra

Epidermal nevi

Erythroplasia of Quyerat

Rhinophyma

Rhytides, facial

Rhytides, non-facial (Er:YAG only, experimental)

Scars, facial

    Acne

    Surgical

    Traumatic

    Varicella

Sebaceous hyperplasia

Solar lentigines, facial

Syringoma

Trichoepithelioma

Xanthelasma

include these areas. Chemical peeling and dermabrasion, though helpful, have often been disappointing in their results in these locations. However, our experience in laser resurfacing has been very rewarding in achieving excellent perioral and periocular results. Though any facial wrinkles may respond excellently to laser therapy, these areas have defined the success of laser resurfacing, primarily because of their difficult response to treatment historically (3, 6, 8, 28, 29).

In general, both wrinkling and photo-damage to the epidermis and dermis are responsive to treatment. As far as epidermal pathology associated with aging is concerned, actinic keratoses, squamous cell carcinoma in situ, lentigines and seborrheic keratoses are all removed with stripping of the epidermal layer. Photodamage of the dermis results in fragmentation of elastin and collagen fibers, most profoundly in the papillary dermis. This is seen clinically as altered surface texture and pallor with crepe-like changes progressing to those of severe photoaging with cream-yellow discoloration and deep creases. These layers of altered dermal tissue may be removed by vaporization

and thermal necrosis and replaced with new healthy collagen developed over a tightened matrix of shrunken collagen. The ability to change these tissues dramatically relates to the depth of damage: the more superficial damage being more responsive. These altered dermal changes result in loose, sagging or folded skin. These folds may be particularly visible under the eyes, on the medial lower cheeks, on the lateral cheeks anterior to the ears, and to a certain extent, at the nasolabial folds. These areas are very responsive to the tightening effects achieved with laser resurfacing (3, 6, 8, 28, 29).

On the other hand, lines of expression such as forehead creases, glabellar furrows, "crow's feet" and nasolabial folds, may be responsive if superficial, but only softened when deep folds or palpable deep creases. Even when these lines completely resolve, they recur much sooner because of the unavoidable effects of muscular contractions compressing and folding the skin with facial expression. This is true of certain perioral lines as well. Dynamic facial lines are best treated with other modalities: botulinum toxin muscle paralysis, bovine collagen injections or other augmentation techniques.

As with any cosmetic procedure, patient expectations are the most important determinant of patient satisfaction. A patient must have realistic expectations as to the improvement that can be achieved. Laser resurfacing can improve, but will not eliminate, all or even most wrinkles. Showing before and after photographs may be helpful. However, photographs of rhytides can often be misleading because of changing light conditions, camera angle, and patient facial expression. If photographs are used, both good as well as less-than-ideal results should be shown to the patient. A detailed discussion of the potential complications and expected postoperative course is imperative to reduce patient anxiety and frequent calls from the patient in the immediate postlaser period.

Patients of any age who are in reasonably good health can undergo laser resurfacing. Screening laboratory tests are generally not necessary as the procedure is most often done under local anesthesia. Contraindications for the procedure are similar to dermabrasion. Patients who form keloids should not undergo laser resurfacing. A reduction in the number of adnexal structures contraindicates laser resurfacing, i.e., skin that has received prior X-ray treatment or patients with scleroderma, as a successful result relies on re-epithelization from normal and intact adnexal structures remaining after laser resurfacing.

Prior isotretinoin treatment has been associated with atypical scarring after dermabrasion or chemical peel, even if the procedure was performed more than 1 year after isotretinoin treatment (30). The frequency of this complication is unknown. Therefore, patients who have received isotretinoin should receive additional warnings about the possibility of scarring from laser resurfacing and the procedure should probably be done more conservatively. We recommend that the patient wait at least 1–2 years before undergoing laser resurfacing after isotretinoin treatment.

Skin that has recently been undermined, as in a facelift or blepharoplasty, has an altered blood circulation for several months. Resurfacing procedures done at the same time as or soon after skin undermining increase the risk of skin necrosis with associated scarring (31, 32). We recommend that laser resurfacing of undermined skin be deferred for 6 months after the original surgical procedure. It is unknown how long after laser resurfacing a patient can safely undergo a procedure that undermines the resurfaced skin, but a wait of 3–6 months seems prudent.

Medications

Many medications are useful to make the procedure safer and more comfortable for the patient. Retin-A has been shown to speed re-epithelization after dermabrasion (33) and chemical peels, and it may work similarly after laser resurfacing. While there are no published controlled trials demonstrating the benefits of tretinoin, we encourage use of Retin-A at the highest tolerable concentration daily for at least 6 weeks before the procedure (34). We use alphahydroxy acids only in patients who are tretinoin intolerant.

Postinflammatory hyperpigmentation is a frequent occurrence after laser resurfacing. A majority of Fitzpatrick type IV patients will develop it as will almost all darker-skinned individuals (3). To reduce the incidence of postinflammatory hyperpigmentation, all patients are encouraged to avoid having a sun tan at the time of the procedure, and type III–VI patients are given hydroquinone, kojic acid or azelaic acid to be used for several weeks before the procedure (34). Our favorite product is Solaquin Forte (ICN Pharmaceuticals, Costa Mesa, CA) which contains 4% hydroquinone and an SPF 15 sunscreen, but irritation occurs in up to 15% of users. As an alternative, we recommend Melanex (Neutrogena Dermatologics, Los Angeles, CA) which is 3% hydroquinone in a liquid vehicle. The ideal time for laser resurfacing is late Fall and in Winter.

In patients with a history of herpes labialis, laser resurfacing can trigger an outbreak that can spread to involve the entire denuded skin surface with resulting increased pain, prolonged healing, and an increased risk of scarring. We have encountered several instances where patients denied any history of herpes labialis, but who developed severe herpes outbreaks after laser resurfacing. Therefore, all patients, regardless of cold sore or fever blister history, are prophylactically given either acyclovir 400 mg orally three times daily, or valacyclovir 500 mg orally twice daily, starting up to 2 days before, and continuing for at least 10 days after the procedure.

After laser resurfacing, there is a layer of necrotic, thermally coagulated dermis that will slough over several days. This material serves as an ideal bacterial culture medium. Therefore, patients are usually given prophylactic antibiotics, such as dicloxacillin 500 mg orally twice daily or, in penicillin allergic individuals, azithromycin 500 mg followed by 250 mg orally daily starting up to 1 day prior to surgery and continuing for a total of 5 days (34). Since oral antibiotics have been introduced, impetiginization of the treated areas has been virtually eliminated.

Some surgeons prescribe a short, 3–4 day, course of oral corticosteroids for the patient perioperatively to reduce the very significant edema that usually occurs during the first 72 hours after the procedure.

ANESTHESIA

Facial resurfacing with a laser requires the use of an anesthetic that effectively blocks the pain that results from vaporizing epidermal and dermal tissue. This is especially important with CO_2 laser resurfacing. While the efficiency of Er:YAG laser ablation produces limited thermal injury, resurfacing with this laser is painful and requires some anesthesia. Though many physicians have attempted to perform CO_2 laser resurfacing using topical anesthetic agents, such as EMLA™, the success of this has been limited. Either only superficial anesthesia is developed, or the occlusion necessary to induce deeper anesthesia results in significant tissue maceration that alters the desired laser-tissue interaction. This topical anesthesia approach has proven too impractical to be useful in CO_2 laser resurfacing, but it has been found to be effective for some in Er:YAG resurfacing.

Local infiltration or regional nerve blocks are preferred for localized areas. Supraorbital, supratrochlear, infratrochlear, infraorbital and mental nerves are easily blocked, providing complete anesthesia of the central face, excluding the upper and lower eyelids, nasal tip and oral commissures. These areas, and also any locations on the lateral and inferior cheeks, temples and along the jawline must be anesthetized with local infiltration. The local anesthetic should be injected into the subcutaneous plane to minimize distortion of the surface rhytides. It may be helpful to mark out the rhytides with gentian violet prior to injecting the anesthetic. Sedatives and analgesics may be administered prior to performing these nerve blocks. Valium™, Versed™, Demerol™, Phenergan™, Halcion™ and Ativan™ have been used in various combinations.

Regional blocks are performed with 1–2% lidocaine with 1:100,000 epinephrine. With proper placement of the anesthetic, as little as 0.5 ml is needed to completely block the nerve. Because the procedure is relatively short, we have found no need to use longer-acting anesthetics such as bupivacaine. For local tissue infiltration, especially around the eyes and for the cheeks, we use a mixture of equal parts 2% lidocaine with 1:100,000, 0.5% bupivacaine, 1 part in 10 of 8.4% $NaHCO_3$, and 75 U of hyaluronidase. The bicarbonate neutralizes the pH and decreases pain of injection and the hyaluronidase improves tissue diffusion. When a large volume of anesthetic is needed, 0.5% lidocaine with 1:400,000 epinephrine can be used to minimize epinephrine-induced tachycardia and to stay within the 7 mg/kg lidocaine total dose limitation.

When full face resurfacing is performed, several choices are available. While regional anesthesia augmented by local infiltration to the eyelids, corners of the mouth and cheeks with some form of oral preoperative sedation may be used, we have found that this does not provide adequate sedation and that patients are uncomfortable during the procedure. Intravenous sedation performed by an anesthesiologist, using appropriate monitoring, is recommended. Versed™ and Propofol™ are commonly used with some analgesic such as Fentanyl™ (Sanofi Pharmaceuticals, New York, NY). While intubation is not re-quired, we have found that the use of a laryngeal mask allows full face resurfacing with intravenous agents alone, without the need for regional and local infiltration.

TECHNIQUE (RHYTIDES) (3, 6, 8, 28, 29)

The skin may be prepared with an antiseptic such as Betadine™ (Purdue Frederick, Norwalk, CT) or Septisol™ (Delasco, Council Bluffs, IA). If alcohol antiseptics are used, they should be allowed to dry completely before starting the procedure. Chlorhexidine should be avoided because of its ocular toxicity, which might be aggravated by laser vaporization. Extensive prepping of the skin prior to laser resurfacing is usually not necessary as the laser sterilizes the surface as it vaporizes (35).

Free-flowing oxygen should be kept away from the field to reduce the risk of fire. The treatment area is wrapped with wet towels. Depending on the area being treated, the patients eyes are covered with laser safety glasses, small opaque goggles or wet eye pads. For resurfacing of eyelids, stainless steel eye shields are placed under the eyelids.

The most commonly requested areas for laser resurfacing are the perioral (Figure 6.1A, B), periorbital (Figure 6.2A–C) and glabellar/forehead regions as isolated units. When treating any of these areas as an isolated treatment, it is important to follow the treated wrinkles out to their end rather than limiting treatment to the cosmetic unit. That means when treating the periorbital area that the "crows' feet" of the lateral canthus area must be followed out to the temporal area as well as to their points over the superior lateral cheeks, and the medial lines over the nasal bridge (Figure 6.2A–C).

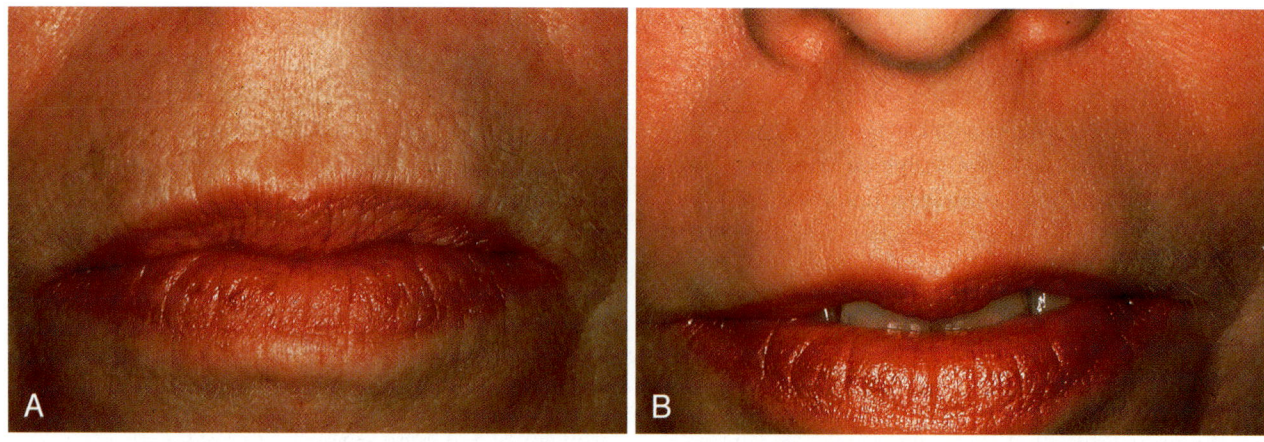

Figure 6.1. Perioral rhytides **A,** before and **B,** one year after UltraPulse™ CO_2 laser resurfacing.

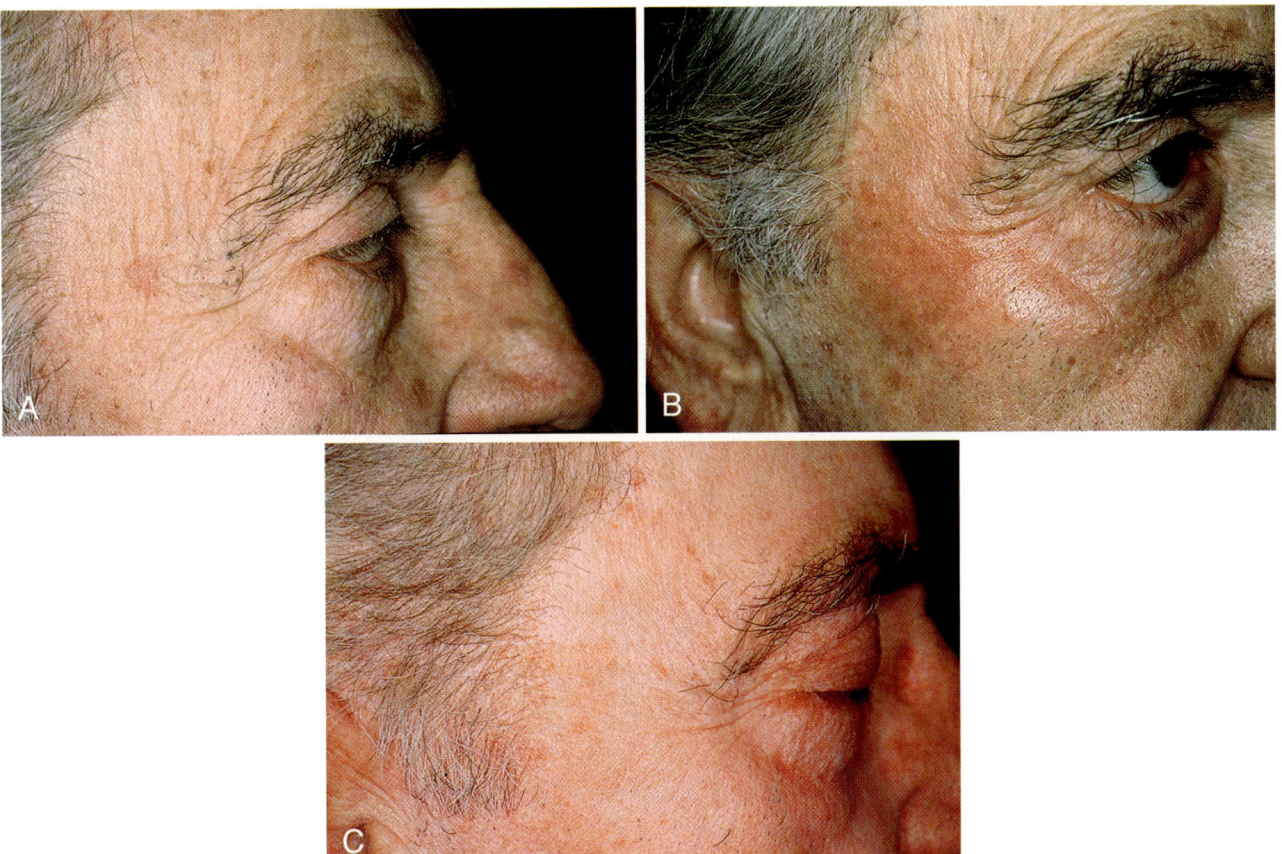

Figure 6.2. "Crow's feet" **A,** before SilkTouch™ CO$_2$ laser resurfacing **B,** six weeks after resurfacing with postinflammatory hyperpigmentation, and **C,** two years after resurfacing of the temple, and one year after resurfacing of the forehead and cheek.

When treating the perioral area alone, the wrinkle lines that often flare laterally off the lower nasolabial fold, and the crescent lines of the medial lower cheek just lateral to the mouth, should also be treated. The treatment should be carried over the jawline to the level of the submental crease. The vermilion border should be treated to remove the fine vertical wrinkles that cross it and cause lipstick to "bleed" into them.

When these areas are treated in this way, the treatment zone extends beyond what is commonly accepted as the anatomical unit of each area for cosmetic purposes. Because of this extension beyond the most visible anatomical markers such as the nasolabial fold and the orbital rim, using a feathering technique with the laser to blend into the untreated skin is important.

When both the perioral and periorbital regions are to be treated, it is preferable to treat the entire face (Figure 6.3A), or at least the full face from the eyebrows down. When this is done, the treatment of the cheeks re-sults in secondary improvement in the other two areas as well. In addition, the erythema and/or transient pigment changes are less visible when present in a more uniform distribution. Permanent hypopigmentation is far easier to camouflage when the entire face is treated.

Patients sometimes request treatment of only the glabellar lines. Though this may be done, the result is not impressive, with very visible erythema of only this location, making it difficult to conceal with makeup or other camouflage. It is preferable to continue the resurfacing across the entire forehead.

In CO$_2$ laser resurfacing, the epidermis of the area to be treated is first removed using a confluent application of single vaporizing laser pulses. The desiccated proteinaceous debris that remains after laser application represents keratinous cellular remnants following intracellular vaporization. This debris must be wiped clear as it will block the laser from reaching its target of dermal tissue underlying this layer, because it no longer has water

Figure 6.3. Full face rhytides in a 60-year-old patient **A,** before, **B,** 3 days after, **C,** 10 days after and **D,** 6 weeks after UltraPulse™ CO_2 laser resurfacing.

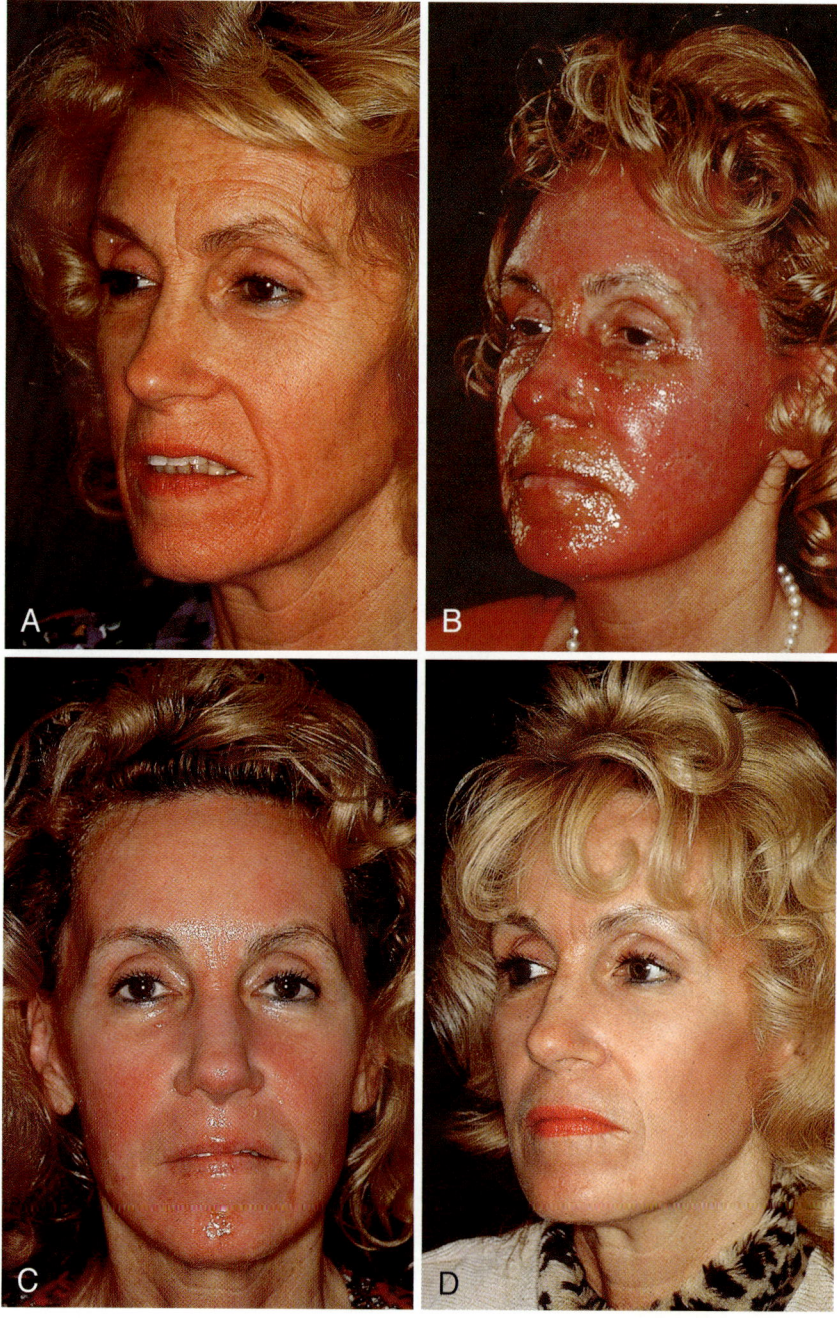

present as a target for the laser. Wiping this layer away with saline not only removes this hurdle, but also acts to rehydrate the underlying tissue. Once this debris has been wiped away, a dry gauze must be used to remove any water remaining on the skin surface as this will absorb the laser energy and block its reaction with dermal tissue. A second laser pass is then performed over the entire area of photodamaged dermis. This is most easily performed in an even, confluent application. However, as multiple passes are performed, the area treated with each pass generally

becomes smaller as more superficially damaged areas are normalized with tissue vaporization. With each additional pass, there is further wrinkle smoothing as well as increased risk of complications because of the greater depth of tissue injury. One of the endpoints of treatment is smoothing away tissue irregularities and visible wrinkle lines so that a smooth and even surface results. This is sometimes accomplished more efficiently by concentrating the laser on high points of tissue on the shoulders of wrinkle lines. This will result in flattening of those high points, both by vaporization as well as collagen contraction. Bleeding is rarely encountered with CO_2 lasers.

The tissue changes color as resurfacing proceeds deeper into the dermis. Entry into the papillary dermis is evident as a pink surface color. The color changes to gray with deeper papillary dermal ablation. Further ablation produces a yellowish hue that corresponds to ablation into the upper reticular dermis and is usually the endpoint of treatment. Additional passes cause a darker yellow to brown color. The color changes are probably related to the buildup of thermally denatured collagen rather some intrinsic property of different dermal layers.

In Er:YAG resurfacing, less tissue is removed per pass. Several passes (up to 4) may be required to remove the epidermis, and as many as a total of 8 or more may be needed to reach the desired endpoint. We recommend wiping away the proteinaceous material at least after the first pass and at the end of the procedure. The endpoint of treatment is effacement of the rhytides and photoaged skin. As more passes are done and resurfacing enters the dermis, however, the amount of residual thermal damage is insufficient to coagulate medium-sized vessels and bleeding may preclude further treatment.

Coherent UltraPulse™

When treating with the UltraPulse 5000™, use of the computer pattern generator (CPG) is preferable because it results in faster, more uniform, and safer treatment as the computer precisely and rapidly places each laser spot within the pattern (36). However, any and all areas of the face may be treated using the 3 mm collimated beam handpiece and using confluent single pulse vaporization with 10% or less overlap.

The CPG scans a 2.25 mm spot across the skin in 1 of 9 different patterns, including a square, parallelogram and hexagon. The shape and size of the scan, and the density of the spots within the pattern are all determined by the operator. No two patients are the same, and as a result no two UltraPulse™ CO_2 laser resurfacing cases are the same. There are, however, certain precepts that can be applied to all cases. The most frequently used CPG patterns are the square and the parallelogram. The largest scan size (scan # 9) is most often used to cover the largest area per scan. The higher the density, the more skin vaporized and the greater the residual thermal damage per pass. We recommend that densities greater than 6 not be used as excessive thermal injury will result. In sensitive, thin-skinned areas, such as periocular skin, lower densities are recommended. Because of lateral heat spread at the dermoepidermal junction, small skip areas will be removed when wiping away the epidermal debris. These small skip areas in the dermis add a protective zone to help prevent heat accumulation that may occur with rapid pulse placement one on top of another. For these reasons, it is far preferable to leave small skip spaces during treatment rather than to overlap too much (37).

Feathering with the laser is accomplished by decreasing both the pulse energy and the density of application of pulses. Performing two concentric peripheral zones of about 10-15 μm each is advisable: start with confluent application of a pulse energy 100-200 mJ less than that used for treatment and gradually decrease the density so that at the end of this zone pulses have a 2-4 mm space of untreated skin between them. The second zone of feathering requires another drop in pulse energy of 100-150 mJ and further gradual spreading of pulses to 5-6 mm apart in an irregular, uneven manner.

Sharplan SilkLaser™

For most resurfacing indications, the "start safe" default laser power settings are a good starting point. The laser parameters are set using a touch screen. The surgeon selects the handpiece, mode (SilkTouch™ or Feather-Touch™), scan size and scan shape and the laser sets the correct scan time and suggests a power setting that is appropriate for most resurfacing cases. The time between scans is set by the surgeon so that he has enough time to move the handpiece between scans and position it for the next scan with intervals of 0.2-0.3 seconds appropriate for relatively short and small scans and 0.4-0.5 needed for long and large scans (38).

The number one determinant of safety and efficacy is the number of laser passes used. One pass with the Silk-Touch™ mode approximates the depth of a medium-depth Jessner's solution plus 35% TCA chemical peel. Two-to-three passes approximate the depth of dermabrasion and four or more passes approach the depth of a deep Baker's phenol peel. The FeatherTouch™ mode requires approximately twice as many laser passes as the SilkTouch™ mode for equivalent clinical results when the laser is set to the recommended start safe settings. Increasing the wattage in the FeatherTouch™ mode will increase the amount of tissue vaporized per pass without significantly increasing the depth of thermal damage. Therefore, higher FeatherTouch™ power settings will reduce the number of laser passes needed.

It is often helpful after the initial 1-3 passes to switch to a smaller scan size to go down the shoulder of each remaining rhytid. The edges of the treatment field receive only one pass to allow for feathering of the edges. Further feathering can be achieved by angling the handpiece away from being exactly perpendicular to the skin surface. This will space out the individual laser passes in the spiral scan farther apart at the edge of the treatment field.

The eyelids should receive a maximum of 1 pass with the SilkTouch™ mode or 2 passes with the FeatherTouch™ mode for an endpoint consisting of a pink to slightly gray surface. The temples, lateral cheeks and jawline in women can receive a maximum of 2 SilkTouch™ passes or 3 FeatherTouch™ passes with a residual light yellow surface color. The rest of the face, including the forehead, glabella, medial cheeks, perioral region and nose, has thicker skin that can usually tolerate up to 3 passes with the SilkTouch™ or 5 passes with the FeatherTouch™ when treating rhytides. Individual deep acne scars on the cheeks, especially in men, may require up to 5 SilkTouch™ or 8 FeatherTouch™ passes to achieve even moderate improvement. After 3 SilkTouch™ or 5 FeatherTouch™ passes using standard resurfacing settings, there appears to be relatively little additional shrinkage, tissue vaporization or added thermal damage.

Er:YAG Laser

Most Er:YAG laser systems pulse at a rate of 10 Hz. The treatment field is covered with moderately overlapping laser pulses, using spot sizes of 3-7 mm, or with some systems a pattern generator can lay down the spots in any shape desired. The pulse energy used is in the 0.5-2 J range depending on the spot size. The settings are adjusted to arrive at an efficient ablative energy fluence. With an energy fluence of 5 J/cm² the epidermis is vaporized away in 4 passes. At 8-12 J/cm², the epidermis is vaporized away with 2 passes (39). Additional passes are carried out until the lesion or rhytid has been effaced, bleeding has been encountered, or a maximum safe number of laser passes has been completed. Each pass will ablate 10-40 μm of tissue depending on the energy fluence used (26). The number of passes used will depend on how deep the laser surgeon needs to go to remove the pathology while staying superficial enough to minimize the risk of scarring and permanent hypopigmentation. Wiping the tissue between passes helps remove the minimal desiccated debris left behind, helps to keep track of the number of laser passes, and may allow for observation

of the tissue to determine the level of ablation. However, there is no color change in the tissue as there is no significant thermal build-up.

OTHER INDICATIONS

Acne scars have traditionally been treated with dermabrasion (40, 41). Moderate improvement can be achieved, but the procedure is quite bloody, and the blood microdroplets can hang suspended in the air for several hours posing a threat to the physician, staff and other patients (42). Laser resurfacing can achieve improvement in acne scars with much less risk to the surgical team. In addition, very precise resurfacing can be done by sculpting the edges of the scars and vaporizing more tissue away only around scar tissue, while resurfacing only superficially in the rest of the cosmetic unit being treated. The procedure is most suited for distensible depressed or elevated acne scars (43, 44). Ice-pick and bound down scars should first be removed with punch excision, punch elevation, or punch grafting: laser resurfacing can be performed 6-8 weeks later (45).

Crateriform varicella scars can be improved with spot laser resurfacing (Figure 6.4A, B). The area around and over the scar is vaporized with one pass of the laser. Additional passes are concentrated along the edge of the scar crater until it has been completely effaced. When done 6-10 weeks after varicella, the scar can be almost totally effaced. Older scars respond, but less completely (46). Postsurgical and traumatic scars can be dramatically improved, especially if resurfaced 6-10 weeks after the surgery or injury (Figure 6.5A, B) (28, 47).

Actinic cheilitis can be successfully treated by performing a laser vermilionectomy using one of the resurfacing lasers (28). This usually requires only one pass with the laser over the vermilion region, including the vermilion border. Postlaser healing has been significantly reduced to approximately 10 days in contrast to the 4 weeks with past conventional CO_2 laser use (48-58). Also, the risk of scarring would be expected to be greatly reduced as the extent of thermal damage is much less. Actinic keratoses unresponsive to conventional treatment with liquid nitrogen and topical 5-fluorouracil can be eliminated by removing the epidermis with one pass using one of the resurfacing lasers. This is especially useful on the dorsal hands and scalp.

Pigmentation irregularities, such as postinflammatory hyperpigmentation and dark circles under the eyes, can sometimes be improved with laser resurfacing. It is very

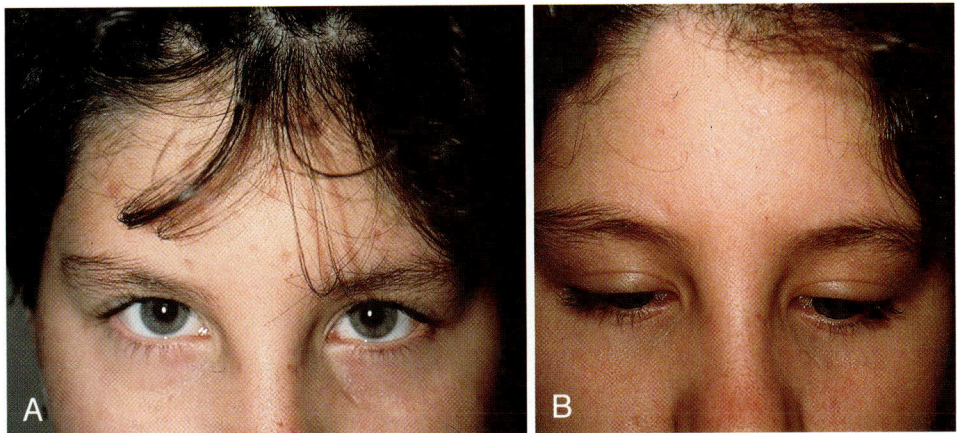

Figure 6.4. Two-month-old varicella scars on a 13-year-old girl **A,** before and **B,** 5 months after SilkTouch™ CO_2 laser resurfacing.

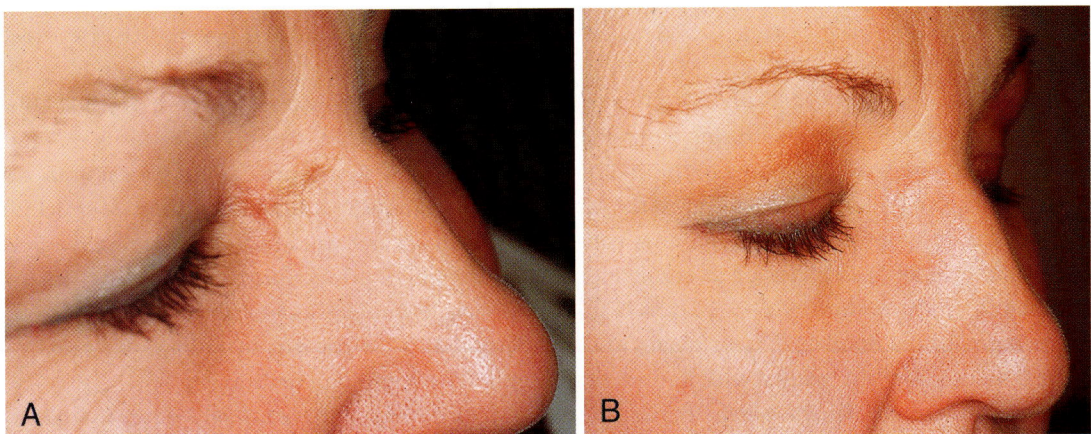

Figure 6.5. Two-month-old full-thickness skin graft **A,** before and **B,** 2 months after SilkTouch™ CO_2 laser resurfacing.

important to use Retin-A and hydroquinones for an extended period of time before and after the procedure. Other lasers more specific for melanin or medium-depth chemical peels are often preferable as they do not require anesthesia and recovery time is much shorter (59–63). Melasma responds variably, similar to other modalities used for its treatment (64).

Rhinophyma (Figure 6.6A, B) (65, 66), epidermal nevi (67, 68), and various small benign growths such as syringoma (69), trichoepithelioma (70), dermatosis papulosa nigra, xanthelasma (71), adenoma sebaceum (72) and sebaceous hyperplasia, have traditionally been treated with the conventional CO_2 laser (73). Using a resurfacing CO_2 laser may reduce the healing time and risk of scarring by reducing the extent of unwanted thermal dam-

age. Sometimes a combination approach can be employed. For example, a rhinophyma can be debulked using the CO_2 laser in the superpulse mode: the procedure is finished by removing the remaining rhinophyma with the resurfacing mode of the laser. When treating epidermal nevi, it is important to cause damage into the papillary dermis with residual hypopigmentation expected. Failure to cause some degree of dermal fibrosis often results in nevus recurrence (67, 68).

Carbon dioxide resurfacing lasers should not be used for nonfacial rhytides because of the very high risk of depigmentation and scarring (74). The Er:YAG laser, with its minimal residual thermal damage, may have a role to play in the treatment of nonfacial rhytides, including the dorsal hands and neck. However, the side-effect

Figure 6.6. Rhinophyma **A,** before and **B,** 7 months after SilkTouch™ CO_2 laser resurfacing.

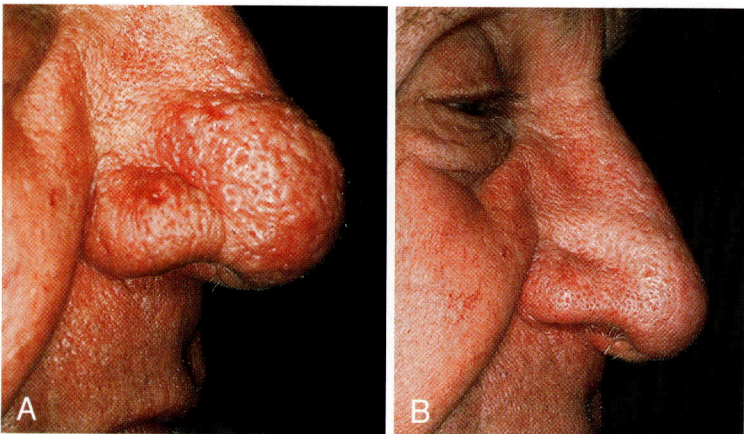

profile of the Er:YAG laser in nonfacial sites remains to be determined.

WOUND CARE

During the first few days after laser resurfacing a significant amount of exudate with some sloughing of thermally denatured collagen exists (Figure 6.3B). The variable amount of edema that develops in the first 48 hours can be controlled with ice packs, head elevation at night, and oral corticosteroids. Reepithialization takes 3–10 days (Figure 6.3C), increasing with the number of laser passes and decreasing if the patient's skin was primed with Retin-A or resurfaced with an Er:YAG laser. We encourage the use of occlusive dressings such as Vigilon™ (Bard Medical, Murray Hill, NJ) during at least the first 24–48 hours as it speeds re-epithialization after regular dermabrasion (75). Continued moist wound healing is achieved with frequent 0.25% acetic acid, normal saline, or cool tap water soaks followed by Aquaphor™ (Beiersdorf, Norwalk, CT) healing ointment application. We have stopped using Polysporin™ (Warner Wellcome, Morris Plains, NJ) and bacitracin ointment and petrolatum: Polysporin and bacitracin ointment cause frequent allergic contact dermatitis in these patients, and petrolatum may cause folliculitis, especially if it is not stopped immediately after re-epithialization is complete (34).

Moderate burning discomfort experienced by some patients during the first 24 hours after laser resurfacing is controlled effectively with ice packs, cold compresses, and acetaminophen alone or with codeine. Patients often develop pruritus during the first few weeks after resurfacing that is usually self-limited and controlled with antihistamines.

A feeling of tightening of the treated skin that may last for several weeks to several months is almost universally experienced by patients. This is generally thought to be a beneficial, rather than an adverse, effect of laser resurfacing.

After re-epithialization, there is a variable period of erythema ranging from 1–4 months in duration (Figure 6.3C, D). Erythema can be successfully camouflaged with cosmetics containing green foundation. Topical steroids are not used in the postoperative period except in cases of pruritus. Sun avoidance after laser resurfacing for the entire period of postlaser erythema should be stressed to the patient to reduce the risk of postinflammatory hyperpigmentation.

Occasionally patients will develop milia 1–3 months after resurfacing. This is far less commonly seen than after dermabrasion. Retin-A pretreatment further reduces milia formation. The milia usually resolve spontaneously. Retin-A can speed their resolution with milia extraction needed only on rare occasions.

RESULTS OF RHYTID RESURFACING

To evaluate the severity of wrinkling and photodamage present, and therefore achieve some degree of predictability of response to resurfacing, a clinical classification and numeric scoring system has been devised (3, 8). Though other wrinkling and photodamage assessment scales exist, the need for a system related purely to visible wrinkling and visible textural changes secondary to solar elastosis was thought to be more relevant to the topic of wrinkle eradication.

Use of this scoring system allows broad classification into mild, moderate and severe categories, and a more objective numerical severity score. Assessing patients both before and after treatment in studies with an average follow-up of about 90 days revealed that the average patient's preoperative score decreased approximately 50% as a consequence of resurfacing (Figures 6.1-6.3) (3, 8, 37, 38). This means that mild wrinkles generally resolve completely and moderate and severe wrinkles improve by one class. These are realistic expectations for the patient, though occasionally even severe wrinkles may completely resolve. The treated area continues to improve up to 1 year after laser resurfacing as collagen remodeling takes place.

In comparison to chemical peels, laser resurfacing is more effective in eradication of wrinkles while preserving normal skin texture and pigment. Superficial chemical peels such as Jessner's solution and alphahydroxy acids remove only a partial thickness of the epidermis and have no appreciable effect on wrinkling (76). Laser resurfacing is generally not done on such a superficial level. Medium depth chemical peels done with solid carbon dioxide or Jessner's solution plus 35% TCA will improve textural irregularities and very superficial wrinkling, but rarely have a significant impact on clinically visible wrinkling (59, 60, 77). This same level of resurfacing can be achieved with a single UltraPulse™ laser pass using a 250 to 350 mJ pulse and 3 mm spot size, or one pass with the SilkTouch™ laser using a 6.5 mm scan size at 15-18 watts. Though this level of chemical peeling is generally predictable and safe, a variable depth of penetration of acids, variable from patient to patient, but also within the same patient varying from one area to another, is possible. This variation in depth of penetration may be related to: the acid quantity applied, the pressure exerted with rubbing the acid into the skin, the degree of cleansing and defatting of the skin surface, the degree of photodamage present, the number and density of adnexal structures, and other unidentifiable factors. Deeper-than-wanted penetration of the acid may cause scarring, hypopigmentation and textural changes. When proper technique is used with laser resurfacing, this depth of resurfacing can be achieved with much greater predictability of depth and little risk of inadvertent deeper penetration with its associated risk.

Deep chemical peels with Baker's phenol solution will remove even deep lines and may result in dramatic clinical improvement, but virtually always result in hypopigmentation and an atrophically smooth, altered surface texture. It is difficult to obtain an even result on the upper lip. Lines present at the vermilion border often persist while the central area of the lip clears completely. In addition, because of the extreme depth of resurfacing, there is an extended period of erythema, often for

6 months or longer, and a significant risk of scarring. The postoperative course for phenol peeling is painful and requires at least 2 weeks for the skin surface to reconstitute itself (78-81).

This depth of Baker's phenol chemical peel injury has not been reported with laser resurfacing, nor is it desired. Because of the combined effects of tissue removed (collagen contraction/skin tightening and new collagen formation/remodeling), comparable degrees of improvement are often achieved with laser resurfacing minus unwanted side effects of hypopigmentation and altered surface texture seen with phenol. Virtually complete pigment loss (depigmentation), as occurs at times with phenol has not yet been reported with laser resurfacing.

Dermabrasion is significantly more difficult to perform from a technical viewpoint than laser resurfacing. It carries additional risks of physician and assistant exposure to blood-borne infectious agents (42). Risks of trauma to the patient from accidental contact of a rapidly rotating wire brush, or diamond fraise catching on loose skin or gauze and being thrown into an eyelid, lip, tooth or other area are possible (41). To achieve obliteration of wrinkle lines with dermabrasion requires a degree of expertise not easily achieved and always remains a challenge on the upper lip and the eyelids. Uneven results and hypopigmentation are common in the perioral area (82), often resulting in improvement of wrinkling centrally across the upper lip, but persisting at the vermilion border. The depth achieved in resurfacing with dermabrasion is usually comparable to that achieved with approximately 2-5 passes of the UltraPulse™ laser using 350 to 500 mJ per pulse, or with 2-3 passes of the SilkTouch™ laser using a 6.5 mm scan size at 15-18 watts.

PRECAUTIONS: SIDE EFFECTS/COMPLICATIONS

Side effects following CO_2 laser resurfacing are frequent and predictable: they are similar to those following chemical peels and dermabrasion, but less common and care-preventable if excellent technique and fastidious postoperative management. They can be divided into five categories: immediate, predictable effects; infectious; eczematous; follicular; scarring and pigmentary changes (Table 6.3).

Erythema lasting 6-12 weeks average is universal and considered part of the normal healing process (Figures 6.3C, D). Erythema and flushing, which develop in the treated site with exertion or emotional upset, are frequent

TABLE 6.3 Side Effects and Complications Associated with Laser Resurfacing

Predictable	Oozing, crusting, swelling (1–2 weeks). Erythema, pruritus, skin tightness (1–4 months)
Infectious	Bacterial, viral, yeast (1–2 weeks)
Dermatitis	Eczema (1–3 months)
Follicular	Acne, acneiform eruption, perioral dermatitis, milia (1–3 months)
Scarring	Atrophic, hypertrophic, keloidal (1+ months)
Pigmentary	Hyperpigmentation (1–6 months). Permanent hypopigmentation (6+ months)

for 1 year after resurfacing. Some individuals have persistent continual erythema lasting up to 12 months. This may be related to the depth of ablation (8, 37, 38, 83).

By far the most common adverse effect of laser resurfacing is postinflammatory hyperpigmentation (Figure 6.2B). Transient hyperpigmentation has been reported in up to 36% of patients (44). It is most often seen in patients with Fitzpatrick's skin type III–VI. The hyperpigmentation is more frequent and severe during the Summer months and year-round in southern areas such as Florida and Southern California. More recent studies demonstrate rates of hyperpigmentation as low as 2.8% in patients pretreated with bleaching creams and Retin-A (84). At the first sign of hyperpigmentation, bleaching creams and Retin-A are restarted (34, 85). Any sun exposure at this time, even through window glass, can be expected to prolong the period of hyperpigmentation, making it more severe. If treatment is started early enough, the hyperpigmentation usually resolves within a few months (34, 85).

Permanent hypopigmentation (Figure 6.7), developing up to 12 months after resurfacing has been reported in 16% of patients and seems less frequent than after dermabrasion or deep chemical peels (82, 84). This hypopigmentation ranges from pale, new "sun-protected" skin to white, depigmented skin. Hypopigmentation is more common in patients who have previously been treated with dermabrasion (44, 86). Patients with significant actinic damage may develop a color mismatch between the pale new skin of the resurfaced area and the surrounding sun damaged areas that may include ephelides and lentigines. This mismatch is minimized by resurfacing the entire face, or at least entire cosmetic units, and feathering the treatment into the surrounding

areas. Rarely, a medium-depth chemical peel of the untreated areas will be needed to even out the skin color. Future sun exposure will also help to blend the resurfaced skin by developing new lentigines and ephelides.

Milia are a result of follicular re-epithelialization compounded by the use of occlusive moisturizers. Acne is a frequent postoperative event, especially in patients with a past history of acne. It usually develops in the first few weeks after resurfacing and responds to standard acne treatment.

Contact dermatitis, noted with the use of some topical anesthetic preparations, does not correspond with patch test findings but resolves with appropriate treatment (3, 8). This occurrence increases the chances of postoperative erythema and hyperpigmentation (34). Eczematous dermatitis occasionally develops in the first 4 weeks after treatment. It responds rapidly to moisturizers and topical midpotency corticosteroids. Infrequently patients develop perioral dermatitis 1 to 3 months after resurfacing of the perioral region. This is easily controlled with tetracycline and is usually self-limited.

In a procedure that removes the epidermis and part of the dermis, infection is a concern (8). Laser surgeons have learned from past experience with dermabrasion and have avoided bacterial infection through the judicious use of antibacterials. Antiviral chemoprophylaxis was originally confined to those with a history of herpes simplex infection, but results suggest that subjects with no past history of infection frequently develop herpes simplex activation in treated areas (3, 8, 87). It is now

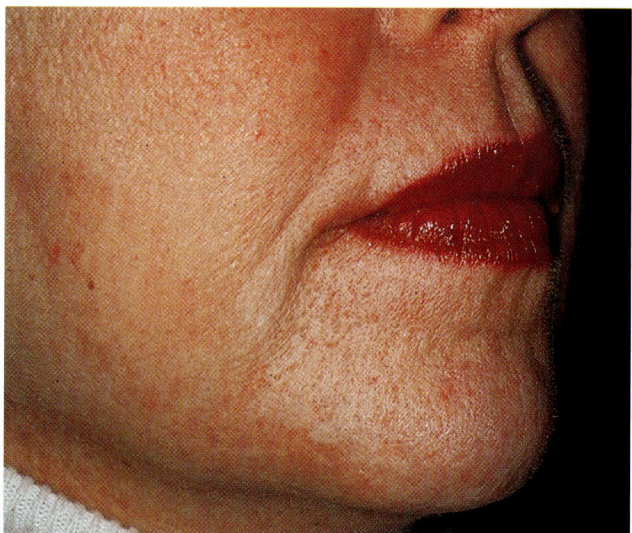

Figure 6.7. Permanent hypopigmentation 6 months after UltraPulse™ CO_2 laser resurfacing.

standard practice to use antiviral prophylaxis in all laser resurfacing patients. Yeast infections have occurred but respond well to treatment (3, 87).

Hypertrophic scarring is seldom seen following laser resurfacing. Scarring from laser resurfacing appears to be rare and, with proper patient selection, being conservative with the number of laser passes and good post-laser wound care, should further reduce the risk (3, 84, 86). It results from a large number of passes or use of excessive energy, and from pulse stacking (overlap of laser irradiated sites, especially after the first pass) resulting in excessive thermal damage (Oral Communication, Fitzpatrick RE, August 1997). It is better to do a touch-up procedure down the road than to go too deeply the first time in an attempt to totally eradicate the offending rhytides. Any areas that may be developing scar tissue should be promptly treated with topical and intralesional corticosteroids, silastic gel sheeting, and pulsed dye laser photocoagulation.

The main advantage of the Er:YAG laser is thought to be the potential for an improved side-effect profile. The procedure is less painful and may be completed under topical anesthesia. Less oozing and crusting and the subsequent erythema results, although dependent on the number of passes, is shorter-lasting than that following CO_2 laser treatment (39, 88). It is unclear if, depth for depth, the duration of healing and erythema are any shorter. It is too early to tell if the rate of permanent hypopigmentation and scarring will be any less after Er:YAG laser resurfacing. When treating superficial lesions, scarring and hypopigmentation would be unlikely to develop as little thermal damage is left behind. However, the endpoint of treatment is often not clear cut and the Er:YAG laser, unlike CO_2 lasers, ablates additional tissue with each laser pass making it possible to ablate all the way into the fat with resulting scarring. Therefore, the number of passes and energy fluence have to be carefully tracked when using the Er:YAG laser.

FUTURE DIRECTIONS

Incisional Laser Surgery and Laser Hair Transplantation (See Chapters 9, 13)

NONABLATIVE RESURFACING

New approaches to laser resurfacing include attempts at achieving selective dermal injury with the epidermis remaining intact. The healing process in the dermis should lead to new collagen deposition and remodeling with the possibility of reducing rhytides. Several methods have been tried with variable results. A carbon-based topical suspension applied to the skin followed by low fluence Q-switched Nd:YAG laser irradiation (89), and the use of a mid infrared (1.32 μm) pulsed (0.2 msec) laser to produce dermal shrinkage while the epidermis is protected with dynamic cooling (90), have both shown moderate improvement of rhytides in small pilot studies. Healing was faster than after CO_2 laser resurfacing.

A bilateral comparison study of CO_2 laser resurfacing and nonablative resurfacing with a Q-switched Nd:YAG laser for the treatment of "crow's feet" demonstrated rhytid improvement in all CO_2 laser-treated sides and in 9 of 11 Nd:YAG laser-treated sides. On the Nd:YAG-treated side, the improvement in 6 patients was less than on the CO_2 laser-treated side, but in 3 patients the improvement was equivalent on both sides (91). These three patients were the only Nd:YAG laser-treated patients with prolonged erythema. The reproducibility of these results awaits a larger patient series with long-term follow-up.

CONCLUSION

Because of its cosmetic implications, CO_2 laser resurfacing has raised a huge amount of interest. Early treatment results have been impressive. As CO_2 laser technology is refined, the side effect and complication profiles of CO_2 laser resurfacing will improve. Many questions remain unanswered, however. How does CO_2 laser resurfacing work? Is thermal damage essential for beneficial results, or is ablation the key to successful treatment? What role do collagen shrinkage and remodeling play? Are short-pulsed CO_2 and Er:YAG lasers effective for resurfacing moderate or severely photodamaged skin and, if so, is the wound healing time actually shorter and is persistent erythema duration shorter than with the longer-pulsed CO_2 lasers? The answers to these and many more questions are essential to better understanding of this rapidly evolving field.

ACKNOWLEDGMENT

This chapter is based in part on a previously published chapter by the authors: Hruza GJ, Fitzpatrick RE, Dover JS. Laser skin Resurfacing. In: Laser in Cutaneous and Aesthetic Laser Surgery. Arndt KA, Dover JS, Olbricht SM, editors. Philadelphia: Lippincott-Raven, 1997:262–290.

REFERENCES

1. David LM, Lask GP, Glassberg E, et al. Laser abrasion for cosmetic and medical treatment of facial actinic damage. Cutis 1989;43:583-587.
2. Fitzpatrick RE, Goldman MP. Advances in carbon dioxide laser surgery. Clin Dermatol 1995;13:35-47.
3. Fitzpatrick RE, Goldman MP, Satur NM, Tope WD. Pulsed carbon dioxide laser resurfacing of photo-aged facial skin. Arch Dermatol 1996;132:395-402.
4. Fitzpatrick RE, Tope WD, Goldman MP, Satur NM. Pulsed carbon dioxide laser, trichloroacetic acid, Baker-Gordon phenol, and dermabrasion: a comparative clinical and histologic study of cutaneous resurfacing in a porcine model. Arch Dermatol 1996;132:469-471.
5. Yang CC, Chai CY. Animal study of skin resurfacing using the ultrapulse carbon dioxide laser. Ann Plast Surg 1995;35:154-158.
6. Chernoff WG, Schoenrock LD, Cramer H, Wand J. Cutaneous laser resurfacing. Int J Aesth Restorative Surg 1995;3:57-68.
7. Chernoff G, Slatkine M, Zair E, Mead D. SilkTouch: a new technology for skin resurfacing in aesthetic surgery. J Clin Laser Med Surg 1995;13:97-100.
8. Waldorf HA, Kauvar AN, Geronemus RG. Skin resurfacing of fine-to-deep rhytides using a char-free carbon dioxide laser in 47 patients. Dermatol Surg 1995;21:940-946.
9. Anderson RR, Parrish RR. Selective photothermolysis: precise microsurgery by selective absorption of pulsed radiation. Science 1983;220:524-527.
10. Green HA, Domankevitz Y, Nishioka NS. Pulsed carbon dioxide laser ablation of burned skin: in vitro and in vivo analysis. Lasers Surg Med 1990;10:476-484.
11. Green HA, Burd E, Nishioka NS, et al. Middermal wound healing. A comparison between dermatomal excision and pulsed carbon dioxide laser ablation. Arch Dermatol 1992;128:639-645.
12. Walsh JJ, Deutsch TF. Pulsed CO_2 laser tissue ablation: measurement of the ablation rate. Lasers Surg Med 1988;8:264-275.
13. Schenk P, Ehrenberger K. Effect of CO_2 laser on skin lymphatics. An ultrastructural study. Langenbecks Arch Chir 1980;350:145-150.
14. Slutzki S, Shafir R, Bornstein LA. Use of the carbon dioxide laser for large excisions with minimal blood loss. Plast Reconstr Surg 1977;60:250-255.
15. Walsh JJ, Flotte TJ, Anderson RR, Deutsch TF. Pulsed CO_2 laser tissue ablation: effect of tissue type and pulse duration on thermal damage. Lasers Surg Med 1988;8:108-118.
16. Hobbs ER, Bailin PL, Wheeland RG, Ratz JL. Superpulsed lasers: minimizing thermal damage with short duration, high irradiance pulses. J Dermatol Surg Oncol 1987;13:955-964.
17. Fitzpatrick RE, Ruiz EJ, Goldman MP. The depth of thermal necrosis using the CO_2 laser: a comparison of the superpulsed mode and conventional mode. J Dermatol Surg Oncol 1991;17:340-344.
18. Fitzpatrick RE, Goldman MP, Ruiz-Esparza J. Clinical advantage of the CO_2 laser superpulsed mode. Treatment of verruca vulgaris, seborrheic keratoses, lentigines, and actinic cheilitis. J Dermatol Surg Oncol 1994;20:449-456.
19. Brugmans MJP, Kemper J, Gijsbers GHM, et al. Temperature response of biological materials to pulsed nonablative CO_2 laser irradiation. Lasers Surg Med 1991;11:587-594.
20. Kauvar AN, Waldorf HA, Geronemus RG. A histopathological comparison of "char-free" carbon dioxide lasers. Dermatol Surg 1996;22:343-348.
21. Hale GM, Querry MR. Optical constants of water in the 200-nm to 200-m wavelength region. Applied Optics 1973;12:555-563.
22. Vogler K, Reindl M. Erbium laser parameters for new medical applications. Biophotonics Int 1996; Nov/Dec:40-47.
23. Walsh JT, Deutsch TF. Er:YAG laser ablation of tissue: measurement of ablation rates. Lasers Surg Med 1989;9:327-337.
24. Walsh JJ, Flotte TJ, Deutsch TF. Er:YAG laser ablation of tissue: effect of pulse duration and tissue type on thermal damage. Lasers Surg Med 1989;9:314-326.
25. Hohenleutner U, Hohenleutner S, Baumler W, Landthaler M. Fast and effective skin ablation with an Er:YAG laser: determination of ablation rates and thermal damage zones. Lasers Surg Med 1997;20:242-247.
26. Kaufmann R, Hibst R. Pulsed Erbium:YAG laser ablation in cutaneous surgery. Lasers Surg Med 1996;19:324-330.
27. Duke D, Khatri K, Grevelink J, Anderson RR. The comparison of a 60 μs pulse duration to a 1 ms pulse duration CO_2 laser system in laser resurfacing. Lasers Surg Med 1997;20(suppl 9):30-31.
28. Hruza GJ. Skin resurfacing with lasers. Fitzpatrick's J Clin Dermatol 1995;3:38-41.
29. Schoenrock LD, Chernoff WG, Rubach BW. Cutaneous UltraPulse laser resurfacing of the eyelids. Int J Aesth Restorative Surg 1995;3:31-36.
30. Rubenstein R, Roenigk HH Jr, Stegman SJ, Hanke WC. Atypical keloids after dermabrasion of patients taking isotretinoin. J Am Acad Dermatol 1986;15:280-285.
31. Hayes DK, Stambaugh KI. Viability of skin flaps subjected to simultaneous chemical peel with occlusive taping. Laryngoscope 1989;99:1016-1019.
32. Hayes DK, Berkland ME, Stambaugh KI. Dermal healing after local skin flaps and chemical peel. Arch Otolaryngol Head Neck Surg 1990;116:794-797.

33. Alt TH. Technical aids for dermabrasion. J Dermatol Surg Oncol 1987;13:638-648.

34. Lowe NJ, Lask G, Griffin ME. Laser skin resurfacing: pre- and posttreatment guidelines. Dermatol Surg 1995;21: 1017-1019.

35. Mullarky MB, Norris CW, Goldberg ID. The efficacy of the CO_2 laser in the sterilization of skin seeded with bacteria: survival at the skin surface and in the plume emissions. Laryngoscope 1985;95:186-187.

36. David LM, Sarne AJ, Unger WP. Rapid laser scanning for facial resurfacing. Dermatol Surg 1995;21:1031-1033.

37. Lowe NJ, Lask G, Griffin ME, Maxwell A, Lowe P, Quilada F. Skin resurfacing with the UltraPulse carbon dioxide laser. Observations on 100 patients. Dermatol Surg 1995;21:1025-1029.

38. Lask G, Keller G, Lowe N, Gormley D. Laser skin resurfacing with the SilkTouch flashscanner for facial rhytides. Dermatol Surg 1995;21:1021-1024.

39. Ziering CL. Cutaneous laser resurfacing with the erbium YAG laser and the char-free carbon dioxide laser: a clinical comparison of 100 patients. Int J Aesth Reconstr Surg 1997;5:29-37.

40. Yarborough JM Jr, Beeson WH. Dermabrasion. In: Beeson WH, McCollough EG, eds. Aesthetic surgery of the aging face. St. Louis, MO: CV Mosby Company, 1986: 142-181.

41. Yarborough JM Jr. Dermabrasion by wire brush. J Dermatol Surg Oncol 1987;13:610-615.

42. Wentzell JM, Robinson JK, Wentzell JMJ, et al. Physical properties of aerosols produced by dermabrasion. Arch Dermatol 1989;15:1637-1643.

43. Apfelberg DB. A critical appraisal of high-energy pulsed carbon dioxide laser facial resurfacing for acne scars. Ann Plast Surg 1997;38:95-100.

44. Alster TS, West TB. Resurfacing of atrophic facial acne scars with a high-energy, pulsed carbon dioxide laser. Dermatol Surg 1996;22:151-154.

45. Abergel RP, Dahlman CM. The CO_2 laser approach to the treatment of acne scarring. Cosmet Dermatol 1995;8:33-36.

46. Young CK. Resurfacing of pitted facial scars with a pulsed Er:YAG laser. Dermatol Surg 1997;23:880-883.

47. Wheeland RG. Revision of full-thickness skin grafts using the carbon dioxide laser. J Dermatol Surg Oncol 1988;14:130-134.

48. Alamillos-Granados FJ, Naval-Gias L, Dean-Ferrer A, Alonso del Hoyo JR. Carbon dioxide laser vermilionectomy for actinic cheilitis. J Oral Maxillofac Surg 1993; 51:118-121.

49. Stanley RJ, Roenigk RK. Actinic cheilitis: treatment with the carbon dioxide laser. Mayo Clin Proc 1988;63: 230-235.

50. Robinson JK. Actinic cheilitis. A prospective study comparing four treatment methods. Arch Otolaryngol Head Neck Surg 1989;115:848-852.

51. Zelickson BD, Roenigk RK. Actinic cheilitis. Treatment with the carbon dioxide laser. Cancer 1990;65: 1307-1311.

52. Dufresne RJ, Garrett AB, Bailin PL, Ratz JL. Carbon dioxide laser treatment of chronic actinic cheilitis. J Am Acad Dermatol 1988;19:876-878.

53. Johnson TM, Sebastien TS, Lowe L, Nelson BR. Carbon dioxide laser treatment of actinic cheilitis. Clinico-histopathologic correlation to determine the optimal depth of destruction. J Am Acad Dermatol 1992; 27:737-740.

54. Ries WR, Duncavage JA, Ossoff RH. Carbon dioxide laser treatment of actinic cheilitis. Mayo Clin Proc 1988;63:294-296.

55. Scheinberg RS. Carbon dioxide laser treatment of actinic cheilitis. West J Med 1992;156:192-193.

56. Whitaker DC. Microscopically proven cure of actinic cheilitis by CO_2 laser. Lasers Surg Med 1987;7:520-523.

57. Frankel DH. Carbon dioxide laser vermilionectomy for chronic actinic cheilitis. Facial Plast Surg 1989;6: 158-161.

58. David LM. Laser vermilion ablation for actinic cheilitis. J Dermatol Surg Oncol 1985;11:605-608.

59. Monheit GD. The Jessner's + TCA peel: a medium-depth chemical peel. J Dermatol Surg Oncol 1989;15:945-950.

60. Brody HJ, Hailey CW. Medium-depth chemical peeling of the skin: a variation of superficial chemosurgery. J Dermatol Surg Oncol 1986;12:1268-1275.

61. Brauner GJ, Schliftman AB. Treatment of pigmented lesions of the skin with alexandrite laser. Lasers Surg Med 1992;12(Suppl 4):72.

62. Fitzpatrick R, Goldman M. Laser treatment of benign pigmented lesions using a 300 nanosecond pulse and 510 nm wavelength. J Dermatol Surg Oncol 1993;19: 341-346.

63. Goldberg D. Benign pigmented lesions of the skin: treatment with the Q-switched ruby laser. J Dermatol Surg Oncol 1993;19:376-379.

64. Taylor CR, Anderson RR. Ineffective treatment of refractory melasma and postinflammatory hyperpigmentation by Q-switched ruby laser. J Dermatol Surg Oncol 1994;20:592-597.

65. Greenbaum SS, Krull EA, Watnich K. Comparison of CO_2 laser and electrosurgery in the treatment of rhinophyma. J Am Acad Dermatol 1988;18:363-368.

66. Wheeland RG, Bailin PL, Ratz JL. Combined carbon dioxide laser excision and vaporization in the treatment of rhinophyma. J Dermatol Surg Oncol 1987;13: 172-177.

67. Ratz JL, Bailin PL, Wheeland RG. Carbon dioxide laser treatment of epidermal nevi. J Dermatol Surg Oncol 1986;12:567–570.

68. Hohenleutner U, Wlotzke U, Konz B, Landthaler M. Carbon dioxide laser therapy of a widespread epidermal nevus. Lasers Surg Med 1995;16:288–291.

69. Apfelberg DB, Maser MR, Lash H, et al. Superpulse CO_2 laser treatment of facial syringomata. Lasers Surg Med 1987;7:533–537.

70. Wheeland RG, Bailin PL, Kronberg E. Carbon dioxide (CO_2) laser vaporization for the treatment of multiple trichoepithelioma. J Dermatol Surg Oncol 1984;10:470–475.

71. Apfelberg DB, Maser MR, Lash H, White DN. Treatment of xanthelasma palpebrum with the carbon dioxide laser. J Dermatol Surg Oncol 1987;13:149–151.

72. Wheeland RG, Bailin PL, Kantor GR, et al. Treatment of adenoma sebaceum with carbon dioxide laser vaporization. J Dermatol Surg Oncol 1985;11:861–864.

73. Olbricht SM. Use of the carbon dioxide laser in dermatologic surgery. A clinically relevant update for 1993. J Dermatol Surg Oncol 1993;19:364–369.

74. Fitzpatrick RE, Goldman MP. Resurfacing of photodamage of the neck using the UltraPulse CO_2 laser. Lasers Surg Med 1997;20(suppl 9):33.

75. Pinski JB. Dressings for dermabrasion: occlusive dressings and wound healing. Cutis 1986;37:471–476.

76. Stagnone JJ. Superficial peeling. J Dermatol Surg Oncol 1989;15:924–930.

77. Brody HJ. Variations and comparisons in medium-depth chemical peeling. J Dermatol Surg Oncol 1989;15:953–963.

78. Stegman SJ. A comparative histologic study of the effects of three peeling agents and dermabrasion on normal and sun damaged skin. Aesthetic Plast Surg 1982;6:123–135.

79. Alt TH. Occluded Baker-Gordon chemical peel: review and update. J Dermatol Surg Oncol 1989;15:980–993.

80. Asken S. Unoccluded Baker-Gordon phenol peels–review and update. J Dermatol Surg Oncol 1989;15:998–1008.

81. Baker TJ, Gordon HL. Chemical peeling as a practical method for removing rhytides of the upper lip. Ann Plast Surg 1979;2:209–212.

82. Falabella R. Postdermabrasion leukoderma. J Dermatol Surg Oncol 1987;13:44–48.

83. Alster TS, Garg S. Treatment of facial rhytides with a high-energy pulsed carbon dioxide laser. Plast Reconstr Surg 1996;98:791–794.

84. Bernstein LJ, Kauvar ANB, Grossman MC. The short- and long-term side effects of carbon dioxide laser resurfacing. Dermatol Surg 1997;23:519–525.

85. Ho C, Nguyen Q, Lowe NJ, et al. Laser resurfacing in pigmented skin. Dermatol Surg 1995;21:1035–1037.

86. Weinstein C. UltraPulse carbon dioxide laser removal of periocular wrinkles in association with laser blepharoplasty. J Clin Laser Med Surg 1994;12:205–209.

87. Sriprachya-Anunt S, Fitzpatrick RE, Goldman MP, Smith SR. Infections complicating pulsed carbon dioxide laser resurfacing for photoaged facial skin. Dermatol Surg 1997;23:527–535; discussion 535–536.

88. Teikemeir G, Goldberg D. Skin resurfacing with the Erbium:YAG laser. Dermatol Surg 1997;23:685–687.

89. Goldberg DJ. Topical carbon suspension potentiated Q-switched Nd:YAG laser resurfacing of rhytides. Lasers Surg Med 1997;20(suppl 9):31.

90. Nelson JS, Milner TE, Dave D, et al. Clinical study of non-ablative laser treatment of facial rhytides. Lasers Surg Med 1997;20(suppl 9):32.

91. Goldberg DJ, Whitworth J. Laser skin resurfacing with the Q-switched Nd:YAG laser. Dermatol Surg 1997;23:903–907.

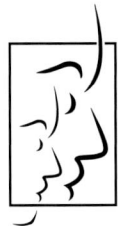

Chapter Seven

Complications of Cutaneous Laser Surgery

Tina S. Alster and Christopher A. Nanni

Cutaneous laser resurfacing has become a popular procedure for the treatment of photodamaged skin, scar revision, and the ablation of epidermal and dermal lesions. Today's high-energy, pulsed or scanned carbon dioxide (CO_2) lasers can generate peak energies of 4-5 J/cm^2 with tissue dwell times shorter than 1 msec (the thermal relaxation time of epidermis), thereby limiting collateral thermal tissue damage. However, CO_2 lasers were not always considered as safe and effective as they are today.

Carbon dioxide lasers were initially designed to operate in a continuous wave (CW) mode, which produced a continuous beam of radiation that was subsequently absorbed by intra- and extracellular water. These continuous wave carbon dioxide lasers were extremely effective in destroying tissue in bulk, but were less useful when ablating thin layers of tissue. Nonspecific thermal buildup and diffusion were the rule when using the continuous wave systems.

The subsequent development of high-energy, pulsed carbon dioxide lasers has revolutionized cutaneous surgery. Current CO_2 laser systems employ the theory of selective photothermolysis to ablate tissue with minimal char formation (1). The CO_2 laser's 10,600 nm wavelength targets intracellular and extracellular water, which is vaporized by high-energy pulses, leaving a narrow zone of residual thermal damage (2-6). Although hypertrophic scarring was a common complication with continuous wave CO_2 laser surgery, the selectivity of modern resurfacing systems has made scarring a rare complication with proper operator technique and patient selection (7-10). Unlike dermabrasion or chemical peeling, the new CO_2 lasers are operator-independent once a certain level of expertise has been reached. The precise depth to which CO_2 lasers ablate tissue with each laser pass gives the operator a high degree of control and consistency. No laser is completely safe, however, and complications may occur even in the most experienced hands. To avoid laser-induced side effects, a thorough knowledge of the potential complications of cutaneous resurfacing is essential. In addition, early treatment interventions for any evolving complications will decrease laser morbidity and improve clinical outcome.

Complications from cutaneous laser resurfacing can be divided arbitrarily into mild, moderate, and severe categories (Table 7.1). Mild complications include prolonged erythema, edema, milia formation, acne exacerbations, allergic or irritant contact dermatitis, burning discomfort, eczematization, and intermittent pruritus (8-13). Moderate complications such as local herpes simplex reactivation, transient post-treatment hyperpigmentation, and irregular delayed hypopigmentation have been reported (8-11, 14-26). The most severe complications include hypertrophic scarring, disseminated infection, and ectropion formation (8-11, 23, 26, 27).

TABLE 7.1 Complications of CO_2 Laser Resurfacing

Mild	Moderate	Severe
• erythema	• transient hyperpigmentation	• disseminated infection
• edema	• localized HSV reactivation	• hypertrophic scarring
• acne exacerbation	• cutaneous candidiasis	• ectropion
• milia formation	• delayed hypopigmentation	
• pruritus or burning discomfort		
• allergic or irritant dermatitis		

TABLE 7.2 Factors Affecting Outcome of CO_2 Laser Resurfacing

Patient	Laser	Operator	Postoperative care
• skin type	• high-energy, pulsed vs. CW scanned system	• experience and training	• staff experience
• medical/surgical history		• familiarity with laser system	• open vs. closed wound technique
• age	• spot/scan size + density	• basic knowledge of laser physics	
• smoking status	• degree of overlap		• presence of infection
• expectations	• tissue dwell time		
• compliance	• maximum energy output		

RISK FACTORS

When a complication results from laser resurfacing, identifying its cause to avoid future unwanted results is important. Morbidity from laser surgery is influenced by operator, patient, laser, and postoperative wound care factors (Table 7.2).

Operator inexperience with resurfacing techniques, or an unfamiliarity with a specific laser system, can result in significant morbidity. A surgeon should be well-educated on laser-tissue interactions before performing resurfacing surgery, including various skin responses at different laser energies and number of passes, which in turn, determines the choice of subsequent laser parameters. Charting an individual treatment course for different patient needs is difficult when unfamiliar with the appropriate tissue response. Being familiar with the laser system to be used is also important for the operator, as several laser systems are available—each with unique physical features and lasing options. A clear understanding of the laser physics behind the high-tech façade should be obtained before resurfacing on live pa-

tients. Laser parameters such as tissue dwell times, pulsed or scanned modes of operation, and appropriate energy levels, should be thoroughly understood for each laser system. Lastly, operator skill is probably the most important factor in determining patient outcome and safety and must be examined critically when a complication occurs.

Patient characteristics such as skin type, medical and surgical history, age, smoking status, expectations, and willingness to be compliant all contribute to laser resurfacing response. Indications and contraindications for resurfacing are determined by a host of patient and lesional characteristics (Table 7.3). Postoperative infection also plays an important role in ultimate patient outcome, and should be managed aggressively to prevent scarring and prolonged healing.

While the laser system used can certainly affect outcome, all available resurfacing laser systems can be operated safely if recommended guidelines are followed (11, 14-16, 19-26). The fact that each system may produce differing depths of tissue ablation, residual thermal damage, and postoperative erythema, does not appear to in-

TABLE 7.3 Relative Indications and Contraindications of CO_2 Laser Resurfacing

Indications	Contraindications
• skin types I & II	• non-facial skin resurfacing
• photodamage	• keloid tendency
• rhytides	• previously radiated skin
• atrophic scars	• concurrent isotretinoin use
• epidermal growths	• active cutaneous infection
• precancerous lesions	
• verrucae	

Secondary indications	Relative contraindications
• dermal lesions	• skin types V-VI
• skin types III-IV	• melasma
• diffuse solar lentigines	• immunocompromised patient
• infraorbital hyperpig-mentation	• prior lower blepharoplasty
• superficial cancerous lesions	

fluence ultimate clinical effect significantly when correct treatment parameters are used (27).

SIDE EFFECTS AND COMPLICATIONS

Postoperative Erythema

The most common side effect of cutaneous CO_2 laser resurfacing is post-treatment erythema (Figure 7.1). Erythema is an expected outcome of laser resurfacing and is seen in all patients for approximately 3-5 months (9-11, 13-16, 19-27). Although the intensity of the erythema varies depending on the CO_2 laser system used, overall duration of erythema is equivalent with all of the currently available resurfacing lasers (27). The depth of tissue ablation is believed to correlate with the intensity and duration of postlaser erythema, with deeper ablation (and residual thermal damage) resulting in prolonged discoloration (4-6, 27).

Treatment Options

Postoperative erythema must run its natural course and, under normal conditions, time and routine postoperative skin care are all that are necessary for its management. Avoidance of irritating substances such as retinoic and glycolic acids and fragrance-containing products until substantive healing has occurred (usually by 4-6 weeks) is helpful in reducing redness (13, 25, 28). Topical ascorbic acid has been shown to be of some help in the management of erythema, but is best applied 4 weeks or more postoperatively to avoid irritation (29). Topical corticosteroids do not appear to help decrease normal postlaser erythema, but will improve erythema caused by a contact dermatitis (12). Camouflage cosmetics and tinted sunscreens are very helpful in masking erythema and should be encouraged during the first several weeks following resurfacing (Table 7.4).

Hyperpigmentation

Post-treatment hyperpigmentation (Figure 7.2) is a common complication of facial resurfacing in 5-83% of patients (8-11, 13-17, 19-26). It is more typically observed within the first postoperative month in individuals with darker skin types and lasts approximately 3-4 months. Overall, it is more noticeable when localized areas are resurfaced, such as perioral or periorbital regions, because the dyspigmentation strongly contrasts with the surrounding skin.

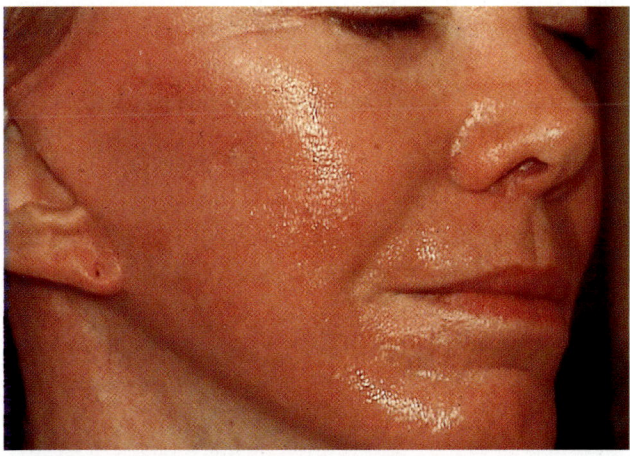

Figure 7.1. Moderate erythema seen 3 weeks after full face laser resurfacing.

TABLE 7.4 Cosmetic Camouflage Options

Trade name	Manufacturer (location)
Maximum Coverage	Estee Lauder (New York, NY)
Continuous Coverage	Clinique (New York, NY)
Cover SPF 20	Natura Bisse (Barcelona, Spain)
Solar Protection Formula	Fallene (King of Prussia, PA)

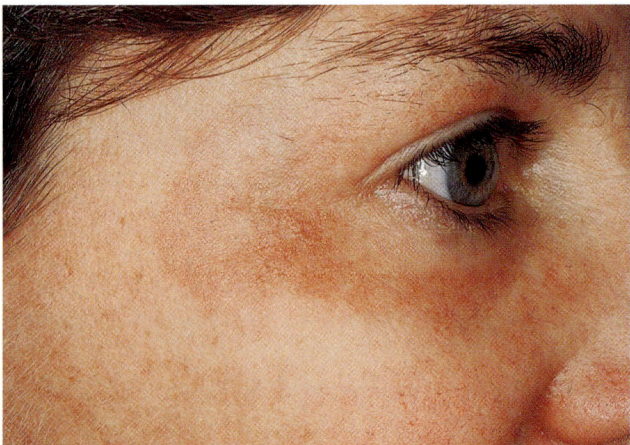

Figure 7.2. Periorbital hyperpigmentation observed 5 weeks following regional CO_2 laser resurfacing.

Treatment Options

Glycolic, retinoic, and azeleic acids, and also hydroquinones and sunscreens, can decrease or limit the severity of hyperpigmentation (9, 17, 24, 28, 30). As skin darkening is observed early after the resurfacing procedure, it is important to intervene at its onset. However, because the newly resurfaced skin is sensitive, the treatment of hyperpigmentation should not be too aggressive to prevent irritation that can lead to further postinflammatory hyperpigmentation. Light in-office glycolic acid peels and nightly applications of glycolic acid cream are generally helpful. Topical azeleic acid can be used on a daily basis with minimal irritation in patients 3–4 weeks postoperatively, and is often used in conjunction with glycolic acid to speed skin lightening. Hydroquinone-containing products, and also kojic and retinoic acids, must be used cautiously during the first few weeks following laser resurfacing because of their potential to irritate and are best used concomitantly with a mild topical corticosteroid.

Hypopigmentation

Although initially thought to be a rare event after laser resurfacing, hypopigmentation has been clearly established as a delayed, and apparently permanent, complication of laser surgery (9, 24, 25) (Figure 7.3). Generally it is not observed until 6–12 months after resurfacing, when postoperative erythema and hyperpigmentation have resolved. Many cases of hypopigmentation are subtle and evident only on examination with indirect lighting. Other cases are obvious and become a cosmetic camouflage challenge for patients. Laser resurfacing patients who have had dermabrasion are at increased risk of postlaser hypopigmentation, presumably by unmasking the tissue changes induced by previous treatment (21). Other than in individuals who have had such prior treatment, however, difficulty remains in predicting those at greatest risk for hypopigmentation: it can be seen in any skin type. Severely photodamaged skin with baseline dyspigmentation and areas of skin lightening should be evaluated carefully in the preoperative period.

Treatment Options

Reassurance and emotional support for the patient is critical. Gradual exposure to ultraviolet light may help to induce pigment production in the hypopigmented areas, or could worsen the condition by accentuating the light (untanned) areas in comparison to normal (tanned) areas. Light glycolic acid peels will often help to decrease any subtle hyperpigmentation of the surrounding skin and to

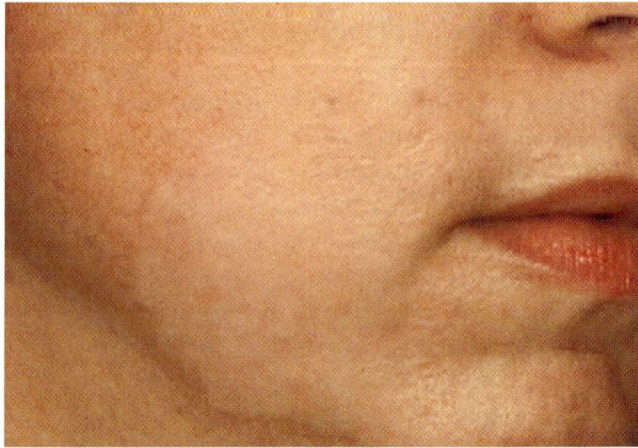

Figure 7.3. Diffuse hypopigmentation on the cheek and jaw observed 9 months after laser treatment.

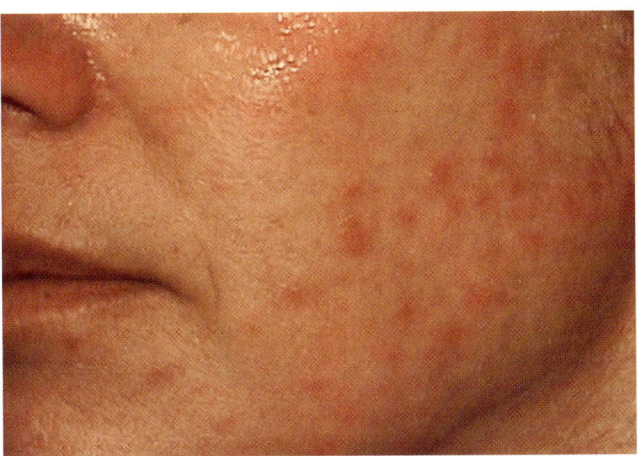

Figure 7.4. Pruritic erythematous papules noted after the use of a topical aloe preparation (allergic contact dermatitis).

improve the overall skin tone. Cosmetic application should be discussed so that the patient is aware of available camouflage options.

Contact Dermatitis

Laser-treated skin is sensitive and may react to a variety of topical irritants and allergens (9, 12). Contact dermatitis, most likely the result of decreased barrier function observed in de-epithelialized skin, is a common complication of cutaneous resurfacing occurring in as many as 65% of patients (8, 12) (Figure 7.4). Initially used during the immediate healing phase, topical antibiotic ointments frequently cause dermatitis, although they more likely cause an irritant response rather than a type IV contact allergy (12). Bland emollients such as plain petrolatum may be less sensitizing and easier for patients to tolerate. Catrix-10 (Donell DerMedex, New York, NY) and Aquaphor (Beiersdorf, Norwalk, CT) used during the initial re-epithelialization process leads to a contact dermatitis in approximately 10% of patients and are usually well-tolerated (25).

Treatment Options

Stopping all possible offending topical agents is essential. Antibiotic ointments, moisturizing creams with fragrances and preservatives, aloe, vitamin E, or other herbal remedies must be avoided or stopped when dermatitis is detected. Low-potency topical corticosteroid ointments or creams may be used to decrease pruritus and inflam-

mation. Cool compresses can also alleviate itching. Sedating oral antihistamines may be necessary in moderate-to-severe cases, especially at night when patients may inadvertently scratch themselves while sleeping.

Acne Flare

Acne and follicular-based papules and pustules may occur postoperatively, especially in acne-prone patients (Figure 7.5) (9). The use of occlusive dressings and emollients during the re-epithelialization process contribute to follicular inflammation and comedones. Mild exacerbations of acne may occur over several weeks postoperatively, even in patients who were not prone to acne before resurfacing.

Treatment Options

Acne will often spontaneously resolve once the use of heavy ointments and occlusive dressings have been discontinued. In patients with strong acneiform tendency and visible acne lesions preoperatively, oral antibiotics should be prescribed before and for 1 month after laser resurfacing. Although heavy emollients and occlusive dressings serve to promote healing during the first 7–10 days after laser resurfacing, it is best to switch patients to a lighter, cream-based moisturizer as soon as re-epithelialization has occurred.

Topical antibiotic *lotions* such as clindamycin or erythromycin may be useful for skin hydration and acne prophylaxis; however, alcohol-based antibiotic *solutions* may

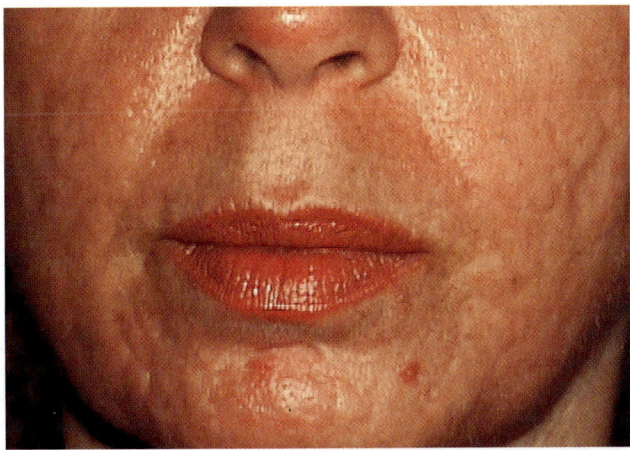

Figure 7.5. Acneiform papules in a patient prone to acne with the use of heavy emollients after laser resurfacing for atrophic scars.

be too drying and irritating in the immediate postoperative period. In patients who are acne-prone and are at increased risk of hyperpigmentation due to darker skin tone, azeleic acid cream may be useful. Azelaic acid has antibacterial properties and the potential to normalize a follicular epithelium, besides the ability to decrease melanocyte activity. Tretinoin and glycolic acid-containing products can be used once skin sensitivity decreases, usually by 4 to 6 weeks. Because resurfaced skin may become irritated by these products, their daily use should be advanced slowly.

Oral isotretinoin has been implicated in the development of hypertrophic scarring after resurfacing procedures and is not recommended shortly before, during, or after laser resurfacing. Cystic acne that is not under control before resurfacing should be treated with oral antibiotics. If acne control is still inadequate, a course of isotretinoin should be administered, followed by a waiting period of 1 year before laser resurfacing is attempted.

Milia Formation

Postoperative milia is attributed to the use of thick emollients and occlusive dressings, but is also observed during the course of normal reepithelialization. Milia formation has been reported in up to 14% of patients (Figure 7.6) (8, 9, 11, 25).

Treatment Options

Postoperative laser resurfacing milia are often superficial and may resolve spontaneously with continued healing. Office-based glycolic acid peels and home use of glycolic

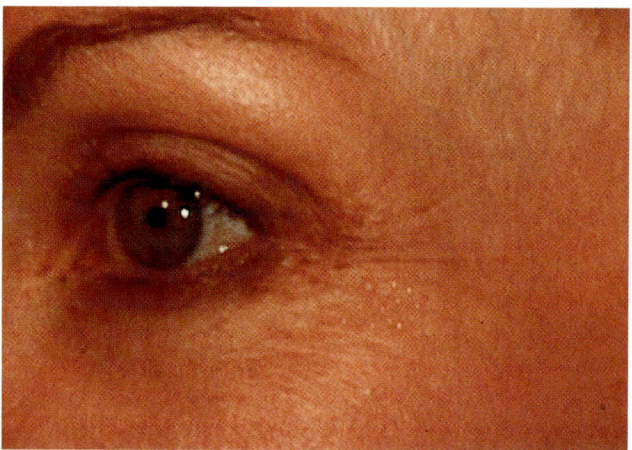

Figure 7.6. Periorbital milia 3 months after laser resurfacing.

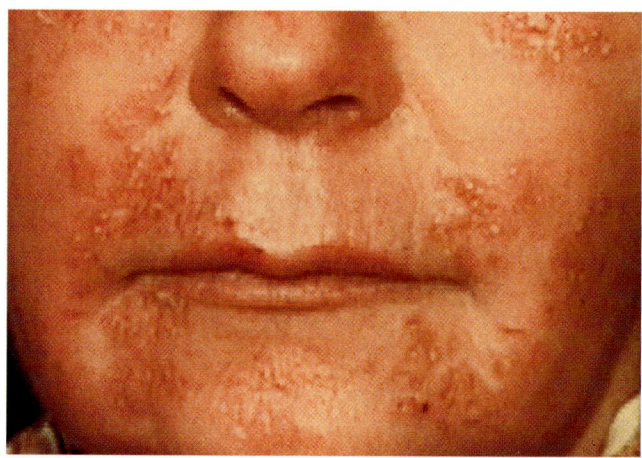

Figure 7.7. Herpes simplex reactivation 1 week after full face resurfacing despite antiviral prophylaxis.

or retinoic acid preparations may also help to prevent or even eliminate milia (9, 25). Manual extraction is an additional simple and effective treatment option for large milia, or for those that have not resolved spontaneously.

Herpes Simplex Infections

Herpes simplex virus (HSV) infections are the most common infections seen as a consequence of laser resurfacing (Figure 7.7) (9, 11, 18). Carbon dioxide laser "trauma" has been reported to cause reactivation of latent HSV in both localized and disseminated forms in up to 7% of patients (9, 11, 18). Herpes simplex virus infections usually develop by the first postoperative week. The prototypic herpetic vesicles may not be visible because of the lack of an overlying epidermis, appearing instead as punctate erosions. Although reactivation and autoinnoculation is the most common way to acquire HSV, viral transmission from a personal contact with active herpes in the postoperative period has occurred and resulted in disseminated infection (11). It is often not possible to predict whether a particular patient will develop HSV after resurfacing based solely upon a history of perioral "cold sores" or "fever blisters" (25). Antiviral prophylaxis is therefore recommended for all patients undergoing laser resurfacing of large cutaneous areas or of the perioral region.

Treatment Options

Oral antiviral prophylaxis is the most effective way to decrease the incidence of HSV infection. Prophylaxis should begin at least 24 hours before resurfacing and continued through the first 7–10 postoperative days during the re-epithelialization process. Although not well studied, standard HSV doses for recurrent perioral/genital infections are usually sufficient for resurfacing prophylaxis. If break-through infections are suspected, the involved area should be cultured and the antiviral dose increased based on individual renal function and clinical lesional appearance. Disseminated cutaneous HSV infection has occurred with maximum dose oral antiviral therapy. A cutaneous disseminated HSV infection is an indication for intravenous acyclovir therapy and aggressive wound care to prevent secondary bacterial infections and scarring.

Other Infections

Bacterial infections such as impetigo have been reported in 3–47% of patients who do not receive prophylactic antibiotics and aggressive postoperative wound care (Figure 7.8) (8–11, 23, 25). More severe cutaneous infections with pseudomonas have also been observed and may be associated with the use of occlusive dressing (31).

Cutaneous candidiasis evident as small, grouped, non-pruritic erythematous papules and pustules are rarely seen (9). Candidal infections should be differentiated from contact dermatitis, bacterial infections, and HSV. These pustules often initially develop around the perioral region and can spread over any resurfaced area that has the moisture to sustain growth. Diabetics, immunocompromised individuals, and those who are using occlusive dressings or heavy emollients for a prolonged period of time are at risk. In addition, women with concomitant

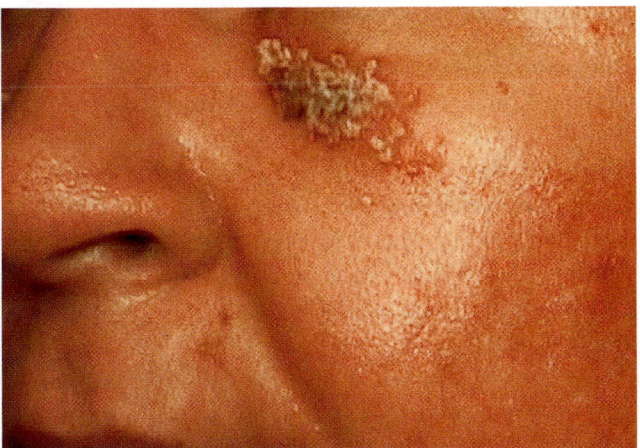

Figure 7.8. Ecthyma (pseudomonal infection) 10 days after laser treatment. Semiocclusive dressings were used postoperatively.

vaginal candidiasis or those individuals with perlèche may be at increased risk for Candida infection post-laser resurfacing (9). A potassium hydroxide examination of the pustules and surrounding skin is helpful in differentiating yeast from other potential pathogens.

Treatment Options

Judicious use of prophylactic antibiotics is suggested when resurfacing large areas or when treating a patient at risk for infection. Oral antibiotics with good staphylococcal and streptococcal coverage are preferred: when good postoperative wound care is practiced, bacterial infections are usually prevented. Being alert to possible pseudomonal infections that may occur with increased frequency in patients using semiocclusive dressings is essential. These infections can be treated with oral ciprofloxacin or appropriate intravenous antibiotics. Acetic acid soaks may also limit pseudomonal infection when used daily. When occlusive emollients or dressings are used, they should be changed regularly, with frequent inspection of the wound base. Once re-epithelialization has occurred (usually 7–10 days), the use of occlusive dressings and/or ointments should be discontinued to limit the moist environment that may breed yeast and bacteria. Prophylactic oral antifungal medications such as fluconazole or itraconazole may be considered in those individuals with risk factors or in those with a delay in wound healing requiring prolonged use of an occlusive dressing or ointment.

Infectious Plume

Infectious cutaneous lesions such as warts and molluscum contagiosum can be effectively ablated with the CO_2 laser. Of concern, however, are the potentially infectious aerosolized viral particles that have been isolated in the CO_2 laser plume (32–34). Laser vaporization of genital warts may place surgeons at a higher risk for nasopharyngeal papillomatosis because human papilloma virus types 6 and 11 that are commonly isolated in genital mucosa also have a predilection for the upper respiratory tract (32).

Treatment Options

The infectivity of the CO_2 laser plume can be virtually eliminated by practicing appropriate operating room safety procedures. The judicious use of a smoke evacuator and facial masks are essential for infection control.

Hypertrophic Scarring

In the hands of an experienced laser surgeon, hypertrophic scarring (Figure 7.9) is a rare outcome of CO_2 laser resurfacing; however, its incidence is expected to rise as less- experienced physicians enter the field (8–11, 14–16, 19–27). To reduce the possibility of scarring, it is essential that proper operative technique is used with appropriate laser settings. Overlapping of scans should be avoided and partially desiccated tissue should be thoroughly removed with wet gauze between laser passes to prevent an excessive thermal buildup in the lased skin.

Patient characteristics contributing to scarring include recent or concurrent isotretinoin use, keloid tendency, and previous radiation treatment, or surgical procedures such as blepharoplasty, dermabrasion, rhytidectomy, and chemical peels (9, 24). Regional variations in tissue response are responsible for increased scarring potential in the perioral, mandibular, and neck areas (9, 35). Proper wound care management, including antibiotic and antiviral prophylaxis, use of healing ointments and dressings, strict avoidance of sensitizing products, and close patient follow-up, is also essential for preventing or limiting scarring.

Treatment Options

Early intervention is ideal in the treatment of any laser complication, but especially important when managing an evolving scar. First-line treatment options include topical and intralesional corticosteroids, silicone gel or pres-

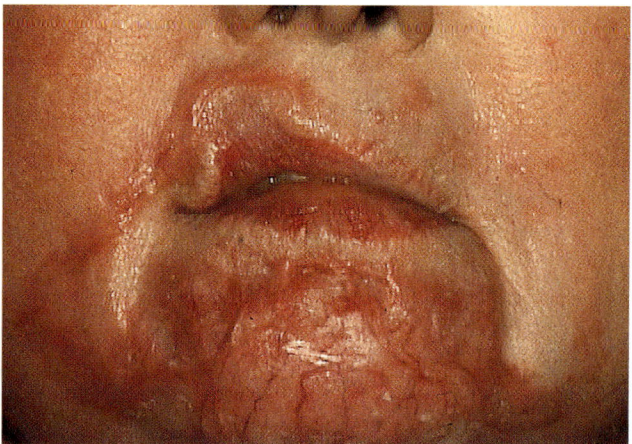

Figure 7.9. Hypertrophic scarring and lip deformity after perioral laser resurfacing in a patient without known risk factors for scarring.

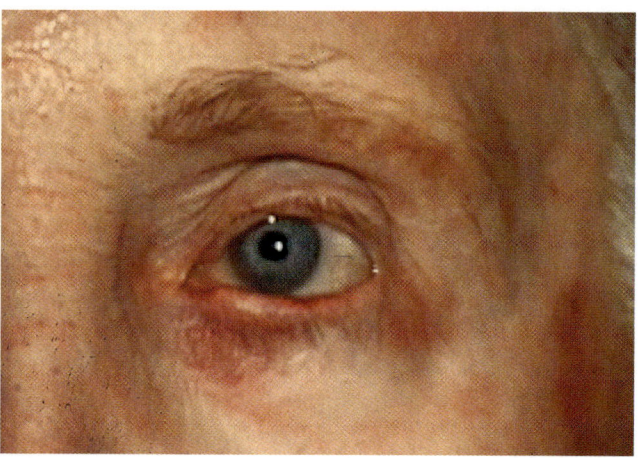

Figure 7.10. Ectropion in a 69-year-old woman with lax infraorbital skin and no prior history of lower blepharoplasty 6 months after laser resurfacing.

sure dressings, and 585-nanometer pulsed dye laser irradiation. The pulsed dye laser is the most effective, convenient, and often least traumatic method to treat erythematous, hypertrophic, or symptomatic (pruritic) scars (35–39). Laser parameters similar to those used in the treatment of vascular lesions are appropriate for these hypertrophic scars. Laser treatments are delivered every 4–6 weeks to allow sufficient healing time between treatments. Scars will typically respond to laser treatment by becoming flatter, less erythematous and pruritic, and more pliable (35–37). Intralesional triamcinolone (3–10 mg/cc) injections can also decrease scar height and symptoms when used alone or in combination with silicone gel sheeting or pulsed dye laser treatment.

Ectropion

Ectropion of the lower eyelid is a severe complication that rarely improves spontaneously and often requires surgical intervention (Figure 7.10). It occurs more commonly in patients who have had a surgical procedure simultaneous with resurfacing, or in patients who have had previous lower blepharoplasties (9, 23, 26). The exact incidence of ectropion formation is not clear from the reported literature, but is rare when proper preoperative patient evaluation and intraoperative technique are employed. An examination of the periorbital skin with baseline evaluation of lower eyelid laxity is essential. It is important to realize that ectropion can result after laser resurfacing-induced collagen tightening from lack of lower lid elasticity, or a lack of redundant skin around the lower eyelid (such as seen after a blepharoplasty). Fibrosis or scarring from resurfacing too vigorously under the eye may also result in a deformity of the lower lid. A "snap test" of the infraorbital skin may be helpful in identifying patients at risk for ectropion. A downward manual pull on the lower lid with release should result in a brisk return of the lower lid to its original position. A delay in lid return should be viewed as a warning sign for potential ectropion development. Fewer laser passes in the infraorbital region and scans with less-densely placed spots may also help to prevent lower lid deformities.

Treatment Options

The use of massage and topical corticosteroids to "soften" the infraorbital fibrosis may reduce the downward pull and thereby improve the appearance of the lower lid skin. Unfortunately, in most cases, surgical repair is required.

SUMMARY

Older continuous wave carbon dioxide lasers have been effective for treatment of a myriad of cutaneous conditions, but remain extremely operator-dependent with a higher risk of scarring. The introduction of the principles of selective photothermolysis has led to the design and manufacture of high-energy pulsed or scanned CO_2 lasers that are highly selective for cutaneous targets with greater margins of safety. Because any laser system can potentially result in scarring and other unwanted complications, adequate operator education and skill, and patient selection and postoperative management, are essential to reduce patient risk.

REFERENCES

1. Anderson RR, Parrish JA. Selective photothermolysis: precise microsurgery by selective absorption of pulsed radiation. Science 1983;220:524–527.
2. Alster TS, Kauvar ANB, Geronemus RG. Histology of high-energy pulsed CO_2 laser resurfacing. Seminar Cutan Med Surg 1996;15:189–193.
3. Cotton J, Hood AF, Gonin R, et al. Histologic evaluation of preauricular and postauricular human skin after high-energy, short-pulse carbon dioxide laser. Arch Dermatol 1996;132:425–428.
4. Kauvar ANB, Waldorf JA, Geronemus RG. A histopathological comparison of "char-free" carbon dioxide lasers. Dermatol Surg 1996;22:343–348.
5. Ross EV, Domankevitz Y, Skrobal M, Anderson RR. Effects of CO_2 laser pulse duration in ablation and residual thermal damage: implication for skin resurfacing. Lasers Surg Med 1996;19:123–129.
6. Trelles MA, David LM, Rigau J. Penetration depth of UltraPulse carbon dioxide laser in human skin. Dermatol Surg 1996;22:863–865.
7. Fitzpatrick RE, Goldman MP. Advances in carbon dioxide laser surgery. Clin Dermatol 1995;13:35–47.
8. Hruza GJ. Skin resurfacing with lasers. Fitzpatrick's J Clin Dermatol 1995;3:38–41.
9. Alster TS. Side effects and complications of laser surgery. In: Alster TS, ed. Manual of Cutaneous Laser Techniques. Philadelphia: Lippincott-Raven, 1997:142–151.
10. Nanni CA, Alster TS. Cutaneous carbon dioxide laser resurfacing: long-term follow-up of 300 patients. Lasers Surg Med 1997;suppl 9:178.
11. Waldorf HA, Kauvar AN, Geronemus RG. Skin resurfacing of fine to deep rhytides using the char-free carbon dioxide laser in 47 patients. Dermatol Surg 1995;21:940–946.
12. Fisher AA. Lasers and allergic contact dermatitis to topical antibiotics, with particular reference to bacitracin. Cutis 1996;58:252–254.
13. Lewis AB, Alster TS. Laser resurfacing: persistent erythema and post-inflammatory hyperpigmentation. J Geriatr Dermatol 1996;4:75–76.
14. Ho C, Nguyen Q, Lowe NJ, et al. Laser resurfacing in pigmented skin. Dermatol Surg 1995;21:1035–1037.
15. Lowe NJ, Lask G, Griffin ME, et al. Skin resurfacing with the UltraPulse carbon dioxide laser. Observations on 100 patients. Dermatol Surg 1995;21:1025–1029.
16. Lask G, Keller G, Lowe N, et al. Laser resurfacing with the SilkTouch flashscanner for facial rhytides. Dermatol Surg 1995;21:1021–1024.
17. Lowe NJ, Lask G, Griffin ME. Laser skin resurfacing: pre- and posttreatment guidelines. Dermatol Surg 1995;21:1025–1029.
18. Monheit GD. Facial resurfacing may trigger the herpes simplex virus. Cosmetic Dermatol 1995;8:9–16.
19. Alster TS. Comparison of two high-energy, pulsed CO_2 lasers in the treatment of periorbital rhytides. Dermatol Surg 1996;22:541–545.
20. Alster TS, Garg S. Treatment of facial rhytides with a high-energy pulsed carbon dioxide laser. Plast Reconstr Surg 1996;98:791–794.
21. Alster TS, West TB. Resurfacing of atrophic facial acne scars with a high-energy, pulsed carbon dioxide laser. Dermatol Surg 1996;22:151–155.
22. Fitzpatrick RE, Goldman MP, Satur NM, Tope WD. Pulsed carbon dioxide laser resurfacing of photoaged facial skin. Arch Dermatol 1996;132:395–402.
23. Weinstein C. UltraPulse carbon dioxide laser removal of periocular wrinkles in association with laser blepharoplasty. J Clin Laser Med Surg 1994;12:205–209.

24. Weinstein C, Alster TS. Skin resurfacing with high-energy, pulsed CO_2 lasers. In Alster TS, Apfelberg DB, eds. Cosmetic laser surgery. New York: John Wiley & Sons, Inc., 1996:9–28.

25. Nanni CA, Alster TS. Complications of carbon dioxide laser resurfacing: an evaluation of 500 patients. Dermatol Surg 1998;24:315–320.

26. Nanni CA, Alster TS. Complications of cutaneous laser surgery: a review. Dermatol Surg 1998;24:209–219.

27. Alster TS, Nanni CA, Williams CM. Comparison of four cutaneous resurfacing lasers: a clinical and histopathologic evaluation. Dermatologic Surgery 1998 (in press).

28. Formica KJ, Alster TS. Cutaneous laser resurfacing: a nursing guide. Dermatol Nurs 1997;9:19–22.

29. Alster TS, West TB. Effect of topical vitamin C on postoperative CO_2 laser resurfacing erythema. Dermatol Surg 1998;24:331–334.

30. Alster TS. Preoperative preparation for CO_2 laser resurfacing. In: Coleman WP, Lawrence N, eds. Skin resurfacing. Baltimore: Williams & Wilkins, 1998:171–179.

31. Sriprachya-anunt S, Fitzpatrick R, Goldman MP, Smith SR. Infections complicating pulsed carbon dioxide laser resurfacing for photoaged facial skin. Dermatologic Surgery 1997;23:527–536.

32. Gloster HM, Roenigk RK. Risk of acquiring human papillomavirus from the plume produced by the carbon dioxide laser in the treatment of warts. J Am Acad Dermatol 1990;23:115–120.

33. Nezhat C, Winer WK, Nezhat F, et al. Smoke from laser surgery: is there a health hazard? Lasers Surg Med 1987; 7:376–382.

34. Sawchuck WS, Weber PJ, Lowy DR. Infectious human papillomavirus in the vapor of warts treated with the carbon dioxide laser or electrocoagulation. J Am Acad Dermatol 1989;21:41–49.

35. Alster TS, Nanni CA, Williams CM. Pulsed dye laser treatment of hypertrophic burn scars. Plast Reconstr Surg 1998 (in press).

36. Alster TS. Improvement of erythematous and hypertrophic scars by the 585 nm pulsed dye laser. Ann Plast Surg 1994;32:186–190.

37. Alster TS, Williams CM. Treatment of keloid sternotomy scars with 585 nm flashlamp-pumped pulsed dye laser. Lancet 1995;345:1198–1200.

38. Alster TS. Laser treatment of hypertrophic scars. Facial Plast Surg 1996;4:267–274.

39. Alster TS, West TB. Treatment of scars: a review. Ann Plast Surg 1997;39:418–432.

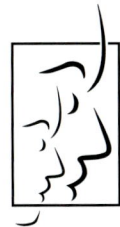

Chapter Eight

Introduction to Laser Incisional Surgery

Jemshed A. Khan

Aesthetic surgery of the face ranks among the most challenging of surgical endeavors. The complex and fragile anatomy, the proximity of vital structures, and the tremendous psychological and social import attached to facial appearance require precise judgement and technique when performing surgical rejuvenation of the face. In recent years the carbon dioxide (CO_2) laser has been adapted for use in blepharoplasty and other periorbital and facial applications. To the benefit of the novice laser surgeon, there is now a significant body of literature, training courses, and experienced surgeons to impart the knowledge and skills developed over the past two decades. It is important for the beginning laser surgeon to recognize that improved results are achieved through superior technical expertise and aesthetic judgment, and are not inherent to the laser.

Though incisional CO_2 laser surgery had been practiced for many years, the continuous wave (CW) CO_2 laser was largely abandoned for aesthetic procedures in the 1980s because it caused significant thermal injury, producing wounds that healed with an unacceptable appearance. The re-emergence of CO_2 laser surgery is attributed to the development of a newer generation of lasers: these produce short pulses of energy avoiding large zones of lateral thermal spread or tissue injury (see Chapter 1 for more details regarding laser-tissue interaction). These lasers permit quick, precise, and nearly bloodless soft tissue incisions while producing a biologically acceptable amount of thermal damage (Figure 8.1).

HISTORIC PERSPECTIVE

The first human laser treatment was performed in 1962 using visible-wavelength ruby and neodymium lasers to create thermal necrosis of a malignant melanoma before excision (1). Treatment of non-pigmented tissues was not feasible until the invisible 10,600-nanometer continuous wave (CW) CO_2 laser was invented by Patel of Bell Laboratories (Murray Hill, NJ) in 1964 (2). Three years later, Polanyi and coworkers reported surgical use of the CO_2

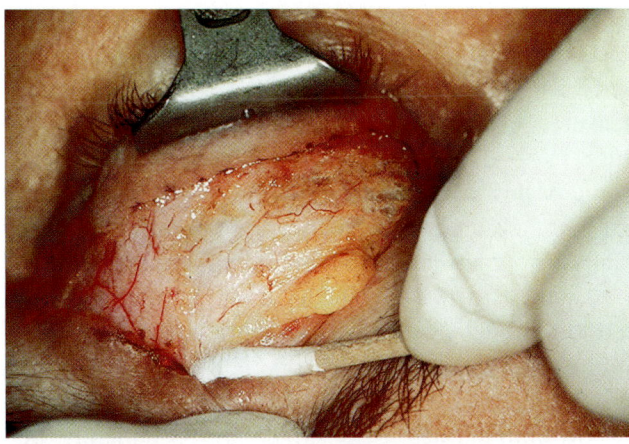

Figure 8.1. The vascular eyelid tissues may be bloodlessly incised with the CO_2 laser allowing for improved identification of anatomic structures.

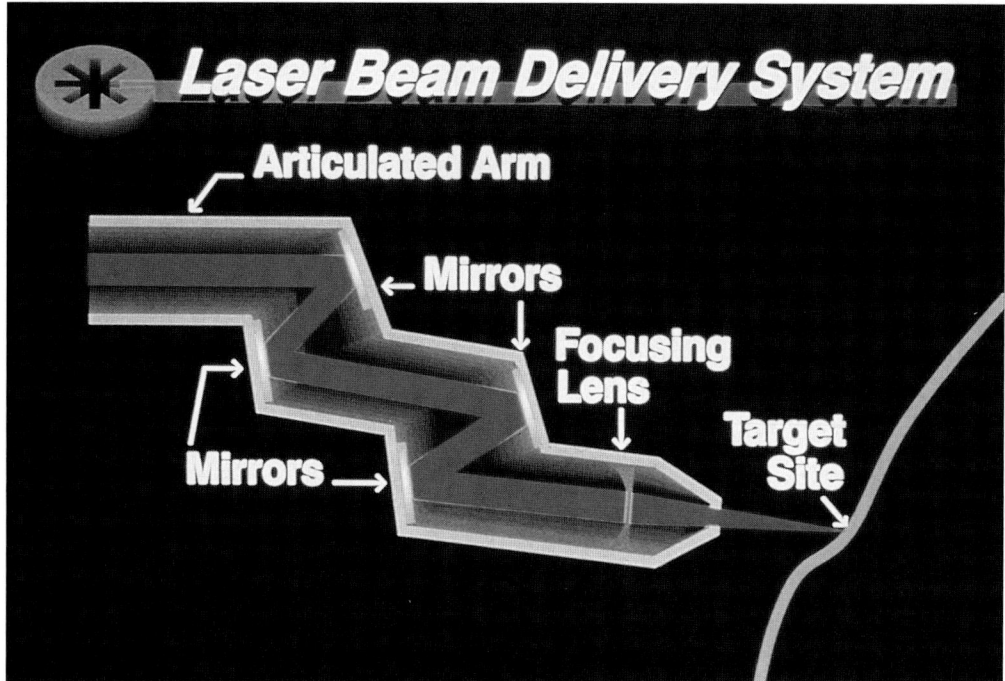

Figure 8.2. The articulated arm delivers the laser beam to a focused handpiece via a series of rigid, hollow tubes and enclosed mirrors.

laser (3). Over the next several years, histologic studies revealed the laser's ability to seal lymphatic vessels, coagulate vessels of up to 0.5 mm diameter, and seal, rather than fray, small nerve endings (4-6).

Initially the CO_2 laser was used through an operating microscope. The beam was directed with a micromanipulator and its location was indicated by a red He:Ne laser (6). This system was cumbersome, and more viable alternatives were sought. Because fiberoptic cables capable of transmitting the 10,600-nanometer wavelength were absent, rigid articulated arm delivery systems were developed: the beam was reflected along a series of mirrors encased in segments of hollow tubing until it was finally delivered to the tissues via a focused handpiece (Figure 8.2) (6). These systems allowed fine surgical control of the beam's path, resulting in more widespread acceptance of incisional energy delivery, and prompting the development of advanced laser incisional procedures.

By the late 1970's, CW CO_2 lasers had found application among gynecologists, otorhinolaryngologists, neurosurgeons, plastic surgeons, and dermatologists. Despite early enthusiasm for CO_2 laser surgery, many plastic and dermatologic surgeons subsequently became disenchanted with this device because unwanted scarring attributed to thermal injury was sometimes

produced (6). The first reports of using the CO_2 laser as an incisional device in the periorbital region appeared in 1980 when Beckman and colleagues described laser-assisted removal of small lesions (7). Incisional eyelid surgery employing CO_2 lasers for more complex procedures was first reported by Baker in 1984, who used the laser for 40 cases of blepharoplasty (8). The prevailing opinion in the 1980s was that CO_2 lasers produced too much thermal damage to be useful in aesthetic surgery (9). Widespread acceptance of incisional CO_2 laser eyelid surgery did not occur until nearly a decade later: advances in laser technology allowed for the production of pulsed lasers, which produced beams nearly an order of magnitude smaller, thus limiting the amount of thermal damage produced. With the availability of this new technology, laser skin resurfacing, once considered highly risky and dangerous, became almost instantly popular and drew even more attention to incisional surgery. Today, many experienced aesthetic surgeons regard with favor the efficiency and decreased operating times associated with incisional CO_2 laser eyelid surgery. Carbon dioxide lasers are used routinely for procedures including entropion repair, ectropion repair, dacryocystorhinostomy, levator resection, enucleation, upper and lower eyelid blepharoplasty, malar lift, rhytidectomy, hair transplantation, endoscopic forehead lift, and others.

PHYSICS OF FREE-BEAM CO$_2$ LASER INCISIONS

Understanding the physics of the CO$_2$ laser and the complex interaction of infrared laser energy and soft tissue are of critical importance to the laser surgeon. Only with sound knowledge of the concepts behind the laser can modifications in laser settings and technique be made to optimize surgical results. The physics of CO$_2$ laser tissue interaction are discussed in detail in chapter 1.

HISTOLOGY OF LASER INCISIONS

The CO$_2$ laser creates a zone of thermal injury along the wound edge. The extent and type of injury depends upon both the thermal gradient created around the wound (Table 8.1) and the length of time that tissue is exposed to the thermal gradient (10,11). When used to make a skin incision, the focused laser beam produces three zones of injury. The central zone represents the actual incision, from which the tissue has been vaporized. Surrounding this is a zone of permanent, or irreversible, thermal damage represented under the light microscope as an area of

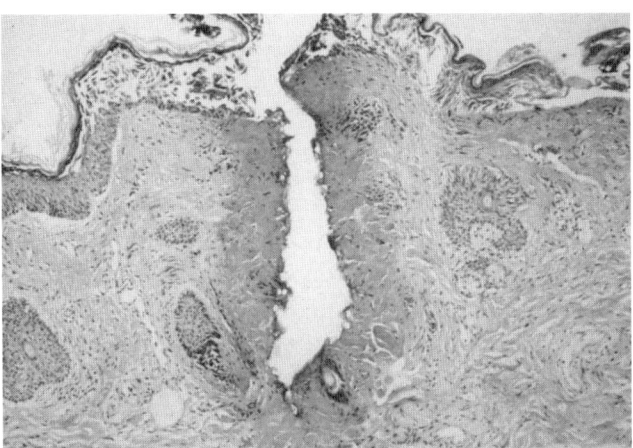

Figure 8.3. A zone of thermal injury approximately 110 μm in width is evident along the edges of this incision made with the UltraPulse™ CO$_2$ laser in human eyelid tissue. Image courtesy of Brian Biesman, MD.

amorphous "ground glass" tissue directly adjacent to the wound edge. Histopathologically this zone represents coagulative necrosis (Figure 8.3) (12). This zone consists not only of necrotic tissue, but also includes denatured, melted, and contracted collagen (Table 8.1). Peripheral to this is a zone of reversible thermal damage created by elevation of the tissue temperature to an insufficient level to cause tissue protein denaturation. Other features characteristic of CO$_2$ laser incisions include infolding of the epidermis and a zone of epidermal injury. These histopathologic observations correlate with the well-recognized delay in the rate of laser wound healing.

Differentiating between CO$_2$ laser beam delivery systems is important because each produces significantly different degrees of histologic injury (Table 8.2). Carbon dioxide laser incisional energy maybe delivered by a continuous wave laser, a mechanically shuttered continuous wave laser, a superpulsed laser, or a radiofrequency-excited pulsed laser. Radiofrequency-excited pulsed lasers differ from continuous wave lasers in that the former actually pulses with a frequency in the low K Hz range. When used as incisional devices, unshuttered and shuttered continuous wave CO$_2$ lasers are associated with large zones of thermal injury, i.e., from 100 μm to as much as 2 mm or more (6). In contrast, when high frequency pulsed lasers such as the Coherent UltraPulse™[3] are used with a 0.2 mm focused handpiece, a much smaller zone of thermal injury, generally in the range of 110 μm is produced (13).

TABLE 8.1 Tissue Effects and Wound Healing at Various CO$_2$ Laser Temperatures

Temperature	Tissue Effects/Wound Healing
37° C	Normal tissue
44–100° C	Thermal tissue damage
55–62° C	Collagen contracts and shrinks
60° C	Type I collagen melts
65–70° C	Collagen relaxes
65–80° C	Tissue collagen welding
70–100° C	Necrosis
75° C	DNA damage
100° C	Vaporization and ablation
> 300° C	Char, carbonization, heat sink effect raises temperature to >600 C, 1–5 mm thermal necrosis

COMPARISON OF CO₂ LASER TO OTHER INCISIONAL METHODS

The value of incisional CO_2 laser surgery has been assessed by histologic comparison with other incisional methods, including scalpel, monopolar electrocautery dissection, and contact laser tips (Table 8.2). The scalpel or scissors incision is still considered by some to be the "gold standard" for skin surgery because no thermal injury is induced (14). This is especially important at the epidermal wound edge where thermal injury may result in more noticeable scarring. However, since scalpel or scissors divide all the vessels traversing the incision, adjunctive thermal cauterization techniques are required. These cautery techniques, which include monopolar, bipolar, and hot-tip devices, result in localized areas of thermal injury. Operating times are prolonged because dissections are interrupted by the frequent necessity to pause, identify, and cauterize individual vessels. The longer operating times and intraoperative hemorrhage lead to bruising, swelling, and tissue distortion (15). Though some authors report that the CO_2 laser offers little advantage over the scalpel (16), a recent survey comparison of scalpel versus CO_2 laser blepharoplasty indicated laser benefits: quicker recovery time and return to usual activities (6.3 vs. 9.1 days), and shorter operating times (four-eyelid blepharoplasty times of 58 vs. 94 minutes) (17).

Monopolar electrocautery incisional techniques present a major advance over cold steel incisions because they simultaneously incise and cauterize soft tissues (18). Monopolar devices produce a sphere of intense coagulation when the conductive tip is in contact with soft tissue. As distance from the tip increases, the current dissipates and the amount of coagulation decreases. Coagulating and cutting modes on monopolar devices differ; a much higher power is delivered by the latter mode. In cutting mode, tissue is vaporized rather than charred. Such devices are not usually used to divide skin because the resultant thermal injury produces a prominent scar (18).

Monopolar electrocautery eyelid surgery should be performed with a needle that is insulated to the tip. In a study performed in rats, extremely sharp needles with etched 1- to 5- micrometer radius tips (Colorado Needle,™ Colorado Biomedical Inc., Evergreen, CO) caused less skin necrosis injury than standard monopolar needle tips (180 μm vs. 250 μm) as shown in Table 8.2 (19). Such fine needle tips also enhance operative dissection of the delicate eyelid structures. The monopolar unit power setting is adjusted upwards if the tip tends to stick or drag through tissues, and is adjusted downwards if there is significant charring or arcing. Dissection is aided by keeping tissues under tension during electrocautery division.

Specific hazards are associated with using monopolar electrocautery for oculoplastic and orbital procedures.

TABLE 8.2 Relative Zones of Thermal Injury Associated With Various Incisional Devices

Device	Settings	Injury zone	Comment
Scalpel	n/a	0 μm	various studies
UltraPulse™ CO₂ 0.2 focused spot (Biesman)	5 W, 15 mJ, 333 pulse/sec, 1 cm/sec speed	110 μm	human eyelid skin
UltraPulse™ CO₂ in CW mode, 0.2 focused spot (Biesman)	6 W, CW mode (i.e., 3000 Hz), 1 cm/sec speed	115 μm	human eyelid skin
Microneedle electrocautery (Farnworth)	Valley Lab, blend 1, 40 W	180 μm	rat skin necrosis
SuperPulse™ CO₂ 0.22 mm focused spot (Schroder)	10 W, 500–700 Hz, 150 μsec pulse	200 μm	pig skin thermal injury
Standard needle electrocautery (Farnworth)	Valley Lab, blend 1, 40 W	250 μm	rat skin necrosis
Shaw scalpel (Farnworth)	220 F	250 μm	rat skin necrosis
Standard needle electrocautery (Schroder)	Valley Lab, blend 2, 50 W	250 μm	pig skin thermal injury
True CW CO₂ (Schroder)	10 W, 0.22 mm focused spot	300 μm	pig skin thermal injury
Contact Nd:YAG (Schroder)	14 W CW, 0.2 mm frosted tip sapphire	350 μm	pig skin thermal injury
Contact CW CO₂ (Fuller)	nonfrosted tip sapphire	300–500 μm	manufacturer data

All measurements are for one side of the incision only.

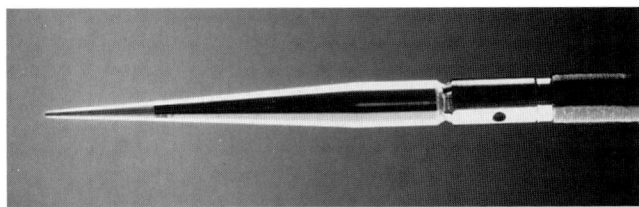

Figure 8.4. Contact sapphire laser scalpel. Image courtesy of Surgical Lasers Technologies Inc., Oaks, PA.

When treating vessels close to the skin surface, the zone of thermal injury and secondary scarring induced by monopolar electrocautery is difficult to control, therefore bipolar cautery is preferable. Deeper vessels may have to be grasped with a metal forceps, which is then touched by the electrocautery tip to allow more direct energy delivery to the vessel. A plastic globe protector should be placed over the cornea when dissecting deep in the eyelid to prevent conduction of current or thermal energy to the corneal surface. In the deep orbit, electrocautery must be used judiciously because of the risk of remote distal injury caused by channeling of current along vessels or nerves (20). Cerebrospinal fluid leaks, visual loss, and third cranial nerve injuries have been attributed to monopolar cautery use during apical orbital surgery (21, 22). Monopolar electrocautery should not be used in patients with pacemakers because the current may reprogram or damage the pacemaker and cause potentially lethal arrhythmias. When compared with pulsed CO_2 laser incisions, the primary drawback of monopolar electrocautery is the degree of thermal injury (Table 8.2). Clinical comparisons of monopolar cautery with CO_2 laser for blepharoplasty surgery suggest that surgery was performed more quickly with the laser and that patients treated with the laser developed less edema, and had a shortened postoperative recovery time (23, 24).

Lasers may be used in free beam (e.g. CO_2) or contact mode (e.g. Nd:YAG). Contact laser tips may be used with a variety of laser wavelengths in order to both incise tissues and create significant thermal injury (Figure 8.4) (25, 26). Comparison of contact tip Nd:Yag, scalpel, and CO_2 skin incisions indicate that the largest zones of injury are associated with the contact tip laser (27). Some contact laser tips have an infrared absorbing surface treatment that converts the laser energy to heat (Surgical Laser Technologies, Montgomeryville, PA) when cautery effects are desired (28). Other tips intended for incisional applications deliver focused laser energy to the target tissue. While the coating, tip optics, and tip geometry may be adjusted to modulate the cutting vs. co-

agulative effect, the zone of tissue necrosis induced by cutting tips, according to manufacturer's literature, is at least 300–500 μm as summarized in Table 8.2. This injury zone is too large to be of benefit for skin incisions, but the contact tip may have applications in some subcutaneous dissections.

Current sapphire cutting tips can reliably deliver CW but not pulsed CO_2 energy because char accumulates on the tip between pulses, and the associated heat damages the tip. When used with the erbium:YAG laser, the rapid pulsing may fracture the tip. Newer tip materials and delivery systems such as ultra-low-expansion glass and synthetic sapphire fibers may overcome current technical limitations.

TRANSITION TO LASER INCISIONAL SURGERY

The transition to laser incisional eyelid surgery requires a commitment to embrace a new knowledge base, master a new set of surgical maneuvers, learn safe laser technique, and acquire laser-safe instrumentation. Carbon dioxide laser surgery is a learned surgical discipline that is demanding and unforgiving, but also rewarding. The importance of seeking a mentor and observing a skilled laser eyelid surgeon cannot be overemphasized. Time spent in such an endeavor is amply rewarded as many finer points of laser surgery are often communicated most effectively in a one-on-one setting.

There are several differences between performing incisional surgery with a laser and using standard instrumentation. Most notable is the lack of tactile feedback from the laser. Traditional surgical techniques provide nonvisual sensations to assist in judging wound depth; in contrast, laser surgery requires visual recognition of tissue planes. An important motor skill for the novice laser surgeon to master is holding and moving the handpiece so that the beam is always focused and perpendicular to the tissue. Surgeons must overcome the natural tendency to increase the distance of the handpiece from the tissues as surgery proceeds. As described in Chapter 1, defocusing even a small amount decreases the power density of the beam exponentially, producing greater thermal injury.

Intraoperative hemostasis is significantly improved when the laser is used to perform eyelid and periorbital surgery. This is important because even a limited amount of hemorrhage rapidly obscures the fine anatomic detail of the delicate eyelid structures. With the ease in visualization of important anatomic structures, eyelid surgery may be performed in a more efficient and precise fashion.

Even subtle color differences between various structures will be discernible (Figure 8.5).

The depth of a laser incision is determined by: the speed at which the handpiece is moved across the target tissue, the focus of the laser beam, the power setting of the laser, and, to a lesser degree, the relative amount of moisture on the skin. The novice laser surgeon must be able to analyze and control the incision depth by relying upon direct visualization to determine the hand speed with which to move the laser across the tissue while maintaining the proper focus. Although the laser seems cumbersome and dangerous at first, the learning curve may be mastered readily by the dedicated surgeon.

When performing laser eyelid incisional surgery, it is important to use appropriate power settings because of the relative thinness of the eyelid dermis and epidermis (Table 8.3), and the proximity of the underlying levator aponeurosis and globe. Recommended power settings will vary with the manufacturer and the model of the laser. Consultation with a surgeon familiar with any given laser is recommended before using the device for the first time. With a 0.2 millimeter-focused hand-piece, energy levels are usually set at 4–6 W in CW mode or 4–5 W and 15–25 mJ in UltraPulse™ mode if the Coherent laser is used. Note that even in "CW" mode the UltraPulse™ laser pro-

TABLE 8.3 Average Thickness of Facial Dermis and Epidermis in Microns at Various Locations (Ranked by Dermal Thickness)

Location	Epidermis	Dermis	Total
Neck	115	138	253
Eyelids	130	215	345
Root of Nose	144	324	468
Cheek	141	909	1050
Lobule of Nose	111	918	1029
Forehead	202	969	1171
Lower Lip	113	973	1086
Upper Lip	156	1061	1217
Mental Region	149	1375	1524

Reprinted with permission from Gonzalez-Ulloa M, et al. Preliminary study of the total restoration of the facial skin. Plast Reconst Surg 1954;13:151–161.

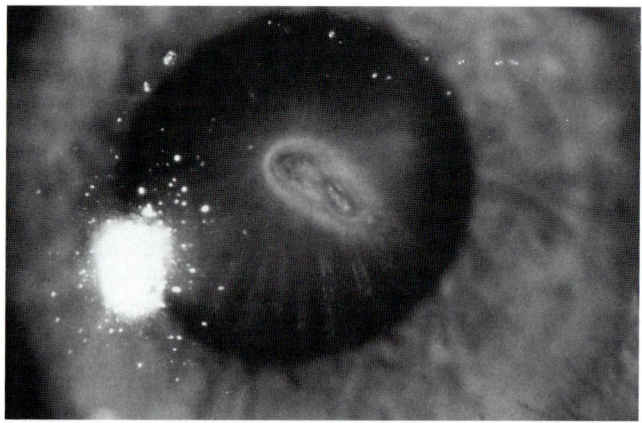

Figure 8.6. A CO_2 laser corneal injury. Courtesy of Oculo-Plastik, Montreal, CA.

duces a pulsed beam with a frequency of 1000–3000 Hz. The ergonomics and small beam size of the Coherent laser make it highly useful as an incisional device.

A number of complications may occur with laser eyelid surgery, including corneal laser burn (Figure 8.6), or frank globe perforation (29). Other complications include premature wound separation (common if blepharoplasty sutures are removed before 9 days), inferior oblique injury, thermal injury, scarring, and levator aponeurosis injury (27). The complications of laser incisional surgery are covered in more detail in another chapter. Once mastered, incisional laser surgery becomes relatively routine and may be applied to almost all eyelid plastic and reconstructive

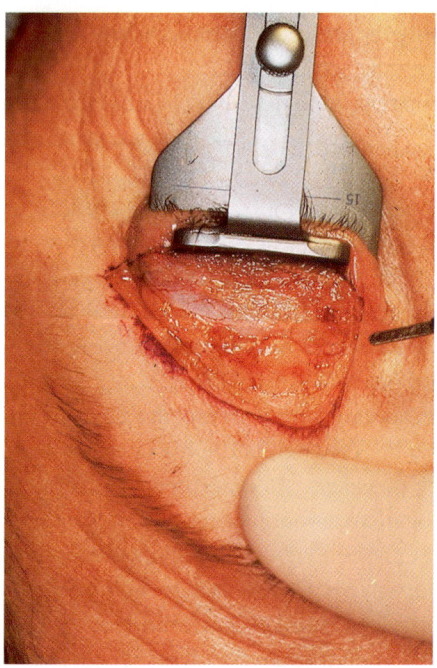

Figure 8.5. Intraoperative photograph demonstrating clear definition of orbicularis muscle, orbital septum (divided), preaponeurotic fat, and the levator aponeurosis. Note the absence of hemorrhage or tissue distortion.

surgeries including entropion, ectropion, ptosis, dacryo-cystorhinostomy, blepharoplasty, and others.

LASER SAFETY

Laser safety is an important part of the transition to laser incisional surgery. A complete discussion of this topic may be found in Chapter 1.

REFERENCES

1. Goldman I. Laser treatment of malignant melanoma. In: Goldman I, ed. Laser cancer research. New York: Springer-Verlag, 1966.
2. Patel CKN. Continuous-wave laser action in vibrational-rotational transitions of carbon dioxide. Phy Rev 1964; 136(A):1187–1193.
3. Polanyi TG, Bredemeier HC, Davis TJ Jr. CO_2 laser for surgical research and medical and biologic engineering. New York: Pergamon Press, 1970.
4. Aschler P, Ingolitsch E, Walter G, Oberhauer RW. Ultrastructural findings in CNS tissues with CO_2 laser. In: Kaplan I, ed. Laser surgery II. Jerusalem: Academic Press, 1976:81–85.
5. Ben-Bassat M, Ben-Bassat J, Kaplan I. An ultrastructural study of the cut edges of skin and mucous membrane specimens excised by carbon dioxide laser. In: Kaplan I, ed. Laser surgery II. Jerusalem: Academic Press, 1976:95–100.
6. Goldman MP, Fitzpatrick RE, eds. Cutaneous laser surgery. St. Louis: Mosby, 1994.
7. Beckman H, Fuller TA, Boyman R, et al. CO_2 laser surgery of the eye and adnexa. Ophthalmology 1980; 87:990–1000.
8. Baker SS, Muenzler WS, Small RG, Leonard JE. Carbon dioxide laser blepharoplasty. Ophthalmology 1984;91:238–243.
9. Wesley RE, Bond JB. Carbon dioxide laser in ophthalmic plastic and orbital surgery. Ophthalmic Surgery 1985;16:631–633.
10. Ross EV, Domankevitz Y, Skrobal M, Anderson R. Effects of CO_2 laser pulse duration in ablation and residual thermal damage. Lasers Surg Med 1996;19:123–129.
11. Fitzpatrick RE. UltraPulse CO_2 laser resurfacing of the facial skin. In: Rabkin MD, ed. CO_2 laser cosmetic blepharoplasty and skin resurfacing. Boston: Ophthalmology Interactive, 1997.
12. Chernoff G. Histology of UltraPulse CO_2 laser incisions. In: Rabkin MD, ed. CO_2 laser cosmetic blepharoplasty and skin resurfacing. Boston: Ophthalmology Interactive, 1997.
13. Biesman BS, Baker SS, Khan JK, Semple J. Histology of CO_2 laser incisions in human eyelid skin. Presented at the annual meeting of the American Society of Ophthalmic Plastic and Reconstructive Surgery, Chicago: October 26, 1996.
14. Hruza GJ, Dover JS. Laser skin resurfacing. Arch Dermatol 1996;132:451–455.
15. David LM, Sanders G. CO_2 blepharoplasty: a comparison to cold steel and electrocautery. J Derm Surg Oncol 1987;13:110.
16. Mittelman H, Apfelberg DB. Carbon dioxide laser blepharoplasty—advantages and disadvantages. Ann Plast Surg 1990;24:1–6.
17. Glassberg E, Babapour R, Lask G. Current trends in laser blepharoplasty. Results of a survey. Dermatol Surg 1995;21:1060–1063.
18. Sherman DD, Dortzbach RK. Monopolar electrocautery dissection in ophthalmic plastic surgery. Ophthal Plast Reconstr Surg 1993;9:143–147.
19. Farnworth TK, Beals SP, Manwaring KH, Trepeta RW. Comparison of skin necrosis in rats by using a new microneedle electrocautery, standard-size needle electrocautery, and the Shaw hemostatic scalpel. Ann Plast Surg 1993;31:164–167.
20. Schaefer M. Drei falle von diathermieschadigungen bei benutzung in der diathermie in der operativen technic. Schweiz Med Wochenschr 1927;8:268–278.
21. Wulc AE, Adams JL, Dryden RM. Cerebrospinal fluid leak complicating orbital exenteration. Arch Ophthalmol 1989;107:827–830.
22. Schietroma JJ, Tenzel RR. The effects of cautery on the optic nerve. Ophthal Plast Reconstr Surg 1990;6:102–107.
23. Shorr N. Lower lid transconjunctival blepharoplasty using the CO_2 laser. Aesthetic Surg Quarterly 1996: Summer.
24. Morrow DM, Morrow LB. CO_2 laser blepharoplasty. A comparison with cold-steel surgery. J Dermatol Surg Oncol 1992;18:307–313.
25. Apfelberg DP, Maser MR, Lash H, et al. Sapphire tip technology for the YAG laser excisions in plastic surgery. Plast Reconst Surg 1989;84:273–279.
26. Putterman A. Scalpel neodymium:YAG laser in oculoplastic surgery. Am J Ophthalmol 1990;109:581–584.
27. Schroder T, Hukki J, Castren M, et al. Comparison of surgical and conventional methods in skin incisions. Scand J Plast Reconst Surg Hand Surg 1989;23:187–190.
28. Fuller TA. Thermal surgical lasers. Oaks, PA: Surgical Lasers Technologies Inc. (monograph), 1993.
29. Shorr N. Avoiding and managing complications of laser blepharoplasty. In: Rabkin MD, ed. CO_2 laser cosmetic blepharoplasty and skin resurfacing. Boston: Ophthalmology Interactive, 1997.

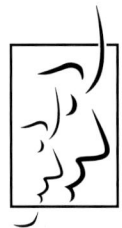

Chapter Nine

Laser-Assisted Upper Blepharoplasty

Brian S. Biesman and Harvey P. Cole III

Aging brings many changes in the periorbital region: descent of the eyebrows, the development of excess eyelid skin (dermatochalasis), degenerative changes of the thin eyelid skin marked by the appearance of fine rhytids, herniation of orbital fat, and drooping of the eyelids. Many of these problems may be corrected by blepharoplasty.

Blepharoplasty is one of the most commonly performed incisional aesthetic procedures in the United States. While this operation is not particularly demanding from a technical standpoint, a thorough understanding of eyelid aesthetics, anatomy, and function is required to achieve satisfactory results. As surgical results are judged by patient satisfaction rather than by restoration of anatomic correctness, having a clear understanding of the individual's motivation for seeking surgery, perception of their own appearance, and expectations of surgery, is necessary. Patients who anticipate a secondary gain, such as improvement in a personal relationship or professional advancement, are not good candidates for aesthetic surgery. The best surgical candidates are those who are able to identify specific aesthetic concerns, who have a reasonable expectation of results, and who do not expect a dramatic change in their lives. Most patients do not desire a marked change in their appearance, but hope for a general improvement that may evoke comments such as "Have you changed your hair style?", "Have you been on vacation recently?", or "Is that a new outfit?". Patients who express an interest in dramatically changing their appear-

ance should be interviewed carefully more than once to ensure that this is indeed their wish.

Patients who make vague statements such as "my eyes look tired," "do whatever you think I need," or "make me look younger," must be carefully evaluated and educated as to the nature of their findings and the potential procedures available to correct them. A large mirror should be used during this discussion to ensure that the patient and surgeon are addressing the same areas of concern. If, following this discussion, the patient is still unable to articulate their concerns and expectations concisely, a second consultation spent reviewing old photographs may be beneficial. A second visit allows the patient and surgeon to develop a stronger relationship with improved rapport and communication, and allows the patient to develop a new level of understanding and appreciation for aesthetic detail. Patients are then often able to identify objective physical findings that they wish to address. In contrast, other patients will express great anxiety about aesthetic defects so slight as to be nearly undetectable, even by a skilled observer. These patients are challenging and usually very difficult to please. The patient's concerns and expectations must be carefully determined during the preoperative evaluation. The use of computerized imaging help patients visualize potential results, but it must be stressed that these images may not provide a realistic picture of the final surgical outcome; they may serve as an educational tool for both the patient and the surgeon to validate each other's expectations (1–4).

Most patients do not wish to look different; instead, they wish to look like a younger and more refreshed version of themselves. This can usually be achieved by addressing dermatochalasis, herniated orbital fat, and laxity of the eyelids. In contrast, elevation of the eyebrows and forehead and changing the position of the lateral canthal angles or eyelid crease is more likely to change a patient's look. Each of these issues must be discussed carefully when making a surgical plan. While guidelines for normal eyebrow or eyelid crease position may be found in medical texts (see Chapters 2 and 9), these are *only* guidelines; each patient's anatomic structure must be evaluated individually using old photographs for comparison when indicated.

During preoperative consultation, other information vital to making surgical decisions should be collected. Each patient's general health status must be carefully assessed, and a careful medical history should include questions about use of over-the-counter medications, which, unbeknownst to the consumer, may contain nonsteroidal antiinflammatory drugs (NSAIDs), e.g., Alka Seltzer™ (Bayer, Morristown, NJ). The patient should also be questioned about a history of thyroid ophthalmopathy and other ophthalmic disorders including dry eye syndrome, contact lens use, the need for regular application of artificial tears, or the presence of periocular skin disease (5). A history of keloid formation or hypertrophic scarring elsewhere should be noted.

Patients sometimes fail to volunteer a history of aesthetic surgical, laser, or chemical peeling procedures either out of reluctance, to test the physician's ability to detect evidence of these procedures, or simply in error. A set of standard photographs should be taken with a camera or digital imaging system that provides adequate visualization of the anatomic region to be treated.

PERIORBITAL AESTHETIC RELATIONSHIPS

It is important to understand the cephalometric dimensions of the periorbital region before performing blepharoplasty surgery. Aesthetic surgeons may be mislead by patients who seem to have dermatochalasis but, in fact, have ptosis of the eyebrows, which is causing compression of the eyelid-eyebrow complex (Figure 9.1). In these cases, skin resection may produce eyebrow ptosis. Similarly, the natural upward slope of the lateral canthus and normal variations in gender and race must be appreciated.

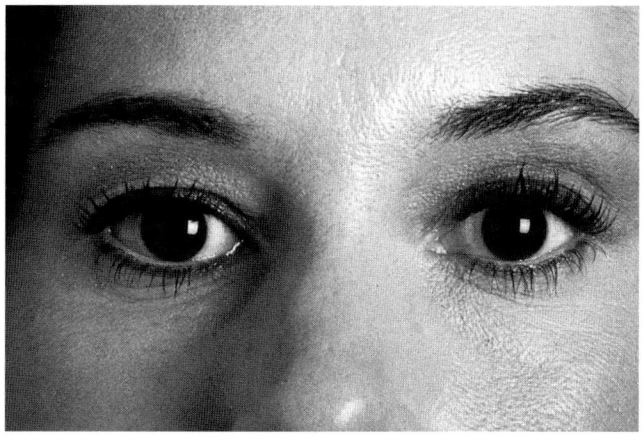

Figure 9.1. A female patient with upper eyelid dermatochalasis, right greater than left. A previously unrecognized right brow ptosis is present.

The normal palpebral fissure measures 9–10 mm in vertical height with the eyes in primary (straight ahead) gaze. The horizontal width of the palpebral fissure is approximately 30 mm, and the lateral canthal angle is approximately 2 mm superior to its medial counterpart. Lowering the lateral canthus can produce a sad, unnatural look. The upper eyelid margin should rest 1–2 mm below the superior corneal limbus; if the superior limbus is visible, suspect either deliberate eyelid elevation or eyelid retraction as is commonly caused by thyroid disease. The lower eyelid margin should rest at the level of the inferior corneal limbus; sclera should never be visible between the inferior limbus and the lower eyelid margin. Lower eyelid position is discussed in greater detail in Chapters 10 and 11. The upper eyelid crease lies 9–11 mm above the lid margin in adult Caucasian females and 8–10 mm above the lid margin in adult Caucasian males (Figure 9.2) (6). There are significant differences in eyelid crease position and contour between Asian and Occidental eyelids (7). Due to the social significance placed on this feature by most Asian societies, these differences must be recognized and respected.

Eyebrows may be straight, curved, or arched. The eyebrow in males normally rests above the orbital rim and is oriented horizontally across its entire length (Figure 9.3). In contrast, the brow in a typical female patient rests further above the orbital rim and has an arched shape with greater elevation temporally than nasally. The peak of the arch is typically located at the junction of the middle and lateral thirds of the eyebrow (Figure 9.4). Although these generalized descriptions of eyebrow position are true in a general sense, in reality a high degree of variability may be observed. Even some female fashion models have eyebrows in a position or configuration more typical of males (8).

The vertical proportions of the midface should also be recognized. If the distance between the upper eyelid margin and eyebrow is divided into thirds, the distance between the upper eyelid crease and the eyebrow should account for two thirds of the total, while the distance from the eyelid margin to the upper eyelid crease should account for the other one third. In other words, the distance from the eyelid crease to the inferior border of the eyebrow should be approximately twice the distance from the eyelid margin to the eyelid crease. If the lid crease-brow distance is decreased, a careful search for ei-

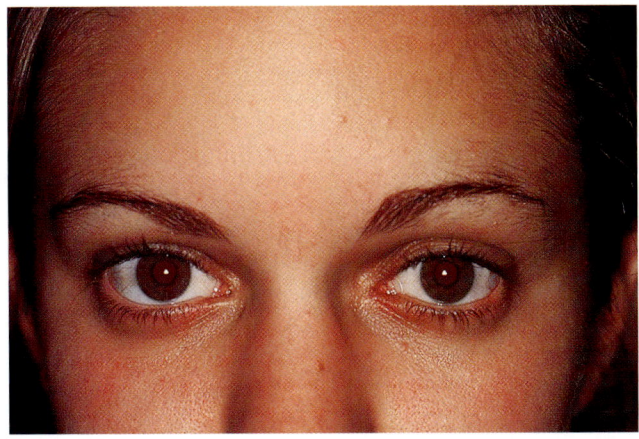

Figure 9.4. Normal position of female brows.

ther ptosis of the eyebrow or elevation of the eyelid crease (indicative of levator aponeurosis disinsertion, see Chapter 11) should be initiated (9, 10).

PREOPERATIVE EXAMINATION

As with any evaluation, the blepharoplasty patient should be examined in a systematic manner. With the patient in an upright position, the forehead is assessed, noting its height above the eyebrows, the presence of horizontal furrows, and actinic damage of the skin. The eyebrows are examined for position, contour, and fullness of the retroorbicularis oculi fat (ROOF) pad, which manifests as a prominence of the superior lateral orbital rim below the eyebrow (Figure 9.5). The lateral portion of the eyelid may also appear full if the lacrimal gland is prolapsed or enlarged (See Figure 1.9).

The position of the globe is noted relative to the orbital rim. In the setting of a flattened malar eminence, a shallow orbit, or axial myopia (near-sighted patient with a long globe), the eye will appear prominent and the upper and lower eyelids may appear retracted. In cases such as these, removal of tissue from the eyelids must be performed with great care: the proptotic appearance of the globe may be emphasized, creating an aesthetically unacceptable staring look and possibly even limiting the ability of the eyelids to close completely. True proptosis (axial anterior displacement of the globe), as may be caused by thyroid ophthalmopathy, orbital tumors, or other less common conditions, may be detected by exophthalmometry measurements. Note that normal exophthalmometry values are sex- and race-dependent (11).

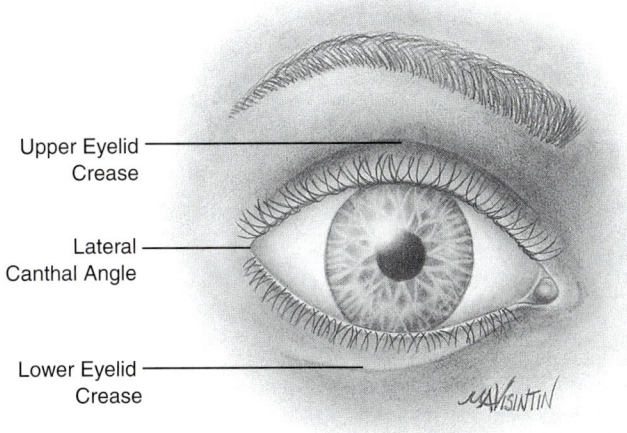

Figure 9.2. Topographic anatomy of the eyelids and periorbital region.

Upper Eyelid Crease

Lateral Canthal Angle

Lower Eyelid Crease

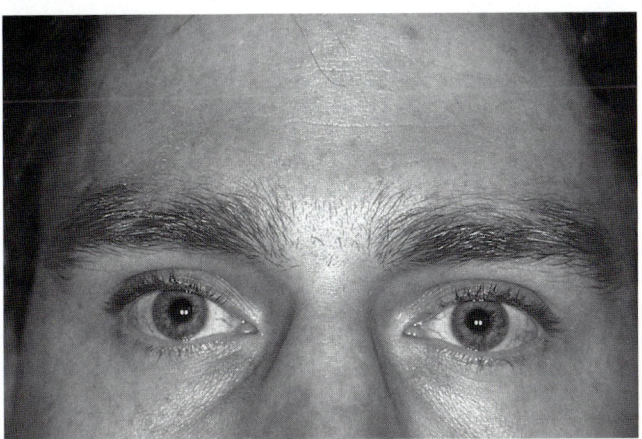

Figure 9.3. Normal position of male brows.

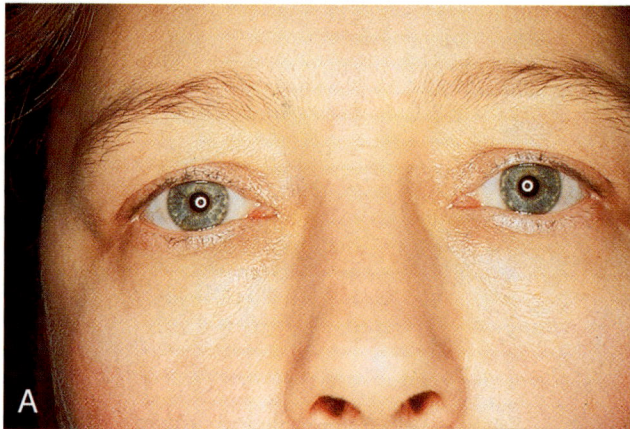

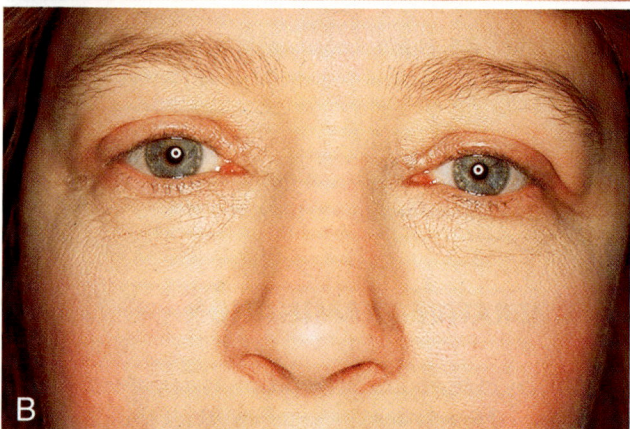

Figure 9.5. A. 37-year-old female with dermatochalasis and fullness of the ROOF fat pads. **B.** Same patient 1 week after laser-assisted upper blepharoplasty and ROOF fat pad reduction.

Attention should then be turned to the upper eyelid. While the examiner holds the brows in fixed position, the eyelid is evaluated for retraction (lid margin above the superior limbus) or ptosis. The eyelid margins are inspected for the presence of redness, crusting, or ulceration, which may indicate active infection or blepharitis. The periorbital skin is explored for evidence of wrinkling, old surgical scars, pigmentary change, and tumors. Webbing or folds in the medial canthus are noted as these will affect the placement of an upper eyelid incision.

The superior sulcus is examined for fullness, indicative of herniated orbital fat, or concavity, which may become exaggerated after blepharoplasty surgery, producing excessive indentation of the superior fornix and a so-called "A-frame" defect (Figure 9.6). The upper eyelid crease is evaluated for position and definition. If the creases are ill-defined or asymmetric, this should be called to the patient's attention as most individuals are more

likely to notice this difference between the eyelids after surgery.

Upon completing analysis of the forehead, eyebrows, and upper eyelid, the lower eyelid is evaluated for its position relative to the cornea, appropriate fullness, pigmentary change within the skin (dark circles), scarring, retraction, laxity of canthal tendons, and the presence of malar bags or "festoons." The significance of these findings will be discussed in greater detail in Chapter 10. Attention is then turned to the globe.

The best-corrected visual acuity is measured at distance (20') with a Snellen chart or, if this is unavailable, at near (14") using a near card. The pupillary size and reaction to light are noted and the extraocular movements are evaluated. Diplopia should be ruled out by asking the patient to fix their gaze on an object, which is moved into the nine cardinal positions of gaze (up and right, straight up, up and left, etc.). While diplopia in extreme positions of gaze is uncommon, it may occur in patients with a history of thyroid ophthalmopathy, many of whom will seek blepharoplasty surgery. The tear film is inspected under magnification, looking for a shortened tear break-up time (>10 seconds is normal), which could indicate a susceptibility to dry eyes after upper blepharoplasty. Fluorescein dye is placed along the internal aspect of the eyelid, and the patient is asked to blink several times to distribute the dye evenly over the ocular surface. Staining will occur in areas where the epithelium has been disrupted as in dry eye syndrome, acne rosacea, Sjögren's syndrome, or other conditions where the eye's ability to maintain its surface is impaired. Fluorescein dye must not be instilled in patients wearing soft contact lenses as it will stain the

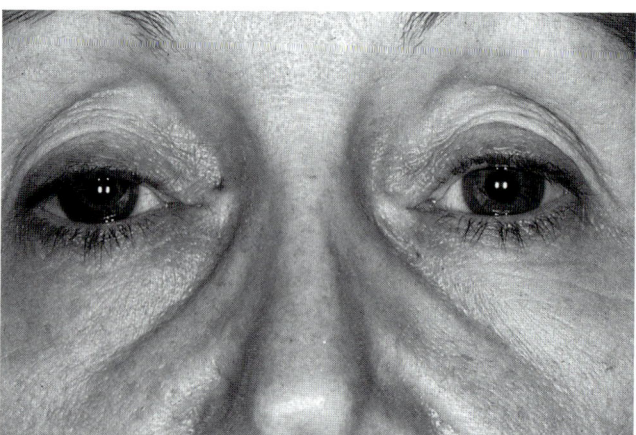

Figure 9.6. A-frame defect. The superior sulcus is deep and the apex of the "A" is clearly visible.

lenses a bright yellow-green color. Basic secretion testing is performed as described in Chapter 11. Intraocular pressure measurement is recommended to detect glaucoma, and fundoscopy is performed to rule out the presence of previously unrecognized intraocular pathology.

If patients complain of visual loss, which may be attributed to upper eyelid dermatochalasis or ptosis, or even eyebrow ptosis, visual field testing may be performed. This test should be performed twice: once with the lids and brows in a relaxed position and again with the ptotic tissues taped into an elevated position simulating the surgical result. To be considered functionally significant by most third-party payers, the visual field must be impaired to within 30° of fixation, or must improve by 20° with elevation of the ptotic structures. The superior visual field should be measured across the entire horizontal meridian, and from 0–60° in the vertical meridian. This may be accomplished via manual or automated testing devices, although automated testing is required in certain areas of the country.

Careful counseling of patients prior to blepharoplasty or any other aesthetic procedure will help eliminate confusion, misunderstandings, and patient disappointment or frustration. A careful discussion about the preparation for surgery, the associated risks and benefits of the contemplated procedure, and the expected postoperative recovery period, is extremely important. The potential complications of surgery should be discussed openly, not avoided or minimized. The surgical consent forms may be sent home with patients for study at their leisure.

ANATOMY OF THE EYELIDS

Upper eyelid anatomy pertinent to the blepharoplasty surgeon is discussed in Chapter 2.

LASER-ASSISTED UPPER BLEPHAROPLASTY

Marking the Incision

While many ways to mark an upper eyelid incision exist, serious problems may be avoided if some basic rules are followed. It is helpful to mark the eyelids with a fine point pen, which may be ordered as a stock item. Alternatively, one may be made using the straight portion of a # 15

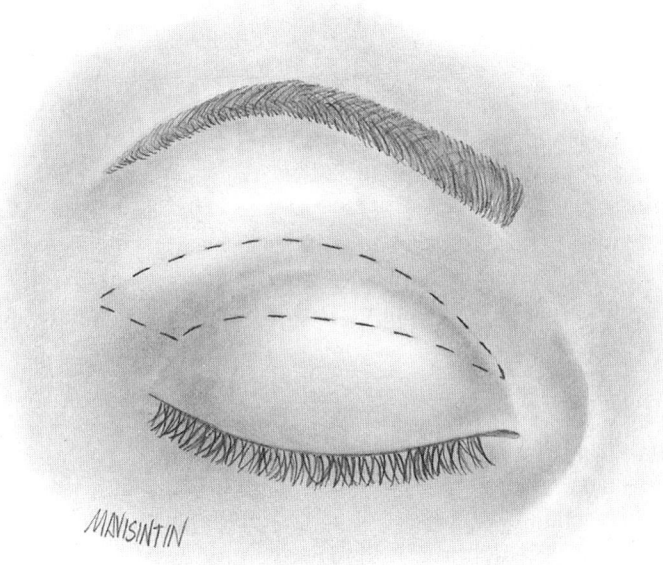

Figure 9.7. Typical upper blepharoplasty incision.

blade to whittle the tip of a standard surgical marking pen to a sharp point. The inferior border of the incision should be placed in the eyelid crease, assuming it has not been distorted by previous surgery, disinsertion of the levator aponeurosis, or other factors. In Caucasian patients, the central portion of the crease is highest while the temporal and nasal ends are lower. In the Asian lid, the crease is more level than arched (7). Nasally, the incision should extend no closer than 5 mm from the superior punctum and generally should not extend medially to a line drawn vertically through this structure. Carrying the incision too far medially can result in cicatricial band formation (webbing). The superior border of the incision should pass no closer than 1 cm below the inferior border of the eyebrow, the approximate point of transition between the thicker skin of the eyebrow and the thinner skin of the eyelid. This will avoid induction of eyebrow ptosis. The amount of eyelid skin to be removed can be estimated: have the patient gently close the eyes as one arm of a smooth forceps is placed in the eyelid crease while the other pinches the redundant skin until the eyelashes just begin to rotate. This marks the maximum amount of skin that may be safely removed. The temporal extent of the incision should not extend lateral to a line drawn vertically through the lateral end of the eyebrow (Figure 9.7, oriented to surgeon's view). Some surgeons prefer to create a W-plasty configuration to the lateral end of the upper eyelid incision to help camouflage the scar (12–14). If brow ptosis is present but not to be corrected per the patient's wishes, the brow should be manually elevated to its appropriate position when marking the eyelids. Failure to do this may result in the resection of too much amount of skin, and subsequent lagophthalmos when the ptotic eyebrow is elevated (14). The eyelids should be marked with the patient in a supine position, and then in a sitting position with a careful evaluation for symmetry. The eyelids should be marked before sedatives are administered.

Incisional Technique

The technique for laser-assisted blepharoplasty was first described and subsequently modified by Baker and others (15–18). The following technique described is derived from Baker's work.

Laser-assisted upper blepharoplasty may be performed with local anesthesia alone, or in conjunction with systemic oral or intravenous sedation. Occasionally patients even request general anesthesia. With advances in anesthetic agents and portable monitoring equipment, deep intravenous sedation can be administered in an office setting. See chapter 4 for additional information about anesthesia for facial aesthetic surgery. To provide local anesthesia, once the patient has been sedated, 1.5–2.0 cc of anesthetic agent is injected subcutaneously in the central upper lid. A 30-gauge needle is used, and care is taken to avoid the orbicularis muscle, which will bleed if engaged. Digital massage is then used to ease distribution medially and laterally throughout the upper eyelid, avoiding multiple punctures in the eyelid skin, and reducing the likelihood of hematoma formation. The actual agent may be lidocaine 2% with epinephrine added at a dilution of 1:100,000 alone, or mixed 1:1 with 0.25–0.75% bupivacaine. If lower eyelid surgery or skin resurfacing is to be performed simultaneously, some surgeons prefer to use lidocaine solution alone to avoid prolonged orbicularis muscle akinesia and subsequent exposure keratopathy.

With no systemic contraindications, dexamethasone (8–10 mg) is administered intravenously to help reduce postoperative swelling. An intravenous antibiotic with good skin flora coverage may also be administered preoperatively, but is not required and has not been proven to reduce the risk of postoperative infection.

The carbon dioxide laser is positioned and adjusted to eliminate tension on the handpiece as the surgeon holds it lightly. This may require proper positioning of the laser or adjustment of counter weights or springs. Executing the fine maneuvers required for blepharoplasty surgery when fighting against an ergonomically unfavorable device is difficult. Incisional periorbital surgery requires the smallest possible laser beam diameter, ideally no more than 0.2 mm. The laser may be operated in continuous wave or high frequency pulse mode. Less lateral thermal damage is produced in the pulsed than the continuous wave mode. The continuous-wave beam produced by the commonly used UltraPulse™ (Coherent Medical, Palo Alto, CA) laser is a high-frequency pulsed beam that creates the same tissue effects as the pulsed-mode beam when making an eyelid incision. Surgeons who prefer to work in continuous-wave mode generally start with a power setting of 5–8 W while those who prefer pulsed mode often begin with an energy setting of 10 mJ/pulse at a power of 10 W. Histopathologic studies performed in our laboratories showed an equal thermal effect on eyelid tissue when the UltraPulse™ laser was operated at settings of 6 W in continuous-wave mode and 15 mJ/pulse and 5 W in pulsed mode (19).

Before making the first incision, laser-safe eye protection is placed. See chapter 1 for a more detailed discussion of appropriate ocular protection (20, 21). With the David-Baker clamp in position and the lid stretched inferiorly, the laser is used to make an incision through skin and orbicularis muscle over the central and nasal portions of the previously marked ellipse. The temporal portion of the incision should extend only through skin to avoid dividing the terminal branch of the lacrimal artery, which passes between skin and orbicularis muscle at the level of the lateral orbital rim (Figure 9.8, oriented to surgeon's view) (8). Incision depth correlates directly with the power setting on the laser, and inversely with the surgeon's hand speed. A single incision through skin and anterior orbicularis, rather than multiple passes, will minimize lateral propagation of laser energy and thermal necrosis while achieving excellent incisional hemostasis. Once the initial incision is complete, a toothed forceps is used to elevate the temporal end of the ellipse so that a skin flap may be dissected with the laser. This is performed easily if traction is kept on the skin flap to help separate it from the underlying orbicularis muscle. Once the lateral orbital rim has been crossed, the incision is deepened to include orbicularis muscle. This dissection should stay above the level of the orbital septum at all times (Figure 9.9, oriented to surgeon's view).

Once the skin muscle flap has been removed, the orbital septum will be clearly visible as a shiny white struc-

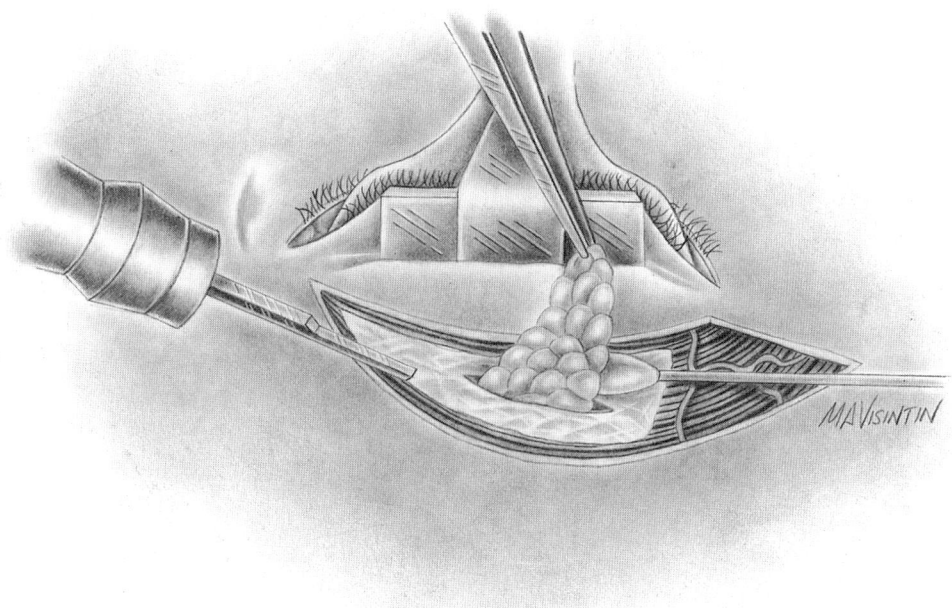

Figure 9.11. The easily herniating preaponeurotic fat is resected with the laser. Clamping the fat pads is not necessary.

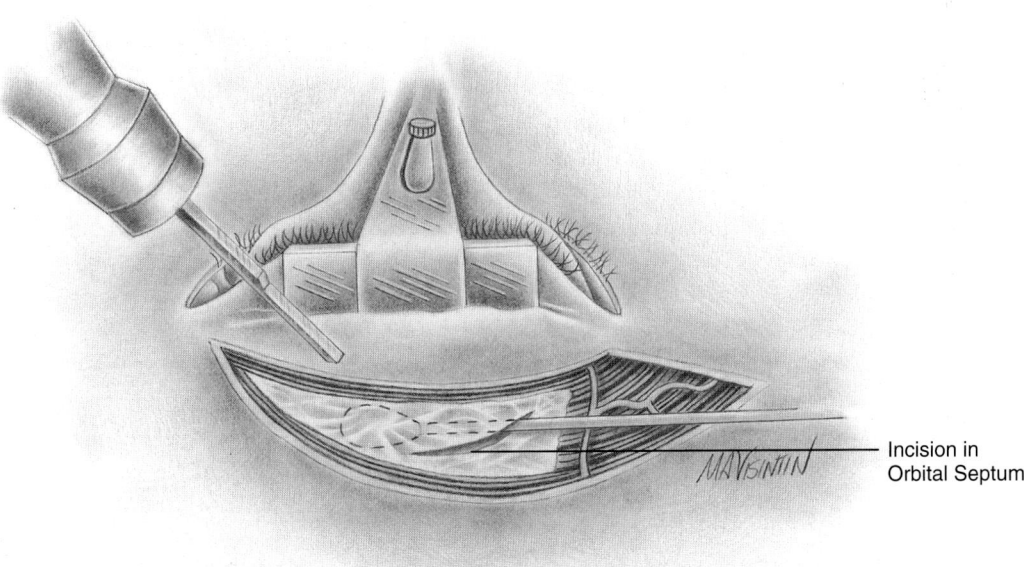

Incision in
Orbital Septum

Figure 9.12. A wet applicator or an antireflective metal instrument is introduced into the wound to protect the underlying levator aponeurosis as the orbital septum is divided with the laser.

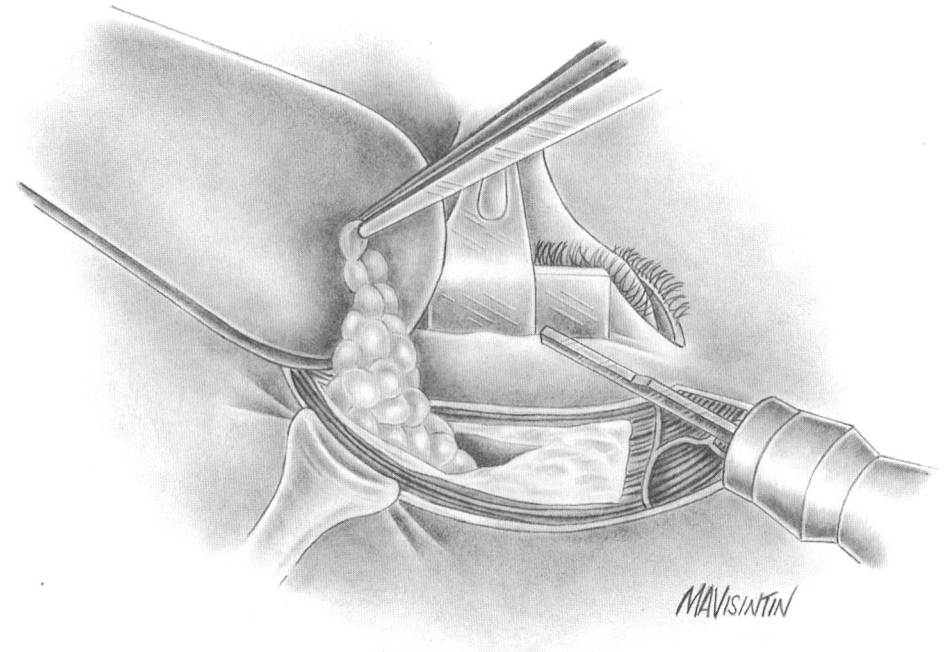

Figure 9.13. The easily herniating medial orbital fat is resected with the laser. Large vessels may be present within this fat pad.

contouring of the ROOF complex may be readily performed with the laser to achieve an optimal aesthetic result. The ROOF complex is contoured to a height of 1–1.5 cm above the orbital rim using a continuous wave energy setting of 10 W. Higher energy is used for this dissection than the eyelid portion of the procedure because of the fibrous nature of the ROOF complex and the presence of the larger vessels contained within. Care should be taken to ensure that this dissection is performed above the level of the superior orbital rim. Medially, the dissection should not extend past the central brow so as to preserve the integrity of the supraorbital neurovascular complex. A thin layer of ROOF fat should be left intact on the undersurface of the orbicularis oculi muscle overlying the orbital rim. Excision of the entire ROOF complex may result in surface irregularities, adhesion of the skin to the underlying periosteum producing an immobile brow, or a combination of these problems. The ROOF complex should be excised with the laser handpiece held in a focused position. Defocusing the beam to shrink the fat is ineffective and produces a significant increase in thermal damage. Significant bleeding may be encountered in the ROOF complex: bipolar cautery should be readily available. The beginning aesthetic laser surgeon should approach this area conservatively and may benefit from ob-

serving a colleague perform this essential blepharoplasty contouring procedure.

Internal tightening of the inferior limb of the lateral canthal tendon may be performed through the lateral end of the upper blepharoplasty incision. Once the upper blepharoplasty has been completed (but before the wound is closed), the laser is set in continuous-wave mode (5–6 W) to dissect down to the supraperiosteal layer along the lateral orbital rim, aiming for the point where the contour of the orbital rim changes from horizontal to a vertical direction. The surgeon demarcates the new location of canthal fixation along the orbital rim approximately 0.5–1.0 cm above the preoperative canthal level. The lateral canthal tendon complex may be palpated "like the strumming of a guitar string" when the lower eyelid is grasped with a large forceps and distracted anteriorly and medially, stretching the tendon. The tendon is readily accessible from this internalized approach. Dissection is carefully performed using the laser and a standard periosteal elevator until all tendon attachments to the orbital rim have been released.

The canthal tendon complex is imbricated with a permanent suture on a small half-circle needle (e.g., 4-0 polypropylene, P-2 needle) and fixated just inside the lateral orbital rim. One author (HPC) has performed this

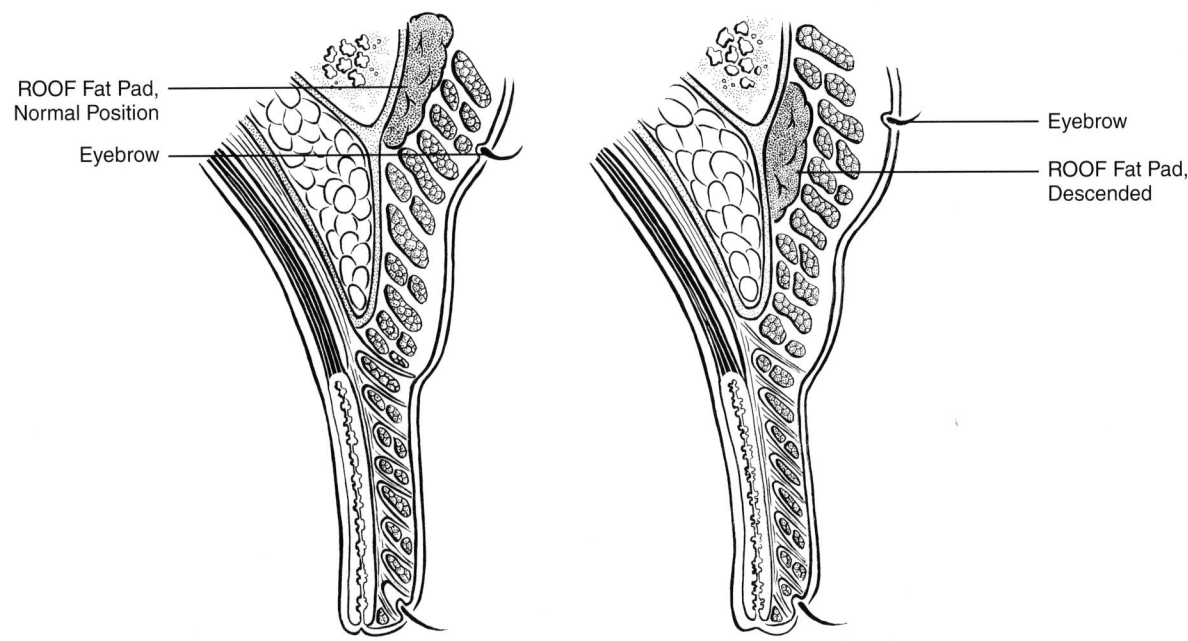

ROOF Fat Pad,
Normal Position

Eyebrow

Eyebrow

ROOF Fat Pad,
Descended

MAVISINTIN

Figure 9.14. A. Sagittal view of eyelid and eyebrow demonstrating normal position of the
ROOF fat pad. **B.** Schematic diagram demonstrating descent of the ROOF fat pad.

procedure on more than 250 patients with excellent postoperative lid position and contour. At 5-year follow-up, the canthal position remains stable. Only minor adjustments in contour and symmetry have been required. There have been no serious complications associated with the internal approach to lateral canthoplasty (20).

Hemostasis must be maintained in a meticulous way throughout the entire procedure to avoid orbital hemorrhage and the possibility of blindness. Most often, this may be achieved by defocusing the laser: where this is not effective, bipolar cautery may be required and should always be available.

Wound closure may be performed in many ways. In cases where the lid crease is not to be emphasized or repositioned, interrupted or running 6-0 or 7-0 permanent monofilament sutures such as nylon or polypropylene may be used. A small cutting needle [P-1 or PC-1 (Ethicon, Somerville, NJ)] works very well, although some surgeons prefer a taper-cut needle, which may cause less trauma to the tissue but dulls more quickly than the cutting needles. Sutures should be passed from skin edge to skin edge without engaging the underlying orbicularis muscle, which may bleed and cause a hematoma. Care should be taken to ensure that the wound is properly aligned across its entire extent. Because of the curvilinear shape of the incision, the vectors of force vary across the entire width of the wound. If interrupted sutures are used, the wound should be aligned by plac-

ing cardinal sutures centrally, nasally, and temporally prior to filling in the areas in between. Care should also be taken to ensure wound edge eversion. Running subcuticular sutures may be used, but the likelihood of bleeding from the orbicularis muscle may be slightly increased with this technique.

If a lid crease is to be created, an interrupted 6-0 undyed polyglactin suture is placed through the skin and orbicularis muscle on the inferior border of the wound, through the levator aponeurosis at the superior tarsal border, and then through orbicularis muscle and skin on the superior border of the wound. Three such sutures are placed: one in the nasal portion of the lid, one in the central portion, and one in the temporal portion. The wound in between these sutures is closed skin edge to skin edge with permanent suture material.

Laser skin resurfacing of the periorbital region or the entire face may be performed simultaneously with blepharoplasty surgery. These procedures are complementary as blepharoplasty recontours the eyelids and removes extra tissues while laser skin resurfacing removes fine rhytids, lines, and actinic damage, and induces dermal collagen production, thus producing an overall rejuvenating effect (Figures 9.14, 9.15).

At the end of the procedure, an ophthalmic antibiotic ointment *without* neomycin is placed on the lids, followed by sponges soaked in iced saline. Patients are instructed to maintain ice compresses as often as possible for the first

Figure 9.15. Before **A,** and 4 weeks after **B,** upper and lower blepharoplasty and full-face laser skin resurfacing.

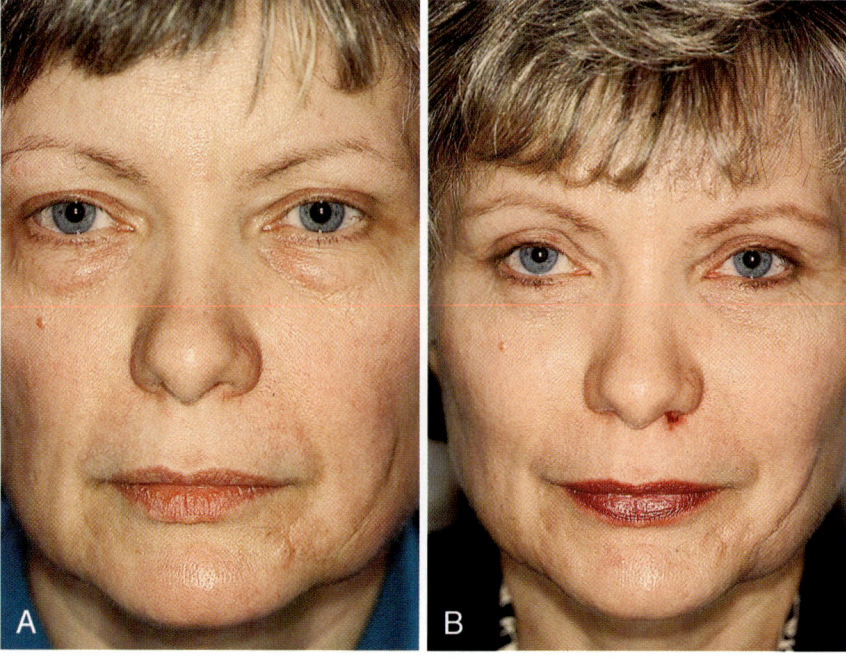

48 hours, to apply antibiotic ointment to the sutures 3–4 times per day, to keep their head elevated during the day and even at night by sleeping on extra pillows, and to avoid heavy bending, lifting, exercise, or other activities that may require a Valsalva maneuver for at least 1 week. Airplane travel should be discouraged to avoid potential exposure to decreased atmospheric pressure, which may allow bleeding to occur. If the patient lives a significant distance from the surgeon, arrangements should be made to have the patient stay in a nearby hotel for the first night after surgery. Patients are contacted by telephone in the evening of the day surgery was performed and are either examined or contacted again by telephone the following day. If persistent bleeding, swelling, significant pain, decreased vision, erythema or discharge from the wounds is reported prompt examination is required. If there are no unanticipated complaints, patients are seen again on postoperative day 6–10 for suture removal. Satisfactory postoperative analgesia may usually be achieved with acetaminophen, although narcotics may be required by some patients. Nonsteroidal antiinflammatory drugs (including ketolorac [Toradol, Roche, Nutley, NJ]) must be avoided to prevent orbital hemorrhage.

Contact lens wear may be resumed 1–2 weeks after surgery. Patients who wear contact lenses should be carefully advised of this preoperatively as many do not have current eyeglasses prescriptions. Cosmetics may be applied to the upper eyelids 1–2 days after the sutures have been removed and concealer may be applied to the lower eyelids to cover ecchymosis within the first several days after surgery. Erythromycin ophthalmic ointment is applied until cosmetic use is resumed. Patients are told to expect 80% of the swelling to resolve over 2 weeks, while the remaining 20% (which is not usually aesthetically significant) make take months to completely resolve. High salt foods or a systemic state of fluid retention may produce increased swelling in the eyelids. Low-level exercise may be resumed after 1 week, and more vigorous activities resumed after 2 weeks.

RESULTS

The advantage of using a laser as an incisional device in blepharoplasty surgery is realized in the immediate postoperative period (Figures 9.16–9.18). Although not yet proven in clinical trials, experienced laser surgeons almost uniformly agree that the postoperative recovery period is shortened when a laser is used to make the soft tissue incisions. While bruising and swelling do occur, the degree and duration are generally less than are produced by standard techniques. This may be related to the shortened procedure time, the intraoperative closure of lymphatics and small blood vessels, or a combination of these factors. Three months postoperatively, there is no discernable difference between patients treated with the laser and those treated with standard techniques (15, 23–26).

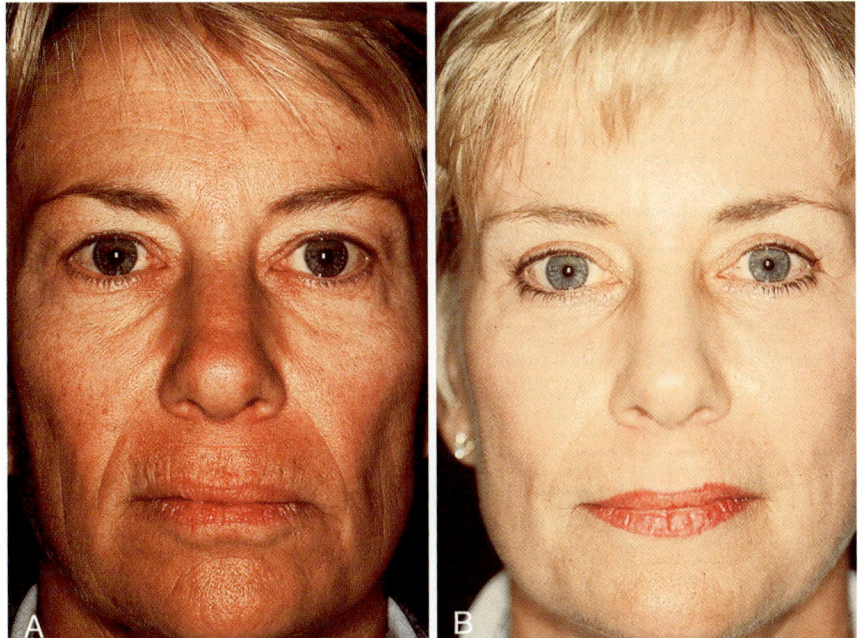

Figure 9.16. Before **A,** and 4 weeks after **B,** upper and lower blepharoplasty and full face laser skin resurfacing.

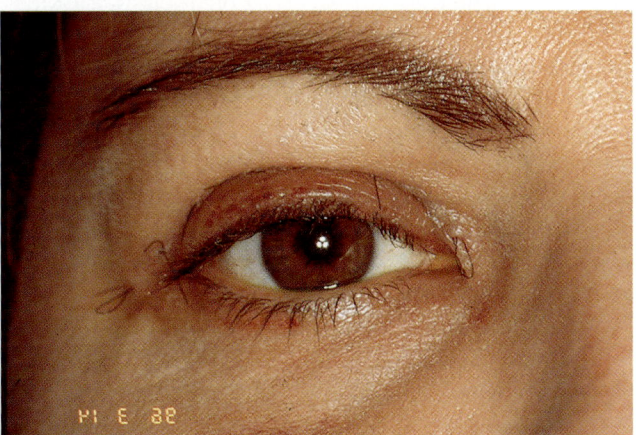

Figure 9.17. Less than 24 hours after upper eyelid laser-assisted blepharoplasty. Ecchymosis and swelling are minimal.

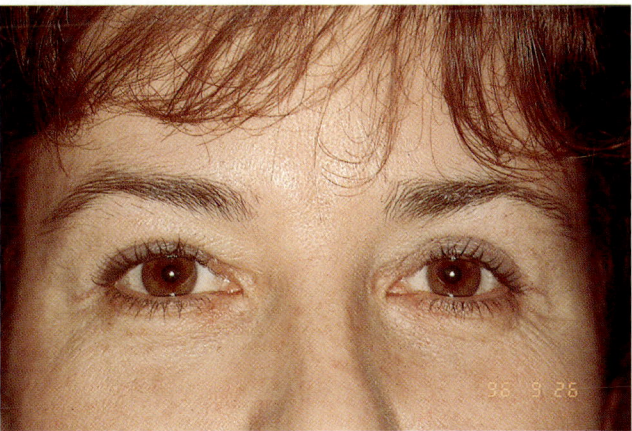

Figure 9.18. Ten days after laser-assisted four-lid blepharoplasty. Only minimal swelling remains.

The complications of blepharoplasty surgery may include bleeding, infection, damage to the globe, inadvertent division of structures such as the levator and, of course, asymmetry or otherwise unsatisfactory results. Complications specific to the use of the carbon dioxide laser include intraoperative fire, laser burn to the eye, ocular adnexa, or operating room personnel, aesthetically unacceptable appearance of the wound, and delayed wound healing. These complications are discussed more comprehensively in Chapter 14. With a clear understanding of eyelid and orbital anatomy, and proper attention to surgical technique and postoperative wound care, the risk of these complications may be markedly reduced.

REFERENCES

1. Putterman AM. Evaluation of the cosmetic oculoplastic surgery patient. In: Putterman AM, ed. Cosmetic oculoplastic surgery, 2nd ed. Philadelphia: WB Saunders, 1993:12-27.
2. Bosniak SL. In: Bosniak SL, ed. Cosmetic blepharoplasty. New York. Raven Press.1990:3-10.
3. Papel ID, Schoenrock LD. Computer imaging. In: Papel ID, Nachlas NE, eds. Facial plastic and reconstructive surgery. St. Louis: Mosby, 1992:110-115.
4. Gorney M. Preoperative computerized video imaging (Letter). Plast Reconstr Surg 1986;78(2):268.
5. Lowery JC, Bartley GB. Complications of blepharoplasty. Survey of Ophthalmology 1994;38:327-350.
6. Callahan M, Beard C, eds. Beard's ptosis, 4th ed. Birmingham, AL: Aesculapius Publishing, 1990.
7. Chen WPD. Comparative anatomy of the eyelids. In: Chen WPD, ed. Asian blepharoplasty: a surgical atlas. Boston: Butterworth-Heinemann, 1995:1-19.
8. Daniel RK, Tirkanits B. Endoscopic forehead lift: aesthetics and analysis. Clin Plast Surg 1990;22(4):605-618.
9. Larrabee WF Jr, Makielski KH. Facial contour analysis. In: Larrabee WF Jr, Makielski KH, eds. Surgical anatomy of the face. New York: Raven Press, 1993:3-12.
10. Lemke BN, Lucarelli MJ. Anatomy of the ocular adnexa, orbit and related facial structures. In: Nesi FA, Lisman RD, Levine MR, eds. Smith's ophthalmic plastic and reconstructive surgery, 2nd ed. St. Louis: Mosby, 1997:3-78.
11. Migliori ME, Gladstone GJ. Determination of the normal range of exophthalmometric values for black and white adults. Am J Ophthalmol 1984;98(4):438-442.
12. Putterman AM. Upper eyelid blepharoplasty. In: Hornblass AH, ed. Oculoplastic, orbital and reconstructive surgery, Vol 1. Baltimore: Williams & Wilkins, 1988: 474-499.
13. Goldberg RA, Charonis GC, Baylis HI, Brazzo BG. Upper and lower eyelid blepharoplasty. In: Nesi FA, Lisman RD, Levine MR, eds. Smith's ophthalmic plastic and reconstructive surgery, 2nd ed. St. Louis: Mosby, 1997: 416-428.
14. Frankel AS, Kamer FM. The effect of blepharoplasty on eyebrow position. Arch Otolaryngol Head Neck Surg 1997;123:393-396.
15. Baker SS, Muenzler WS, Small RG, Leonard JE. Carbon dioxide laser blepharoplasty. Ophthalmology 1984;91: 238-243.
16. Baker SS. Carbon dioxide laser upper lid blepharoplasty. Am J Cosmetic Surg 1992;9:141-145.
17. Biesman BS. Precautions in the use of the laser for blepharoplasty. Plast Reconstr Surg 1997;99(1):275-277.
18. Morrow DM, Morrow LB. CO_2 laser blepharoplasty: a comparison with cold steel surgery. J Dermatol Surg Oncol 1992:18:307-313.
19. Biesman BS, et al. Pulsed versus continuous wave incisions with the UltraPulse carbon dioxide laser: a histopathologic study. Presented at the ASOPRS fall meeting, Chicago, 1996.
20. Ries WR, Clymer MA, Reinisch L. Laser safety features of eye shields. Laser Safety Surg Med 1996;18:309-315.
21. David LM, Baker SS. David-Baker Eyelid Retractor. Am J Cosmetic Surg 1992;9:147-148.
22. Ullmann Y, Levi Y, Ben-Izhak O, et al. The surgical anatomy of the fat in the upper eyelid medial compartment. Plast Reconstr Surg 1997;99(3):658-661.
23. Goldberg RA. The carbon dioxide laser in oculoplastic surgery and sliced bread. Arch Ophthalmol 1996; 114(9):1131-1133.
24. Weinstein C. UltraPulse carbon dioxide laser removal of periocular wrinkles in association with laser blepharoplasty. J Clin Laser Med Surg 1994;12(4):205.
25. Glassberg E, Babapour R, Lask G. Current trends in laser blepharoplasty: results of a survey. Dermatol Surg 1995; 21:1060-1063.
26. Shorr N. Lower lid transconjunctival blepharoplasty using the CO_2 laser. Aesthetic Surg Quarterly, 1996; Summer:101.

Chapter Ten

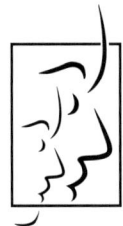

Lower Eyelid Blepharoplasty and Periorbital Rejuvenation

Daniel E. Buerger and Brian S. Biesman

Rejuvenation of the lower eyelid requires reversing changes typically associated with an "aged" or "tired" appearance. These changes may include herniation of orbital fat, laxity of the canthal tendons with subsequent change in lid position, actinic damage of the skin with thinning, loss of elasticity, fine wrinkling and pigmentary change of the skin, dark circles in the infraorbital region, and hypertrophy of the pretarsal portion of the orbicularis oculi muscle. Many of these changes are associated with the aging process, while others may represent familial traits. Lasers play a significant role in lower eyelid and periorbital rejuvenation.

Procedures commonly used to achieve periorbital rejuvenation include upper eyelid blepharoplasty, elevation of the eyebrows, removal of anterior orbital fat from the lower eyelid using a transcutaneous or transconjunctival approach, recontouring of inferior orbital fat, elevation of the suborbicularis oculi fat (SOOF), resurfacing of the skin using chemical agents, CO_2 or Er:YAG lasers and, occasionally, treatment of dermal hyperpigmentation with other lasers. Upper eyelid blepharoplasty, treatment of eyelid malposition, and forehead and eyebrow rejuvenation are discussed in other chapters and will not be considered here further.

ANATOMIC RELATIONSHIPS

Understanding the anatomic relationships of the structures in the lower eyelid and anterior orbit is of paramount im-

portance when performing lower lid blepharoplasty to achieve the desired results without unwanted complications. The anatomy of the lower lid and orbit was discussed in Chapter 2, but because of the importance of this topic, a few salient points will be reviewed. It is helpful to conceptualize the eyelids as structures composed of three layers, or lamellae. The anterior lamella is composed of skin and orbicularis oculi muscle. Immediately posterior to this layer is the orbital septum, the middle lamella of the eyelid. Division of this structure can result in internal eyelid scarring with subsequent retraction or ectropion (1). The posterior lamella of the eyelid consists of the tarsus, conjunctiva, and lower eyelid retractors; the lower lid tarsus is 4 mm in height. The orbital septum fuses with the lower lid retractors approximately 4 mm below the inferior tarsal border. Behind the orbital septum, located within the anterior orbit, is the orbital fat. Clinically, the orbital fat is separated into three pockets: medial, central, and lateral (2, 3), but anatomically, there are no divisions (4, 5). The lateral fat pad is further divided into two separate pockets, one slightly posterior and lateral to the other (6). The medial and central fat pads are separated by the inferior oblique muscle, which may be identified, and even damaged, when fat is excised in this area. The central and lateral fat pads are separated by a fascial plane, the arcuate expanse of the inferior oblique muscle. This structure may be divided with impunity during surgery, better exposing the lateral fat.

The orbicularis oculi, along with the platysma, frontalis muscles, and other muscles of facial expression, is

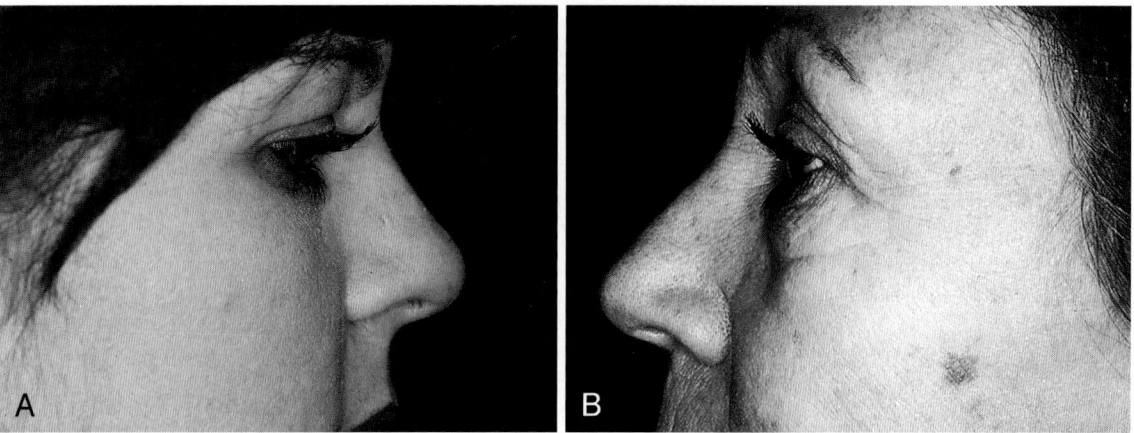

Figure 10.1. A. Young patient with single, convex curve of the lower lid and upper cheek.
B. Aging changes become apparent as a double convex curve: the orbital fat
herniates forward and the upper cheek fat descends.

invested in the inner layer of the superior cervicofacial fascia known as the superficial musculoaponeurotic system, or SMAS (7, 8). This fascial layer plays an important role in surgical rejuvenation of the face. Superficial to the SMAS in the infraorbital area is an area of thickened subcutaneous fat extending from the malar region to the nasolabial crease, and a line marking the constant dermal insertion between the skin and the SMAS where the levator labii muscles become very superficial. This area of thickening is known as the malar fat pad and in youth is adherent to the overlying skin and underlying SMAS. With aging, it remains closely adherent to the overlying skin while the deeper attachments to the SMAS are lost, allowing it to descend in a plane anterior to the SMAS. Ultimately, the descended malar fat pad accentuates the nasolabial fold, a well recognized sign of aging. There are no vital structures within the SMAS itself as the muscles of facial expression and their accompanying neurovascular supply are found deep to this layer.

Successful periorbital rejuvenation requires an appreciation for midfacial contour, and the changes which occur in this region with aging. The youthful appearance on profile is a single convex curve including the lower lid and upper cheek (Figure 10.1A). Because of degeneration of elastic fibers in both the dermis and the SMAS with age and gravitational effect, the skin and subcutaneous fascia of the forehead, lower face, and neck are believed to slide down over the deeper fascia, which contains the facial muscles (9). The malar fat pad is one of two areas on the face where gravity exerts an effect on the skin, but not the fat. As the superficial structures descend, the inferior orbital rim is exposed and a "bulge" is created on the infraorbital portion of the cheek. When viewed adjacent to the

fullness produced by herniated orbital fat just above the inferior orbital rim, the aging face has a double convex appearance (1) (Figure 10.1B). Patients often attribute the signs of midfacial aging solely to the herniated orbital fat and may thus present requesting blepharoplasty surgery. While removal, redistribution, or recontouring of orbital fat and lower eyelid skin play a role in the management of midfacial aging, these maneuvers alone do not address all of the age-related changes that occur midface.

PREOPERATIVE ASSESSMENT

As discussed in earlier chapters, the preoperative consultation should be used to establish open communication and good rapport with patients in order to ensure that their understanding and expectations are appropriate. Patients seeking aesthetic surgery of the lower lids will often complain of "baggy" eyelids, dark circles under their eyes, a tired appearance, or wrinkles. At times, the presenting complaint is even more vague, such as wanting to look younger or wanting "an eye job." One can use a mirror, digital imaging system, or standard photograph to help patients call attention to areas of concern in order to understand the source of dissatisfaction. Aging changes of the periorbital region and midface may often be better assessed when comparison to old photographs is made.

Preoperative Evaluation

A careful ophthalmic examination is performed as outlined in Chapter 11. The lower eyelid position is noted with the eye in primary gaze to rule out inferior scleral show, which may be indicative of eyelid laxity, proptosis, eyelid retraction, or previous surgery. The skin of the entire face should be examined. Cutaneous changes including fine wrinkles, thinning skin, scars, pigmentary changes and excess skin, are noted. The relative amount of excess skin in the lower lid is determined as the patient gazes upward with the mouth open, stretching the lower lid skin maximally. Any excess skin measured in this position may be sacrificed without fear of producing lid retraction or cicatricial ectropion (11).

Dark circles under the eyes may be produced by shadows cast by herniated tissues, by pigment in the epidermis or the dermis, or a combination of these factors. Removal of herniated fat will reduce the shadowing effect, but will not improve pigmentary changes within the skin. Laser skin resurfacing will improve the appearance of eyelids containing epidermal pigment, but will generally not have an effect on dermal pigment. Dermal pigment has been treated by excision of the involved skin and, with varying degrees of success, using the Q-switched ruby laser (12).

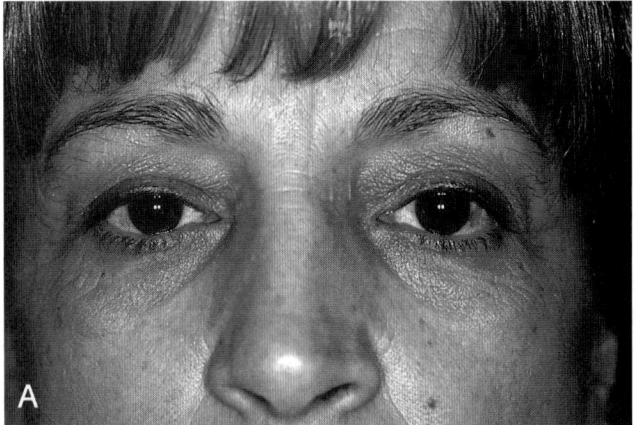
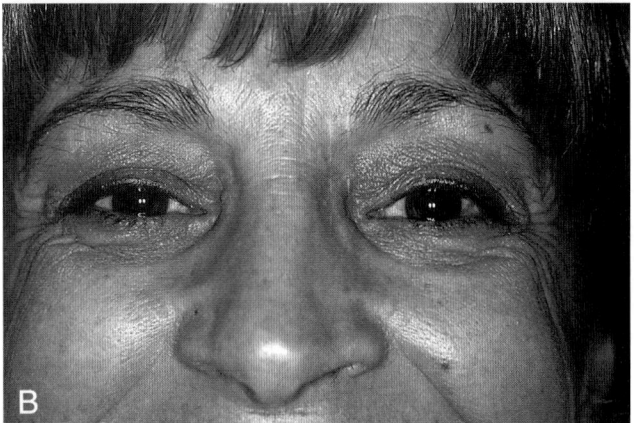

Figure 10.3. This patient presented for lower lid blepharoplasty. **A.** The excess tissue of the lower lid is caused by hypertrophy of the orbicularis muscle and not herniated fat. **B.** Notice how this is accentuated when the patient smiles.

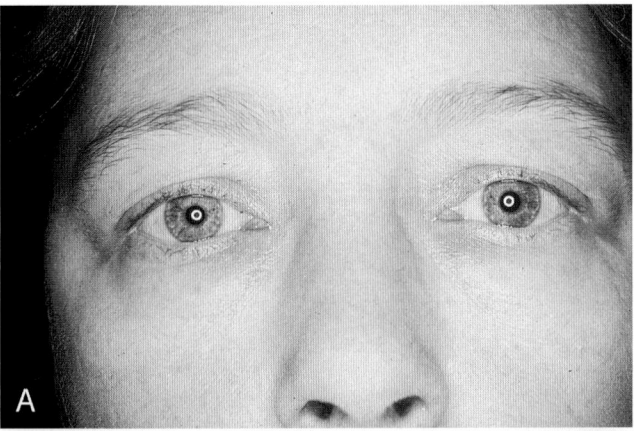
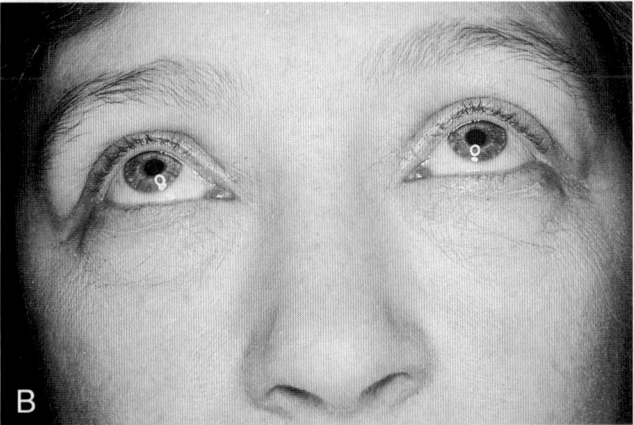

Figure 10.2. Evaluation of the lower eyelid fat. **A.** The patient looking straight ahead, and **B.** in upgaze. Note how the fat becomes more prominent with upgaze.

It can be difficult to differentiate between dermal and epidermal pigment, although in some situations the Wood's lamp may be of benefit in making this distinction (13).

Herniated inferior orbital fat is best assessed with the eyes in upgaze (Figure 10.2). To differentiate fat from edema, retropulsion of the globe is performed. This maneuver will increase the fat herniation, but not change the appearance of the edema (11). Herniated fat is a static condition in the lower portion of the eyelid, which must be differentiated from hypertrophy of the orbicularis oculi muscle, a dynamic condition that appears as an exaggerated bulge in the pretarsal and superior preseptal area when the patient smiles (11) (Figure 10.3). Lower eyelid laxity is assessed by the pinch or snap tests described in Chapter 11. Failure to recognize lower lid laxity increases the risk of postoperative eyelid malposition (14, 15).

The upper cheek below the orbital rim is inspected for the presence of malar festoons or "bags," which result from attenuation and degeneration of the orbicularis of the lower lid, weakening of the orbitomalar ligament (16), sagging of the skin, and anterior bulging of the suborbicularis oculi fat (SOOF) (17). True festoons must be differentiated from an extension of orbital fat into the recess of Eisler, a potential space between the orbital septum and anterior face of the maxilla, because of a low insertion of the orbital septum below the orbital rim (18). When gentle pressure is applied to the globe, the extraorbital extension of orbital fat will increase in size while festoons will remain unchanged. Treatment of festoons usually requires a combination of approaches and can not be accomplished solely with blepharoplasty. Various modifications of external blepharoplasty have been recommended (19, 20, 21) and will not be discussed here. Baker has successfully treated festoons with an aggressive laser resurfacing technique. He treats the inferior preseptal skin with no more than 2 passes with the UltraPulse (Coherent Med-

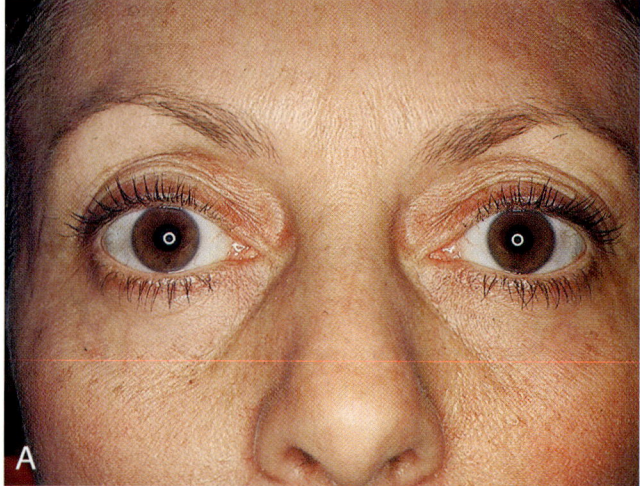

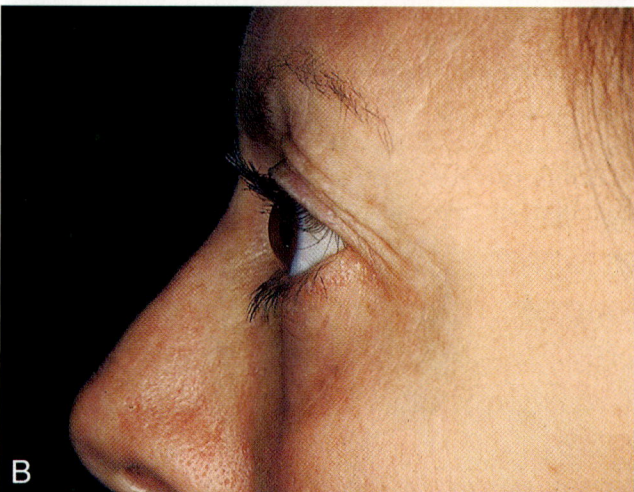

Figure 10.5. A, B. This patient requested lower lid blepharoplasty. She has prominent globes produced by a flat malar eminence. Lower blepharoplasty alone would accentuate her eyes.

ical, Palo Alto, CA) laser [energy = 300 mJ/pulse, power = 60 W, CPG pattern 4, size 7, density 5 (30% overlap of spots)] or 1 pass with the Sharplan SilkTouch (Sharplan Lasers, Allendale, NJ) laser (6 mm spot, power = 16 W). Baker then treats the portion of the festoon overlying the orbital margin and anterior face of the maxilla until no further shrinkage of tissue is noted. Six-to-eight passes are usually required with the UltraPulse laser (energy = 300 mJ/pulse, power = 60 W, CPG pattern 3 size 5, density 5) and 3-5 passes required with the SilkTouch laser (6 mm spot, power = 18 W). Because of the extensive thermal damage produced, the wounds heal somewhat slowly but the clinical results can be excellent (22) (Figure 10.4).

The projection of the malar eminence is assessed relative to the globe by viewing the patient's profile sitting upright and gazing straight ahead. Patients with shallow

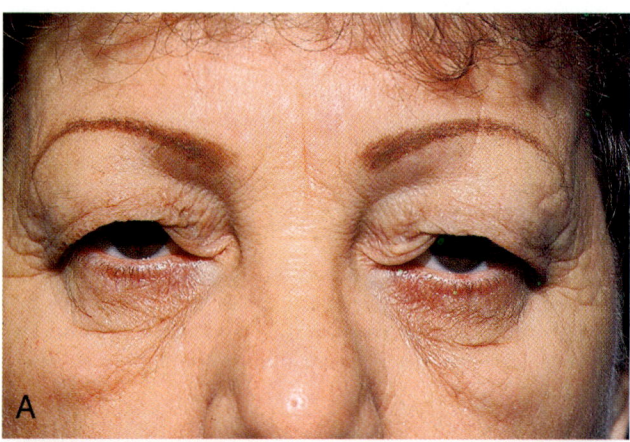

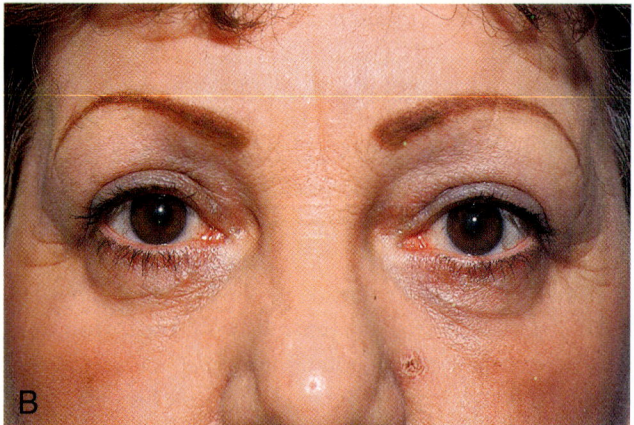

Figure 10.4. A. Preoperative appearance of a patient with mild to moderate malar festoons. Note also the significant dermatochalasis of the upper eyelids. **B.** The same patient 2 months postoperatively after upper lid blepharoplasty, full face Er:YAG laser treatment, and CO_2 laser treatment to the malar region. Note the reduction of the malar fullness (Courtesy of SS Baker).

orbits, large globes, or flattened cheeks often have prominent eyes, which will appear protuberant if orbital fat or lower eyelid skin is removed. These patients should undergo malar augmentation in addition to (or in lieu of) blepharoplasty surgery (Figure 10.5).

The traditional approach to the treatment of herniated orbital fat is resection and/or recontouring of fat via transconjunctival or transcutaneous approach. An alternative procedure has been proposed by Hamra and others that releases the arcus marginalis with redistribution of fat (10, 23). This redistribution of fat beyond the infraorbital rim under the orbicularis muscle achieves a reduction in the double convex appearance of the aging midface without producing a hollowed, "operated" appearance to the lower eyelids. While this procedure is used successfully by some, it has not replaced the standard approach to blepharoplasty surgery and will not be discussed here.

TRANSCONJUNCTIVAL LOWER EYELID BLEPHAROPLASTY

The clinical applications for transconjunctival removal of herniated fat continue to expand (24, 25). Transconjunctival lower eyelid blepharoplasty is a versatile procedure that may be performed in conjunction with chemical peels, laser skin resurfacing, lid tightening procedures, and/or resection of excess skin. When used along with laser skin resurfacing, the transconjunctival approach can produce a more natural-appearing, aesthetically acceptable result than can generally be produced transcutaneously, with a reduced risk of postoperative lower lid retraction (14).

Lower eyelid transconjunctival blepharoplasty is easily performed using the CO_2 laser as an incisional device. In the opinion of many experienced eyelid surgeons, the laser offers significant advantages over cold steel and electrocautery. The bloodless field provides easier identification of eyelid and orbital structures, and also less postoperative ecchymosis and edema. As a result, operative times are reduced, and the postoperative recovery period is shortened (26–29).

Laser-assisted transconjunctival blepharoplasty may be performed in an office or an operating room setting. While a combination of topical and local anesthetics alone provides sufficient anesthesia for some patients, most prefer systemic anxiolytic or sedative agents. Appropriate monitoring is required if intravenous sedation is administered. More details on the anesthetic requirement for this procedure may be found in Chapter 4.

A topical anesthetic (proparacaine 0.5% or tetracaine 0.5%) should be instilled into the inferior conjunctival fornix. If intravenous sedation is not available, then the palpebral conjunctiva and inferior fornix can be anesthetized first with 4% lidocaine topically applied with a soaked cotton-tipped applicator for 1–2 minutes prior to injection. Otherwise, deep intravenous sedation is obtained prior to local injection. The commonly preferred local anesthetic agent is 2% lidocaine with 1:100,000 epinephrine, delivered either alone or as a 1:1 mixture with 0.25–0.75% bupivacaine. The addition of bupivacaine not only provides longer sensory anesthesia, but also longer paralysis of the orbicularis oculi muscle, impairing the eyes' ability to close completely for several hours after surgery. Hyaluronidase may be added if desired. The injection is given transconjunctivally with a 27- or 30-gauge needle directed at, or just posterior, to the orbital rim. One milliliter of anesthetic is injected into each of the three fat pockets. Pupillary dilation may occur if the nerve to the inferior oblique muscle and its accompanying parasympathetic fibers are anesthetized.

Surgical Technique

The patient is prepared and draped in the standard fashion, while appropriate laser safety precautions are observed. The goal of the initial portion of the procedure is to expose the orbital fat. This may be accomplished easily if the lower eyelid is retracted anteriorly and inferiorly by the assistant while the surgeon gently places the end of the laser-safe bone plate (Jaeger plate) into the inferior fornix with his/her non-dominant hand. The bone plate is used to both protect the eye and to gently move the globe posteriorly, allowing the orbital fat to herniate into the inferior fornix. The Jaeger plate must not be allowed to rest against the inferior orbital rim as this will prevent the fat from moving forward into the surgical field. The inferior fornix is now exposed with the orbital fat clearly visible as a smooth mound behind the conjunctiva and lower eyelid retractors.

The laser is set at 6–8 W continuous wave (CW) or 10 mJ/pulse, 10 W power in pulsed mode and the 0.2 mm focused handpiece is used to make an incision directly into the orbital fat, posterior to the orbital septum. The incision is placed midway between the inferior tarsal border and the base of the inferior fornix, and extends from the base of the caruncle to the lateral canthus (Figure 10.6). If the incision is made less than 4 mm below the lacrimal punctum and canaliculus, these structures may

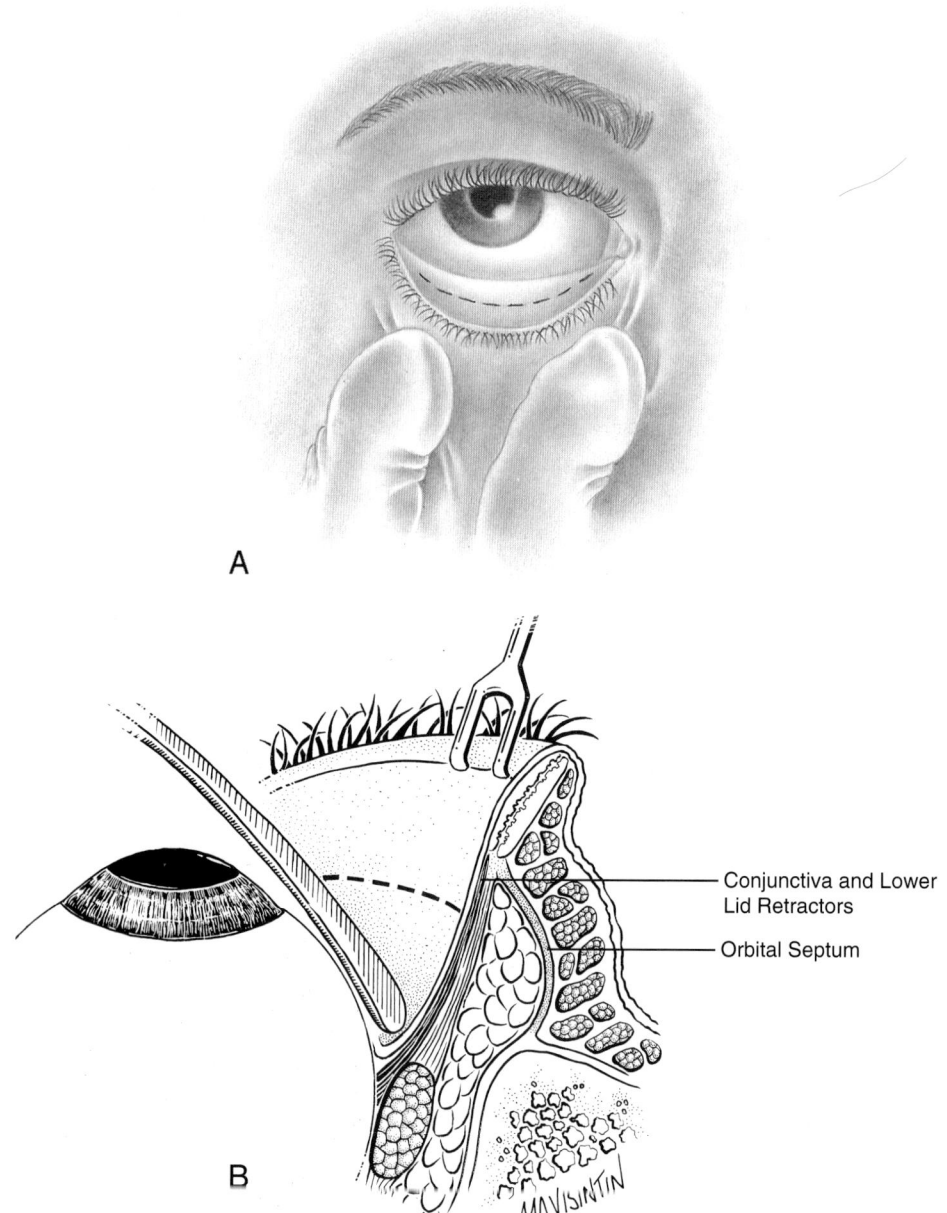

Figure 10.6. Exposure of the inferior fornix with traction inferiorly on the right lower lid. **A.** The dotted line shows the area where the incision will be performed. **B.** The sagittal view of the inferior fornix as the surgery is set to begin. The bone plate is placed into the inferior fornix to protect the globe and produce anterior herniation of the orbital fat.

be damaged. The laser should be held in a focused position when making the incision and directed anteriorly and inferiorly, aiming toward the inferior orbital rim. Once two-to-three passes have been completed in the same incision, the orbital fat should present itself into the wound (Figure 10.7).

An alternative approach places an incision 2–3 mm below the inferior tarsal border (where the lower lid retractors and septum are fused) dissects anteriorly, and continues inferiorly in the plane between orbital septum and orbicularis oculi muscle (30). This approach presents the orbital fat in an orientation that may be more familiar to the surgeon accustomed to the transcutaneous approach, but requires division of the septum and thus forfeits one major advantage of the transconjunctival approach. Theoretically, a higher incidence of lower eyelid retraction should result following this approach, but this has not been reported.

The second step of transconjunctival blepharoplasty is to resect the herniating orbital fat. This portion of the procedure is begun by placing a laser-safe vein (Desmarres) retractor in the wound with the blade anterior to the orbital rim. The skin below the retractor must not be allowed to roll posteriorly (toward the globe) as it may present into the surgical field, where it is at risk for inadvertent damage. The dissection is facilitated if the assistant holds the retractor in one hand and uses the other to apply gentle posterior pressure on the Jaeger plate. The central fat pocket, with its surrounding fascial investments, is then easily visible in the midportion of the wound (Figure 10.8). The fibrovascular tissue surrounding the fat may be carefully stripped away from the fat pad itself using blunt dissection with the laser handpiece or a cotton-tipped applicator. Large vessels are closed by defocusing the laser or, if necessary, with a bipolar cautery. The fat should be gently teased into the wound to avoid tearing vessels in the posterior orbit (24, 31). When the fat prolapsing anterior to the orbital rim has been isolated, it is inspected on all sides for the presence of vessels that may not be closed by the laser. It is transected with the CO_2 laser taking care *never* to direct the beam posteriorly as this may result in injury to the globe or extraocular muscles (32). Defocusing the laser to sculpt or shrink the fat should be avoided as this directs additional laser energy into the orbit, producing increased thermal damage. Inadvertent laser burns of the lower eyelid skin can be avoided: the fat pad is held against the retractor and gently moved from side to side while the laser is directed against the central portion of the retractor and held in a stationary position. Every effort should be made to remove each fat pad with a single cut rather than in a piecemeal fashion to reduce the total amount of laser energy applied to the orbit. Removing fat which does not easily prolapse anterior to the orbital rim may produce a "hollow" appearance to the lower lid (24). Because surgery is performed with the patient in a supine position, the lid often has a slightly concave appearance at the conclusion of the procedure. When the patient is returned to an upright position, the concavity disappears.

Attention is then turned to the white-colored medial fat pocket, which occupies the nasal aspect of the wound (Figure 10.9). The medial fat pocket is isolated and

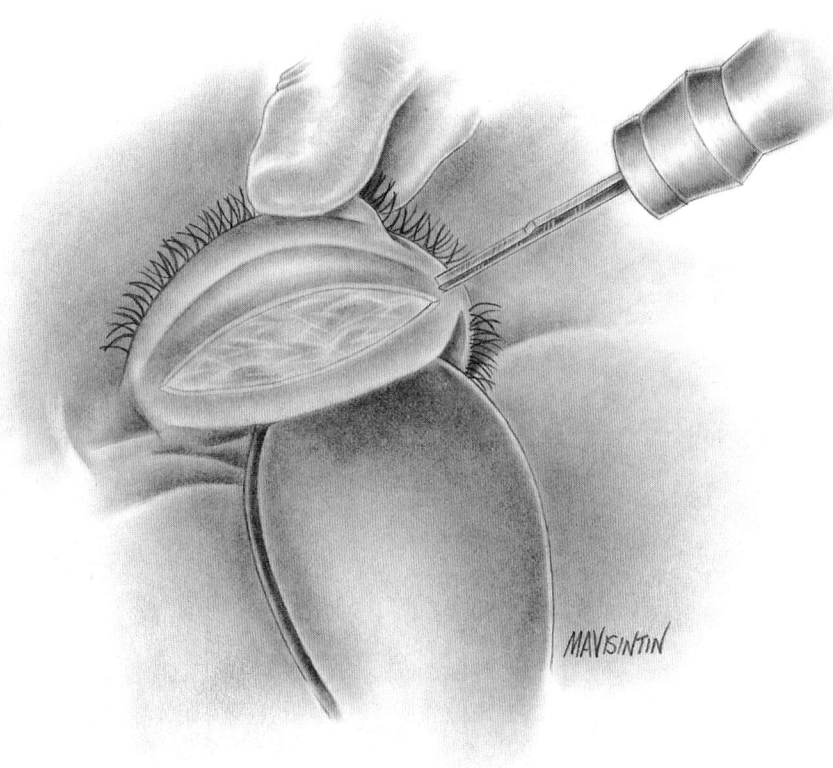

Figure 10.7. The incision extends from the lateral aspect of the caruncle to the lateral canthus.
As the lower lid retractors are incised, the fat bulges into the wound.

Figure 10.8. The central fat pad is isolated from the surrounding fascial attachments and held against the laser-safe Desmarres retractor. The laser is used to excise the fat pad at the level of the inferior orbital rim.

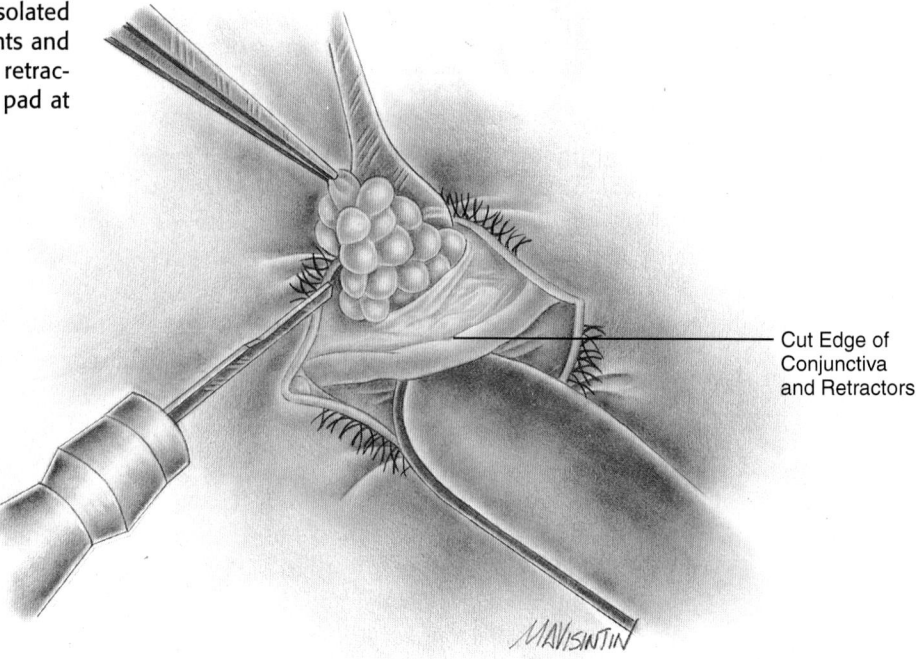

Cut Edge of
Conjunctiva
and Retractors

Figure 10.9. The location of the three fat pads in the lower lid as seen during transconjunctival blepharoplasty. Note the location of the inferior oblique muscle between the medial and central fat pads of the right lower lid.

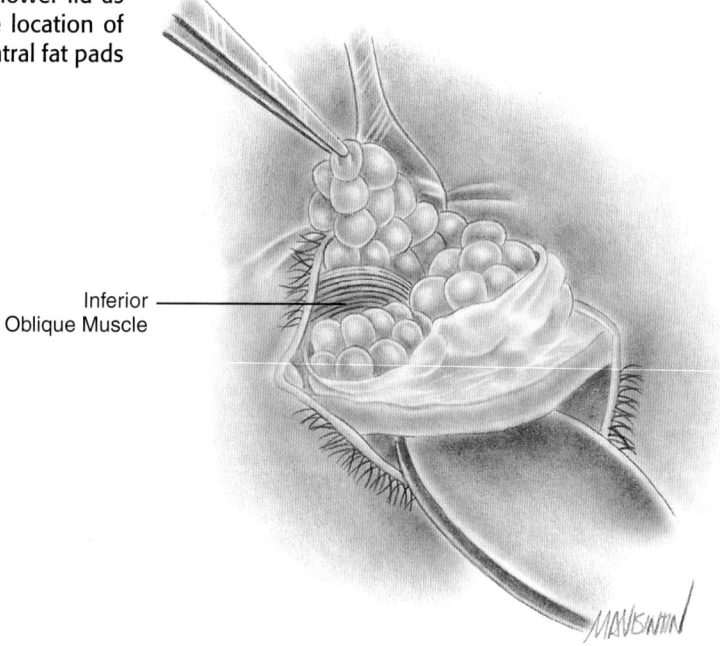

Inferior
Oblique Muscle

inspected for the presence of large vessels that are more likely be found in this fat pad than the others. The inferior oblique muscle may be apparent during this dissection and should be avoided. If the muscle does not present itself, it should not be aggressively sought out. In many patients the medial fat is also divided into two compartments, and the herniating portion of each is resected (33).

The temporal portion of the eyelid is then inspected and the lateral fat pocket is identified. As discussed earlier, this pad is usually divided into two compartments: one next to the central fat pad and the second located more posterior and lateral to the first. The more posterior portion of this fat pad is often overlooked by the inexperienced blepharoplasty surgeon (6). The arcuate expanse of the inferior oblique may be divided to aid in exposure of the lateral fat. The anterior portion of the lateral fat is then exposed and excised, allowing easier access to the posterior portion of the fat pad. The cut edge of the lower eyelid retractors is grasped with a toothed forceps and pulled superiorly and slightly posteriorly, delivering the fat pad into the surgical field. The posterior portion of the lateral fat pad is usually tightly adherent to the lower eyelid retractors and enveloped in an opaque, fibrous capsule that may initially obscure it from view. The fat pad is delivered into the wound as this capsule is divided by directing the laser beam in a plane parallel and just anterior to the lower eyelid retractors (Figure 10.10). Once the posterior portion of the lateral fat pad has been removed, an instrument should pass easily to the inferior lateral orbital rim without encountering fat.

The goal of the third and final step of the procedure is to reposition the lower eyelid and inspect the eyelids for symmetry. Once the fat resection is complete, the Jaeger plate is removed. The Desmarres retractor is used to pull the lower lid anteriorly and superiorly to ensure that the wound edges do not overlap, leading to the development of a cicatricial entropion. With the eyes closed, gentle pressure is applied to both globes, prolapsing the remaining orbital fat anteriorly. Each lower lid is examined for evidence of residual herniating fat and is then compared to its fellow lid to ensure symmetry. Finally, the wounds are carefully reassessed to ensure complete hemostasis. Suturing the wound is not required, but the edges must not overlap or cicatricial entropion may result.

At the end of the procedure, two drops of tobramycin-prednisolone acetate 1% solution are instilled in each eye, and ice compresses or gauze soaked in iced saline are applied to the eyes. The patient is monitored in the recovery area to ensure that there is no evidence of bleeding or diplopia. Patients who complain of nausea should receive metaclopramide, ondansetron (Zofran), or a similar agent to prevent retching and its associated valsalva effect. Before discharge, signs and symptoms of orbital hemorrhage are reviewed with the patient and their family, and the surgeon's telephone and pager number are provided for use in case of an emergency. Patients who live a significant distance from the surgeon's office are encouraged to stay in a local hotel for 24 hours.

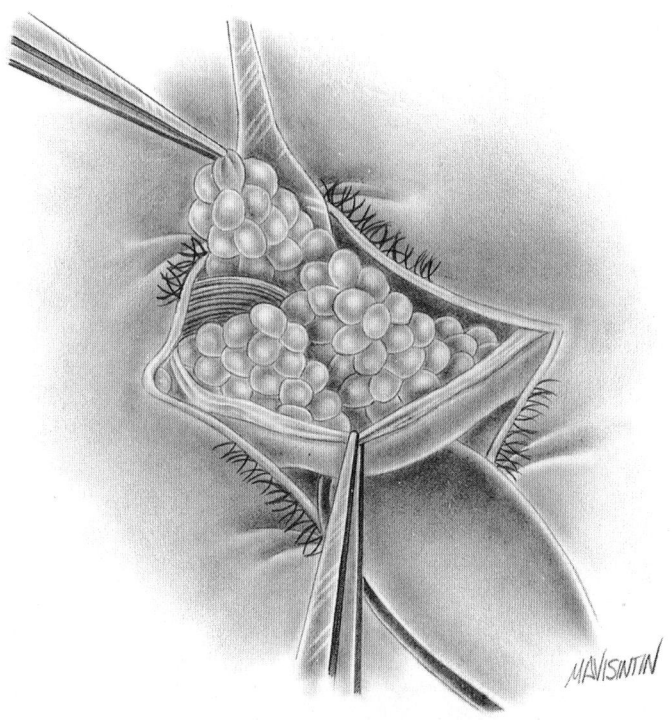

Figure 10.10. The second part of the lateral fat pocket is located posterior to the other portion and is located just anterior to the lower lid retractors. The laser is aimed parallel to the retractors to open the fascia surrounding the pocket.

Postoperative Instructions

Patients are instructed to apply ice compresses as often as possible for the first 48 hours after surgery. Crushed ice in a bag, a reusable "ice mask" made specifically for the eyes, or a bag of frozen peas or corn wrapped in a clean cloth may be used. To reduce postoperative swelling further, a short course of oral steroids may be administered, although it is usually not necessary. Patients are encouraged to keep their head elevated at all times for the first week, including sleeping on extra pillows. The steroid-antibiotic drops are continued 4 times a day for 1 week. Ointment preparations are avoided after the transconjunctival approach because of the risk of ointment cysts or granulomas associated with their use (34, 35). Contact lens use may be resumed 1–2 weeks after surgery. Patients are instructed to avoid heavy bending, lifting, and exercise for the first week after surgery. Low-level exercise may be resumed after 1 week and more vigorous activities after 2 weeks. Flying should be avoided for 1 week. If laser resurfacing was performed in conjunction with a

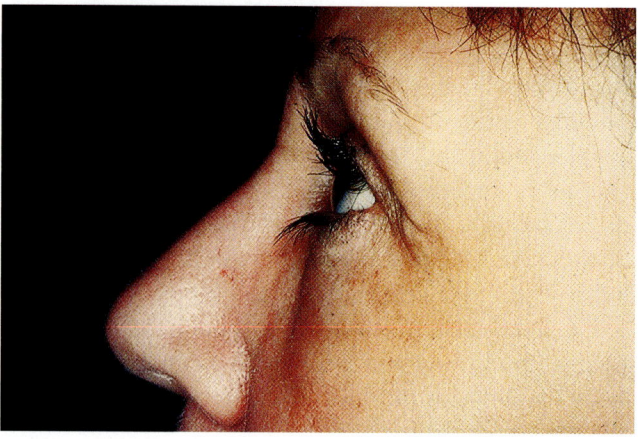

Figure 10.12. Six months postoperative after upper and lower lid blepharoplasties and full face CO_2 skin resurfacing. Preoperative appearance is Figure 10.1B.

lower lid blepharoplasty, these wounds are managed in the standard way.

Results

Transconjunctival laser-assisted blepharoplasty is extremely well accepted by patients (Figure 10.11). A cutaneous incision is avoided, and the risk of eyelid retraction, cicatricial ectropion, or "scalloping" of the lateral lid is essentially eliminated if the orbital septum is preserved. As seen after liposuction, the skin usually contracts and conforms to the contour of the underlying tissues following transconjunctival blepharoplasty. Patients with extensive actinic damage or loss of elasticity of the skin in the periorbital region may benefit from concomitant laser skin resurfacing (Figure 10.12).

TRANSCUTANEOUS LOWER EYELID BLEPHAROPLASTY

The initial description of CO_2 laser-assisted lower eyelid blepharoplasty used the transcutaneous approach (36). As current trends in blepharoplasty surgery favor the transconjunctival approach, often in combination with chemical peels or laser skin resurfacing, the transcutaneous approach is less often used. The primary disadvantage of this approach is the need to divide the skin and the orbital septum, increasing the risk of scarring and lower eyelid retraction or "scalloping," common stigmata of blepharoplasty surgery. Proponents of the external ap-

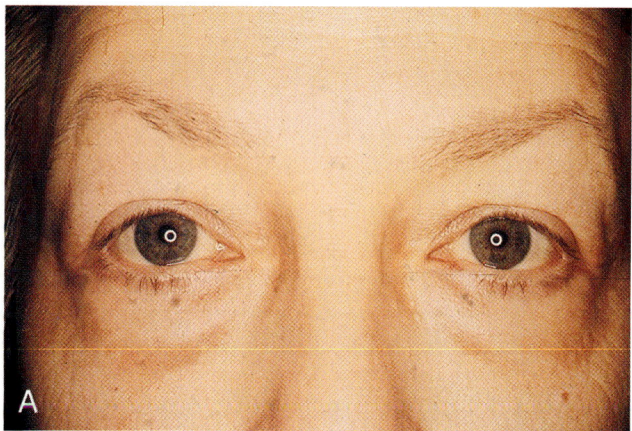

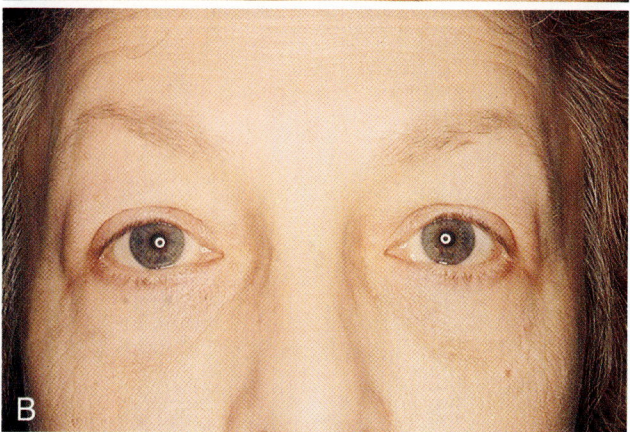

Figure 10.11. A. Preoperative, and **B.** 1 month postoperative after a transconjunctival lower lid blepharoplasty.

proach cite the benefit of excess skin removal (37), but in fact, the 'excess' skin of the lower lid usually conforms to the contour of the underlying orbital tissues. Fine wrinkling, dyschromia, or other signs of actinic damage and aging will not be improved with the removal of excess skin, and chemical peeling or laser resurfacing are still required. However, these techniques may not be safely performed simultaneously with transcutaneous blepharoplasty because the transcutaneous approach affects the cutaneous vascular supply. Transcutaneous lower blepharoplasty is currently recommended for patients with severe lower eyelid dermatochalasis or clinically significant hypertrophic orbicularis oculi muscle. Even in these cases, fat removal may be accomplished via a transconjunctival approach followed by transcutaneous excision of excess skin and muscle, leaving the orbital septum intact (38, 39).

The lower lid is anesthetized as described earlier with the addition of local anesthesia for the anterior lamella. The anterior lamella may be anesthetized via direct subcutaneous infiltration, or an infraorbital nerve block may be performed through the conjunctiva, skin, or gingival buccal mucosa (See Chapter 4). If a traction suture is to be placed through the lower eyelid margin, the margin itself should also be infiltrated.

Surgical Technique

Prior to injecting the anesthetic agent, an incision site is marked 2–3 mm inferior to the lash line, beginning below and just lateral to the lacrimal punctum. The patient is prepared and draped in standard laser-safe manner, and metal eye protection is placed. A 4-0 silk traction suture is placed through the central lower lid margin and fixed to the drape superiorly while the assistant places digital traction inferiorly on the lower eyelid. The CO_2 laser is set on continuous wave mode at 6 W, or ultrapulse mode at 10 W and 10 mJ/pulse, and the 0.2-millimeter focused handpiece is used to make an incision through skin and orbicularis muscle. The anterior inferior tarsal border is visible in the wound. A skin-orbicularis muscle flap is then elevated to the level of the inferior orbital rim, using the laser to separate the muscle from the underlying orbital septum, and taking care not to buttonhole the skin. The septum is opened along the entire length of the incision, similar to an upper lid blepharoplasty (see Chapter 9), to expose the underlying orbital fat.

The laser-safe Desmarres retractor is used to retract and protect the skin-muscle flap inferiorly as the fat pads

are identified, isolated from surrounding fascial attachments, and resected with the CO_2 laser. Again, only that fat which herniates anterior to the orbital rim is resected. If vessels larger than 1.0 mm in diameter are encountered, they should be closed with electrocautery prior to division with the laser. Hemostasis must be meticulously maintained: then the redundant skin and orbicularis muscle are excised. The wound is closed with a running 6-0 or 7-0 nylon suture, which may be removed 6–7 days after surgery.

Postoperative Care

The postoperative care and instructions following transcutaneous lower lid blepharoplasty differ from the regimen described above in two ways. First, an ophthalmic antibiotic ointment such as erythromycin is applied to the wound 3 times a day and into the inferior conjunctival fornix at bedtime. Second, contact lens wear may be resumed as early as a few days after surgery, although it is still preferable to wait until after the first postoperative week.

COMPLICATIONS

Complications of laser blepharoplasty may be divided into complications of incisional blepharoplasty and complications of laser incisional surgery. The most common complication of lower lid blepharoplasty, regardless of technique used, is inadequate excision of fat and the need for additional surgery (14, 15, 38, 40). Other complications include lower lid retraction, ectropion, injury to the inferior oblique muscle or other extraocular muscle resulting in diplopia, hemorrhage, infection, damage to the canaliculi, chemosis, and incisional irregularities from hypertrophic scarring and granuloma formation (15, 38, 40–43). Blindness from hemorrhage is the most feared complication, and with particular emphasis on meticulous hemostasis, this complication is extremely rare (44). A more comprehensive discussion of complications is found in Chapter 14. Complications will be reduced with particular attention to the anatomy of the lower lid and surrounding structures and proper laser use.

PERIORBITAL LASER SKIN REJUVENATION

Laser skin resurfacing plays an important role in periorbital rejuvenation, either alone or as an adjunct to blepharoplasty. Blepharoplasty, whether performed via an internal or external approach, will not address fine periorbital wrinkles or actinic damage. These undesirable changes respond well to skin resurfacing using either the CO_2 or Er:YAG lasers. These lasers produce similar effects, but differ somewhat in their indications for use (45–50). Pass for pass, the CO_2 laser ablates more tissue than the Er:YAG by a factor of approximately 4 (for the first and second passes; this number probably decreases as more passes are made), and is thus a more efficient tool. It also produces a greater amount of residual thermal damage in the dermis than the Er:YAG laser, a fact believed to be responsible for the visible tissue "shrinkage" and tightening that is noted during treatment (51, 52). It is not clear whether this phenomenon is temporary or permanent. Thermal injury of the dermis is responsible for the prolonged period of postoperative erythema associated with CO_2 laser treatments, but may also be responsible for the increased dermal collagen production and often dramatic clinical results that are achieved (53, 54, 55). In contrast, the Er:YAG laser produces very little thermal damage with each pass, and the duration of postoperative erythema is reduced (52). Also reduced are the beneficial effects associated with dermal injury. The Er:YAG laser is thus best suited for use in young patients with mild actinic damage and only very superficial wrinkles. With greater numbers of passes (10–12), a larger zone of thermal damage and therefor a more significant clinical effect may be produced, but the recovery time will also be prolonged. Such treatments may defeat the purpose of using a laser that produces less thermal damage and a shortened recovery period.

If transcutaneous lower eyelid blepharoplasty is performed, skin resurfacing with either laser should be delayed for 3–6 months. The upper eyelid may be resurfaced either before or after blepharoplasty surgery. If the upper lid is to be resurfaced with the CO_2 laser after blepharoplasty, the area between the incision and brow is usually treated; otherwise, the entire lid may be treated. Care must be taken in the medial canthal area as excessive resurfacing in this region may produce webbing.

The periorbital area may be treated on its own or in conjunction with full face skin resurfacing. If only the periorbital area is to be resurfaced, the treatment area is outlined to ensure symmetry. The usual treatment extends superiorly to the eyebrow, medially to include the medial canthus, inferiorly respecting the orbital rim, and laterally either partially or entirely to the hairline. If prominent malar festoons are to be treated, the treatment zone is extended inferiorly to include the superior portion of the cheek.

Anesthesia is generally provided with subcutaneous infiltration in the area to be treated. Regional nerve blocks can also be performed in the periorbital area as described in Chapter 4. Topical anesthesia alone may be adequate for superficial treatments with the Er:YAG laser.

Periorbital skin resurfacing with the CO_2 laser can be performed with either the 3- millimeter collimated handpiece or a computer pattern generator handpiece such as the CPG (Coherent) or the FeatherTouch (Sharplan). Treatment is usually begun in the pretarsal area with the eyelashes retracted out of the surgical field with a cotton-tipped applicator or similar device. The eyelid skin is the thinnest in the body and must be treated delicately to reduce the chances of post-treatment scarring. When using the 3-millimeter collimated handpiece (Coherent), the energy is set to 500 mJ. Treatment with the Coherent CPG can be performed with a square pattern (#3) with 30%–40% overlap of spots at an energy setting of 300 mJ and power of 60 W. When using the FeatherTouch (Sharplan) a typical power setting is 16–18 W. These parameters are not uniform and must be determined case-by-case. Independent studies performed by Dailey et al (56) and Biesman (unpublished data) demonstrate treatment to the level of the reticular dermis when two passes are made at these settings. When the CPG handpiece is used, the direction of tissue contraction may be controlled and should be directed parallel to the lower eyelid margin to avoid producing an ectropion. Conversely, when treating the upper eyelid, the direction of skin contraction can be oriented vertically. The dessicated debris should be completely removed with saline-soaked gauze after each pass with the CO_2 laser. Some surgeons prefer decreasing the energy or power settings when working on the eyelids to avoid over-treatment. As long as sufficient energy and power are used to ablate tissue, this strategy will be successful. Generally, no more than two passes should be made on the eyelid skin with any of the available devices, except occasionally in the hands of an experienced laser surgeon.

Periorbital skin resurfacing with the Er:YAG laser is usually performed at a fluence of 4–5 J/cm^2. Most surgeons prefer a spot size no larger than 5 mm when treating the periorbital region. Scanning handpieces are also now available for the Er:YAG laser. Four-to-six passes are usually made with the Er:YAG laser in the periorbital region, although the needs of each patient must be addressed individually. Because of the explosive ablation produced by the Er:YAG laser, it is generally not necessary to debride the skin after each pass has been completed or at the conclusion of treatment. The skin tightening produced by CO_2 resurfacing is not seen when the Er:YAG is used. The endpoint of treatment with the CO_2 and Er:YAG lasers is discussed in Chapter 6.

The postoperative care of resurfaced skin as outlined in Chapter 6 also applies to blepharoplasty. Performing skin resurfacing concomitantly with blepharoplasty does not prolong the healing period or increase the risk of complications relative to resurfacing alone.

REFERENCES

1. Hawes MJ, Dortzbach RK. The microscopic anatomy of the lower eyelid retractors. Arch Ophthalmol 1982; 100:1313-1318.
2. Castanares S. Blepharoplasty for herniated intraorbital fat: anatomical basis for a new approach. Plast Reconstr Surg 1951;8:46.
3. Lemke BN, Lucarelli MJ. Anatomy of the ocular adnexa, orbit, and related facial structures. In: Nesi FA, Lisman RD, Levine MR, eds. Smith's ophthalmic plastic and re-constructive surgery, 2nd ed. St. Louis: Mosby, 1997:3-78.
4. Barker DE. Dye injection studies of intraorbital fat components. Plast Reconstr Surg 1977;59:82-85.
5. Yousif NJ, Sonderman P, Dzwierzynski, et al. Anatomic considerations in transconjunctival blepharoplasty. Plast Reconstr Surg 1995;96:1271-1278.
6. Putterman AM. The mysterious second temporal fat pad. Ophthalmic Plast Reconstr Surg 1985;1:83-86.
7. Mitz V, Peyronie M. The superficial musculoaponeurotic system (SMAS) in the parotid and cheek area. Plast Reconstr Surg 1986;58:80-88.
8. Reuss W, Owsley JQ. The anatomy of the skin and fascial layers of the face in aesthetic surgery. Clin Plast Surg 1987;14:677-682.
9. Owsley JQ. Anatomy of the head and neck for aesthetic surgery. In: Owsley JQ, ed. Aesthetic facial surgery. Philadelphia: WB Saunders Co, 1994:7-24.
10. Hamra ST. Arcus marginalis release and orbital fat preservation in midface rejuvenation. Plast Reconstr Surg 1995;96:354.
11. Putterman AM. Evaluation of the cosmetic oculoplastic surgery patient. In: Putterman AM. Cosmetic oculoplastic surgery, 2nd ed. Philadelphia: WB Saunders, 1993: 12-26.
12. Lowe NJ, Wieder JM, Shorr N, et al. Infraorbital pigmented skin: preliminary observations of laser therapy. Dermatol Surg 1995;21:767-770.
13. Rubin MG. Photoaged and photodamaged skin. In: Manual of chemical peels superficial and medium depth. Philadelphia: JB Lippincott, 1995:7-8.
14. Goldberg RA, Charonis GC, Baylis HI, et al. Upper and lower eyelid blepharoplasty. In: Nesi FA, Lisman RD, Levine MR, eds. Smith's ophthalmic plastic and recon-

structive surgery, 2nd ed. St. Louis: Mosby, 1997: 416-435.
15. Palmer FR 3rd, Rice DH, Churukian MM. Transconjunctival blepharoplasty: complications and their avoidance: a retrospective analysis and review of the literature. Arch Otolaryngol Head Neck Surg 1993:119:993-999.
16. Kikkawa DO, Lemke BN, Dortzbach RK. Relation of the SMAS to the orbit and characterization of the orbitomalar ligament. Ophthal Plast Reconstr Surg 1996;12: 77-88.
17. Brazzo BG, Nesi FA. Evaluation of the cosmetic patient. Chapter in Nesi FA, Lisman RD, Levine MR, eds. Smith's ophthalmic plastic and reconstructive surgery, 2nd ed. St. Louis: Mosby, 1997:290.
18. Zide BM, Jelks GW. The eyelids. In: Zide BM, Jelks GW, eds. Surgical anatomy of the orbit. New York: Raven Press, 1985:25.
19. Adamson PA, Tropper GJ, McGraw BL. Extended blepharoplasty. Arch Otolaryngol Head Neck Surg 1991:117:606-609.
20. Byrd HS. The extended browlift. Clin Plast Surg 1997; 24:233-246.
21. Furnas DW. Festoons, mounds, and bags of the eyelids and cheek. Clin Plast Surg 1993;20:367.
22. Baker SS. Laser assisted reduction of festoons. Ophthal Plast Reconstr Surg. In press.
23. Hamra ST. The role of orbital fat preservation in facial aesthetic surgery: a new concept. Clin Plast Surg 1996; 23:17-28.
24. Seckel BR. Aesthetic laser surgery: a text and videotape atlas. Boston: Little Brown and Company, 1996: 136-138.
25. Zarem HA, Resnick JL. Expanded applications for trans-conjunctival lower lid blepharoplasty. Plast Reconstr Surg 1991;88:215-220.
26. David LM, Sanders G. CO_2 laser blepharoplasty: a comparison to cold steel and electrocautery. J Dermatol Surg Oncol 1987;13:110-114.
27. Morrow DM, Morrow LB. CO_2 laser blepharoplasty: a comparison with cold-steel surgery. J Dermatol Surg Oncol 1992;18:307-313.
28. Mittelman H, Apfelberg DB. Carbon dioxide laser blepharoplasty: advantages and disadvantages. Ann Plast Surg 1990;24:1-6.
29. Lask G. Laser may be faster and better than scalpel for blepharoplasty. Skin and Allergy News 1992;23:20.
30. Perkins SW, Dyer WK 2nd, Simo F. Transconjunctival approach to lower eyelid blepharoplasty: experience, indications, and technique in 300 patients. Arch Otolaryngol Head Neck Surg 1994;120:172-177.
31. Putterman AM. Transconjunctival approach to resection of lower eyelid herniated orbital fat. In: Putterman AM. Cosmetic oculoplastic surgery, 2nd ed. Philadelphia: WB Saunders, 1993:228-235.

32. Biesman BS. Precautions in the use of the laser for blepharoplasty. Plast Reconstr Surg 1997;99:275–277.

33. Ullmann Y, Levi Y, Ben-Izhak O, et al. The surgical anatomy of the fat in the upper eyelid medial compartment. Plast Reconstr Surg 1997;99:658–661.

34. Buerger DE, Woog JJ. Unpublished data.

35. Heltzer JM, Ellis DS, Stewart WB, et al. An eyelid lipogranuloma following sutureless transconjunctival blepharoplasty dressed with topical ointment. Presented at the American Society of Ophthalmic Plastic and Reconstructive Surgery Annual Scientific Symposium, San Francisco, 1997.

36. Baker SS, Muenzler WS, Small RG, et al. Carbon dioxide laser blepharoplasty. Ophthalmology 1984;91:238–244.

37. Adamson PA, Strecker HD. Transcutaneous lower blepharoplasty. Facial Plast Surg 1996;12:171–183.

38. Baylis HI, Long JA, Groth MJ. Transconjunctival lower eyelid blepharoplasty: technique and complications. Ophthalmol 1989:96:1027–1032.

39. Flanagan JC. Internal lower eyelid blepharoplasty with mini skin excision. Presented at the Wills Eye Hospital Annual Conference, Philadelphia, 1997.

40. Trelles MA, Baker SS, Ting J, et al. Complications in carbon dioxide laser lower blepharoplasty. Ann Plast Surg 1996;37:465–468.

41. Mullins JB, Holds JB, Branham GH, et al. Complications of the transconjunctival approach: a review of 400 cases. Arch Otolaryngol Head Neck Surg 1997;123:385–388.

42. Jordan DR, Anderson RL, Thiese SM. Avoiding inferior oblique injury during lower blepharoplasty. Arch Ophthalmol 1989;107:1382–1383.

43. Trelles MA, Garcia L. Complications in laser transconjunctival lower blepharoplasty [letter]. Ann Plast Surg 1997:39:105–106.

44. Stasior OG. Blindness associated with cosmetic blepharoplasty. Clin Plast Surg 1981;8:793–795.

45. Biesman BS. Cutaneous facial resurfacing with the carbon dioxide laser. Ophthalmic Surg Lasers 1996;27:685–698.

46. Dover JS, Hruza GJ. Laser skin resurfacing. Semin Cutan Med Surg 1996;15:177–188.

47. Goldbaum AM, Woog JJ. The CO_2 laser in oculoplastic surgery. Surv Ophthalmol 1997;42:255–267.

48. Kaufmann R, Hibst R. Pulsed erbium:YAG laser ablation in cutaneous surgery. Laser Surg Med 1996;19:324–330.

49. Miller I. The erbium laser gains a role in cosmetic surgery. Biophotonics International 1997;May/June:38–42.

50. Teikemeier G, Goldberg DJ. Skin resurfacing with the erbium:YAG laser. Dermatol Surg 1997;23:685–687.

51. Alster TS, Kauvar AN, Geronemus RG. Histology of high-energy pulsed CO_2 laser resurfacing. Semin Cutan Med Surg 1996;15:189–193.

52. Hohenleutner U, Hohenleutner S, Baumler W, et al. Fast and effective skin ablation with an Er:YAG laser: determination of ablation rates and thermal damage zones. Laser Surg Med 1997;20:242–247.

53. Bernstein LJ, Kauvar AB, Grossman MC, et al. The short- and long-term side effects of carbon dioxide laser resurfacing. Dermatol Surg 1997;32:519–525.

54. Cotton J, Hood AF, Gonin R, et al. Histologic evaluation of preauricular and postauricular human skin after high-energy, short-pulse carbon dioxide laser. Arch Dermatol 1996;132:425–428.

55. Gardner ES, Reinisch L, Stricklin GP, et al. In vitro changes in non-facial human skin following CO_2 laser resurfacing: a comparison study. Lasers Surg Med 1996;19:379–387.

56. Dailey R, et al. Presented at the American Society of Ophthalmic Plastic and Reconstructive Surgery Annual Scientific Symposium, Chicago, October 1996.

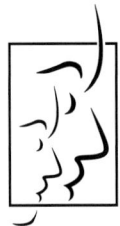

Chapter Eleven

The Carbon Dioxide Laser in Repair of Eyelid Malposition: Ptosis, Ectropion, Entropion

Sterling S. Baker and Brian S. Biesman

Many advantages conferred by using the carbon dioxide laser in blepharoplasty surgery apply to the correction of eyelid malposition. The incisional phase of the surgery is accomplished in a virtually bloodless field that eases intraoperative identification of lid and orbital structures and also definition of lid pathology. The excellent hemostasis achieved with the CO_2 laser results in decreased intraoperative time and improved appearance in the immediate postoperative period.

PTOSIS

Blepharoptosis or "ptosis" is present when the upper eyelid is downwardly displaced. The upper eyelid normally covers 1–3 mm of the superior cornea with gaze fixation at distance and the eyes directed forward in primary position. The vertical distance between the eyelids, known as the interpalpebral distance measures 9–11 mm in the nonptotic adult assuming a normal lower eyelid position. If a light source is directed at the patient, a pinpoint corneal light reflection will appear centrally and may be used as a reference point to judge eyelid position, both pre- and intraoperatively. The distance between the corneal light reflex and the upper eyelid margin is known as the margin reflex distance 1 (MRD_1), and usually measures 2 mm or greater in the nonptotic adult. The MRD_1 is a particularly sensitive measurement for detecting the presence of ptosis, but will not be accurate in patients with vertical strabismus (hyper- or hypotropia), enophthalmos, or conditions in which the globe is displaced.

Elevation of the normal upper eyelid is accomplished by the combined contraction of the levator palpebrae superioris and Müller's muscle. The levator muscle is the primary elevator of the upper eyelid, and its force is transmitted to the tarsal plate via a broad, strong aponeurosis. Fibers of the levator aponeurosis also inserted cutaneously to form the eyelid crease, and it is commonly believed that an absence of these fibers is responsible for the smooth, "single lid" contour seen in Asian patients (Figure 11.1). See Chapter 1 for more detailed information on the anatomy of the upper eyelid. When ptosis is severe enough to impair vision, the occipitofrontalis muscle is recruited to elevate the brows so that the eyelids are elevated. Ensuring that the frontalis muscle is relaxed is important to when evaluating eyelid position as bilateral ptosis may be masked, or a unilateral ptotic lid may be made to appear normal while the fellow nonptotic lid appears retracted.

Etiology

Ptosis may be congenital or acquired, unilateral or bilateral, symmetric or asymmetric. The etiology of congenital ptosis is unknown, but the pathophysiology involves a

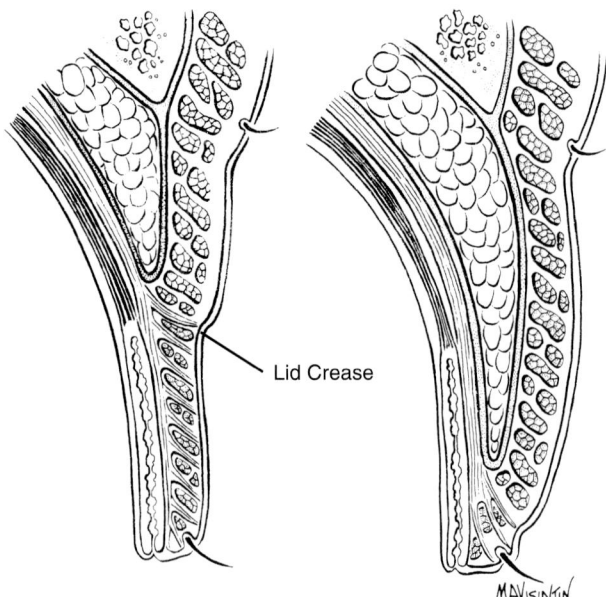

Figure 11.1. Insertion of fibers from the levator aponeurosis into the skin.

TABLE 11.1 Classification of Levator Function

Levator Function	Classification
10–15	Excellent (normal)
>8	Good
5–7	Fair
<4	Poor

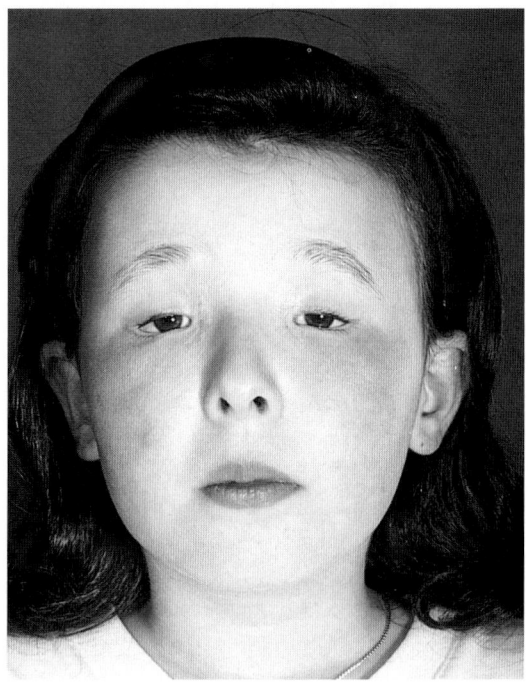

Figure 11.2. Congenital ptosis. The lid crease is poorly defined.

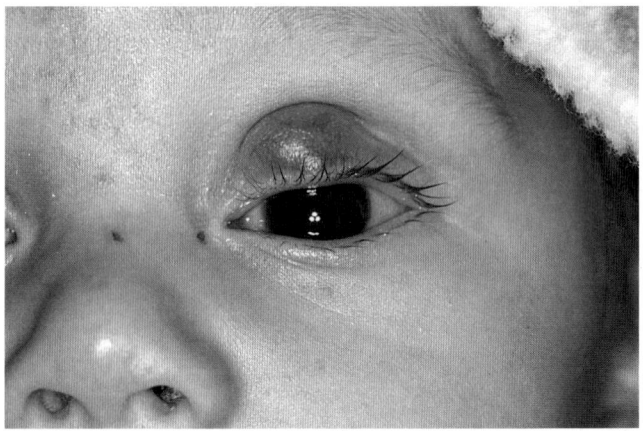

Figure 11.3. Mechanical ptosis caused by an eyelid hemangioma.

developmental dystrophy of the levator muscle without associated neurologic abnormalities. In one variant of congenital ptosis, aberrant innervation produces a condition in which stimulation of the motor branches of CN V results in elevation of the ptotic lid (1). Patients with congenital ptosis may be classified by degree of drooping: mild, moderate, or severe, and by the relative function of the levator muscle: excellent-to-good, fair, and poor-to-none (Table 11.1). Indications for surgical repair of congenital ptosis include induced astigmatism resulting from the eyelid position relative to the cornea, amblyopia arising from occlusion of the visual axis, development of a "chin up" head position, or cosmetic disfigurement (Figure 11.2). The psychosocial implications of an abnormal appearance must not be underestimated.

Acquired ptosis usually occurs in adults and, unlike congenital ptosis, represents a heterogeneous group of disorders that can be divided into five groups: neurogenic, myogenic, traumatic, mechanical, and aponeurogenic (2). Neurogenic ptosis may be caused by any condition affecting the third cranial nerve throughout its pathway: vascular lesions, tumors, and inflammation. Horner's syndrome is perhaps the most recognized cause of neurogenic ptosis. Patients with myogenic ptosis may display abnormal function of several extraocular muscles, including the levator palpebrae superioris. The more common causes of myogenic ptosis include chronic progressive external ophthalmoplegia, myotonic dystrophy,

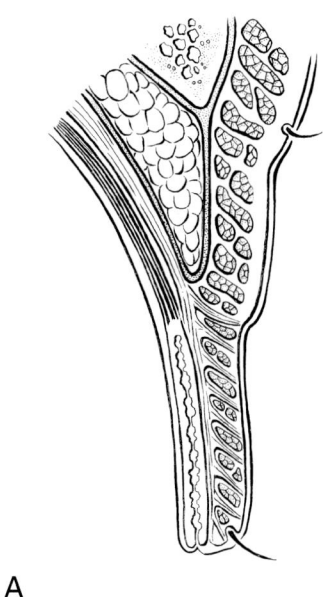

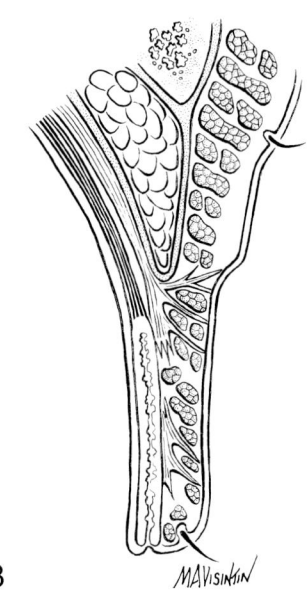

A   B

Figure 11.4. A. Schematic drawing demonstrating normal position of the levator aponeurosis with its cutaneous and tarsal insertions. **B.** Schematic drawing demonstrating disinsertion of the levator aponeurosis with subsequent retraction and elevation of the eyelid crease. (Figures adapted from unpublished drawings by Julie Woodward, MD.)

myasthenia gravis, and oculopharyngeal dystrophy. Traumatic ptosis refers to lowering of the eyelid after blunt eyelid trauma. The ptosis may be partial or complete, and is felt to be related to disinsertion of the levator aponeurosis from the tarsal plate. Traumatic ptosis may resolve spontaneously up to 6 months following an injury. Mechanical ptosis occurs when tumors or swelling force the lid closed. Some more common tumors inducing ptosis include hemangiomas, seborrheic keratosis, and neurofibromas (Figure 11.3). Aponeurotic ptosis is the most common form of ptosis encountered in most clinical practices and occurs when the levator aponeurosis becomes unable to effectively transmit the force of a normal levator muscle to the tarsal plate (Figure 11.4 A and B). Signs of aponeurotic ptosis include good levator function (at least 12 mm), thinning of the eyelid, elevated or absent lid crease, deepening of the superior sulcus and, in certain cases, ptosis of the eyelashes and contraction of the occipitofrontalis muscle manifested by elevation of the eyebrows (Figure 11.5) (3-5).

Surgical repair of acquired ptosis may be performed in severe cases when the visual axis is impaired, or in milder cases for aesthetic reasons (3, 6). Procedures for the correction of ptosis have included transcutaneous or transconjunctival resection of the levator muscle and/or its aponeurosis, and transconjunctival resections of conjunctiva, Müller's muscle, and tarsus (7, 8). Today, the most common approach to correction of acquired ptosis involves transcutaneous repair of the levator aponeurosis

(5, 9-17). Although CO_2 laser incisional periorbital surgery (18) was initially greeted with tepid enthusiasm (19-23), it has subsequently gained wide acceptance (24-27). The CO_2 laser is particularly beneficial in levator aponeurosis surgery as the bleeding normally associated with eyelid incisions can easily obscure the subtle differences that distinguish an attenuated levator aponeurosis from adjacent tissues planes, such as the orbital septum. In addition, with improved hemostasis, surgical times are shortened and less tissue swelling and distortion occur intraoperatively, improving the predictability of the final surgical result. Laser-assisted levator aponeurosis repair

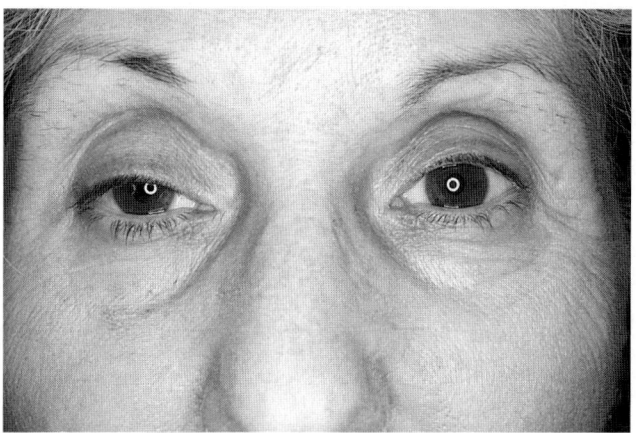

Figure 11.5. Acquired ptosis caused by disinsertion of the levator aponeurosis.

has been adapted from established blepharoplasty techniques, and may be used for congenital or acquired ptosis. For the correction of mild to moderate ptosis, some surgeons prefer to use an internal approach with resection of conjunctiva, Müller's muscle, and occasionally tarsus. The CO_2 laser does not play a useful role in these procedures.

LASER-ASSISTED REPAIR OF THE LEVATOR APONEUROSIS

Preoperative Evaluation

The preoperative evaluation of patients with acquired ptosis should always begin with "across the room" external examination, observing the amount of ptosis present and adopted compensatory mechanisms, such as upward tilting of the chin or elevation of the eyebrows. Visual acuity is measured and recorded before manipulation of the eyelids or eyes. The external examination should include measurement of the palpebral fissures with the brows relaxed, excursion of the eyelid from extreme downward gaze to extreme upward gaze with the eyebrow fixed (referred to as *levator function*), distance of the eyelid crease from the lid margin (noting the position of the eyelashes and the contour of the superior sulcus), and palpation of the lid to assess relative thickness. The pupils should be evaluated to rule out Horner's syndrome, and the extraocular movements should be assessed, paying particular attention to the superior rectus, which arises from the same mesodermal complex as the levator (28). Limited function of the superior rectus muscle may predict abnormally decreased levator function. The tear film is inspected under magnification, and baseline tear production is measured to determine the potential for symptomatic dry eyes after surgery. The basic secretion test is performed by placing 1–2 drops of topical anesthetic (proparacaine hydrochloride, tetracaine hydrochloride) in the inferior fornix and then blotting the fornix dry with a cotton-tipped applicator. One end of a Schirmer strip (Whatman #15 filter paper, Figure 11.6) is placed in the inferior fornix for 5 minutes. A normal result is 10 mm or more of the wetting of the filter paper. Bell's phenomenon should be evaluated by forcibly opening the eyelids as the patient resists the examiner by squeezing the eyes closed. Most patients will demonstrate an upward rotation of the globes for protection of the cornea when the eye is closed. If this phenomenon is absent, or if the patient has dry eye syndrome, a more con-

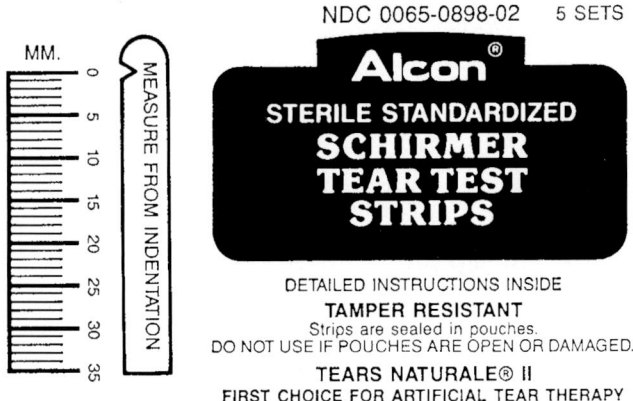

Figure 11.6. Filter paper used for Schirmer testing.

servative operation should be planned. Finally, patients should understand that postoperative revision of the eyelid position may be necessary in a significant percentage of patients.

Surgical Steps

The procedure is begun with marking of the proposed incision site on the upper eyelid. If skin is to be removed, an ellipse is marked as in preparation for blepharoplasty surgery (see chapter 9, Upper Eyelid Blepharoplasty). In patients who have a dehisced levator aponeurosis with a deep superior sulcus and little dermatochalasis, an incision may be made only through the upper eyelid crease. If intravenous sedation is to be administered before injecting the local anesthetic, a short-acting agent, such as propofol, should be used to maximize the patient's ability to cooperate during surgery. Oxygen may be given during the period of sedation, but should be discontinued before operating the laser (See chapter 1 for laser safety precautions). Two percent lidocaine solution with 1:100,000 epinephrine added may be used alone or as a 1:1 mixture with plain 0.75% bupivacaine to achieve local anesthesia. While the bupivacaine provides a greater duration of anesthesia, if lower eyelid surgery is being performed simultaneously, the prolonged orbicularis muscle paralysis may result in corneal exposure or abrasion because of the inability to close the eyes well. When the anesthetic is injected, it should be delivered through a 30-gauge needle into the subcutaneous space, taking care not to engage the underlying orbicularis muscle, which may bleed, producing a hematoma. Two-to-three milliliters of anesthetic agent are injected into a single site in the central-lateral part of the eyelid and is distributed throughout the lid using digital massage. Hyaluronidase is not added to the anesthetic solution: it can expedite enough intraorbital diffusion to compromise levator muscle function, making the endpoint of surgery difficult to assess. The apex of the lid curve is then marked at a point directly above the pupil as the patient's gaze is fixed at distance. This mark will guide the placement of the central suture when the aponeurosis is advanced onto the tarsal plate, thereby maintaining an appropriate lid contour. The above steps may be performed in the holding area or the operating room itself.

With the patient's head placed at the end of the operating table, the skin is prepared with a laser-safe agent and wet towel drapes are applied. Supplemental oxygen is discontinued and a David-Baker lid clamp (27) is fastened into position on the upper eyelid (Figure 11.7) with the blade in the superior cul de sac and the lid on minimal traction. The globe and plate may be lubricated with several drops of topical anesthetic such as proparacaine hydrochloride or tetracaine hydrochloride. The laser is then brought into the surgical field and set in the continuous wave mode at 6 W or in the superpulsed ("ultrapulsed") mode at 10 mJ, 10 W. A 0.2 mm focused delivery system is recommended. A laser safe-smoke evacuation system is activated, and laser safety principles are scrupulously observed.

With the laser handpiece held perpendicular to the skin in a focused position, the eyelid incisions are made through skin and orbicularis muscle. A skin-muscle flap is elevated from the preseptal area and, if necessary, hemostasis is obtained by defocusing the laser or using bipolar cautery (Figure 11.8). The superior margin of the tarsus is visible at the inferior wound edge. A horizontal plexus of vessels, the peripheral arcade, lies beneath the levator aponeurosis on the surface of Müller's muscle, and may be visible if the levator aponeurosis is disinserted from the tarsus. This structure is normally obscured by the opaque levator aponeurosis. With careful inspection, the distal margin of the levator aponeurosis may be visualized as a thickened, white band (Figure 11.9). Recognition of the aponeurosis may be enhanced by having the patient look upward and downward. If the aponeurosis is successfully identified at this time, it may be simply advanced and sutured into place onto the anterior superior portion of the tarsal plate. The superior third-to-half of the tarsal plate is exposed by using the laser set at 3 W to reflect the overlying pretarsal orbicularis muscle. This dissection is helped by grasping the inferior edge of the wound with a

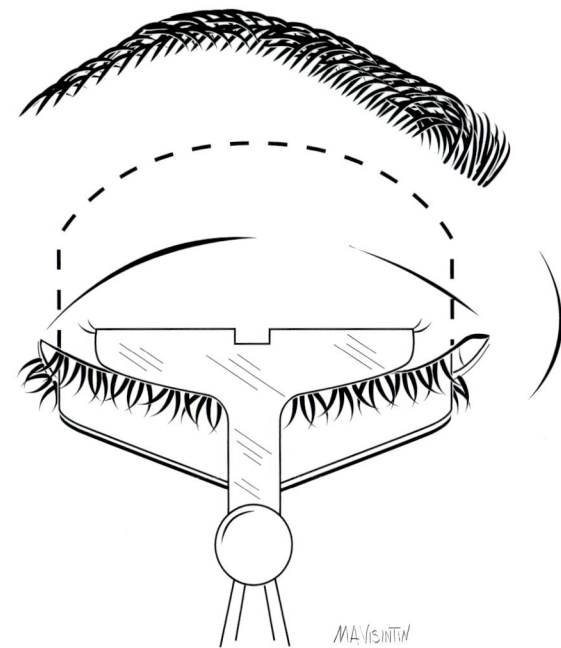

Figure 11.7. Schematic drawing of David-Baker clamp in place. In contrast to most metal eye shields, this device protects the entire superior fornix. (Figure adapted from unpublished drawings by Julie Woodward, MD.)

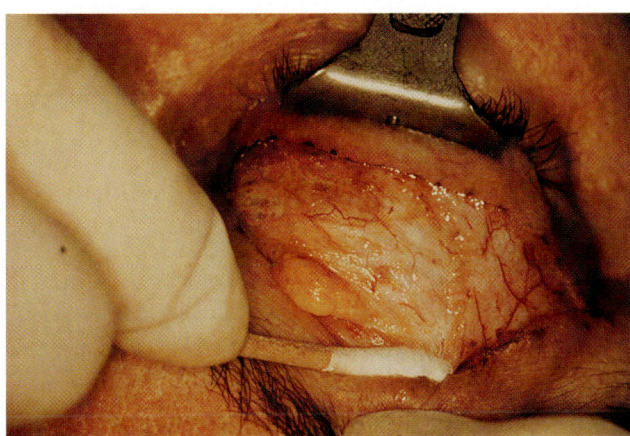

Figure 11.8. The skin muscle flap has been elevated, exposing the orbital septum. A small opening in the septum has allowed prolapse of the preaponeurotic fat pad.

toothed forceps, and distracting it perpendicularly to the plane of the eyelid while the laser is directed inferiorly at an angle of 45–60° (Figure 11.10). The tarsus soon becomes visible as a white or yellow-white structure. The lid clamp is removed and a suture is passed in a partial-thickness style approximately 3 mm below the superior tarsal border at a location corresponding to the apex of the eyelid curvature. Note that this position does not

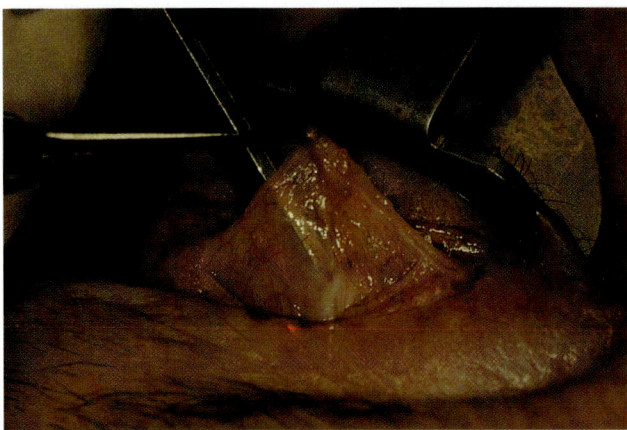

Figure 11.9. The levator aponeurosis is identified, in this case, after opening the orbital septum.

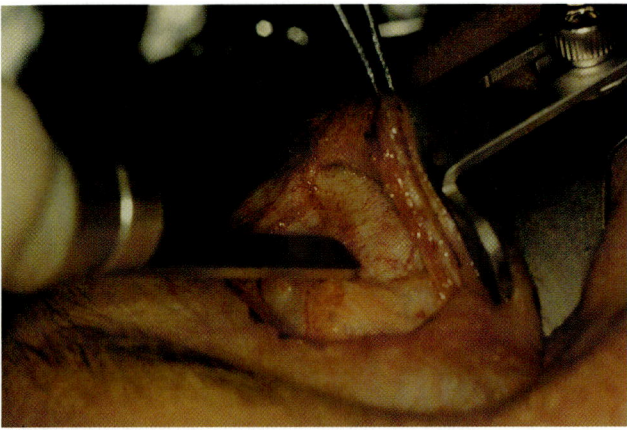

Figure 11.10. The orbicularis muscle has been reflected from the tarsal plate.

correspond to the center of the eyelid, but to the junction of the medial and middle thirds of the eyelid. The suture may be passed horizontally or vertically: acceptable alternatives for suture material include 6-0 polygalactin, 6-0 silk, 5-0 or 6-0 polypropylene, and others (Figure 11.11). A spatulated needle (Ethicon S-14 or equivalent) should be used to avoid lacerating the tarsal plate. After the needle is retrieved, the lid should be everted to rule out inadvertent full-thickness suture placement. Each needle is then passed through the disinserted inferior edge of the levator aponeurosis and tied temporarily with a slip knot. The operating room lights are directed away from the patient, and the upper eyelid position and contour are assessed with both eyes open and gaze fixed at a distant point. Also observe the lid position with the fellow eye occluded to eliminate the possibility of excessive neuromuscular output driven by a fellow ptotic lid. According

to Hering's law, corresponding muscles receive equal motor innervation, and thus a ptotic lid drives excessive innervation to both levator muscles (29). The lid is set at its desired position by adjusting the location of the sutures. Additional sutures may be placed in the medial and lateral portions of the tarsus (corresponding to the medial and lateral limbus) to adjust eyelid contour as needed (Figure 11.12).

If the superior vascular arcade is not clearly visible once the skin-muscle flap is removed, the levator aponeurosis is still attached to the tarsus and must be exposed. This is accomplished by dividing the orbital septum as described in Chapter 9, Upper Eyelid Blepharoplasty. The yellow preaponeurotic fat is bluntly dissected from the underlying levator aponeurosis using cotton-tipped applicators or the laser handpiece. Some orbital fat may be removed if desired, although not necessary. In most cases of acquired ptosis, the removal of preaponeurotic fat should be conservative.

Once the orbital fat has been swept aside, the levator palpebrae superioris muscle and its aponeurosis should be clearly visible. The superior transverse (Whitnall's) ligament may be visible in the superior orbit posterior to the orbital rim. The aponeurosis is followed distally and inspected for evidence of attenuation or fatty degeneration. Fatty infiltration of the levator aponeurosis may be mistaken for preaponeurotic fat by the unsuspecting surgeon, leading to an inadvertent resection of the levator. The aponeurosis is reflected from its underlying attachment to Müller's muscle and conjunctiva using the laser at a setting of 2 W in the continuous wave mode. With appropriate eye protection in place, the laser is directed in a plane parallel to the conjunctiva and used to separate the levator

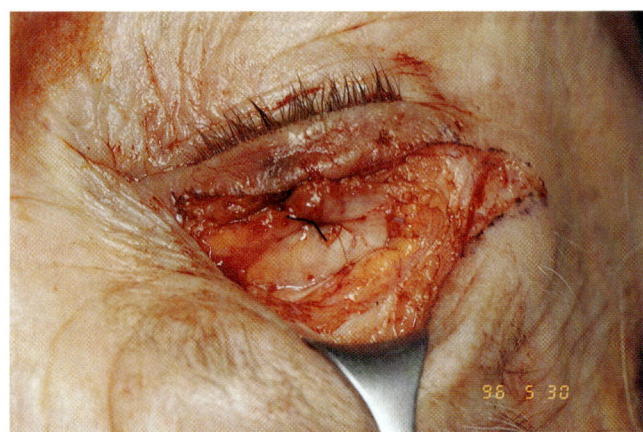

Figure 11.11. The levator has been sutured to the tarsus with a 6-0 silk suture.

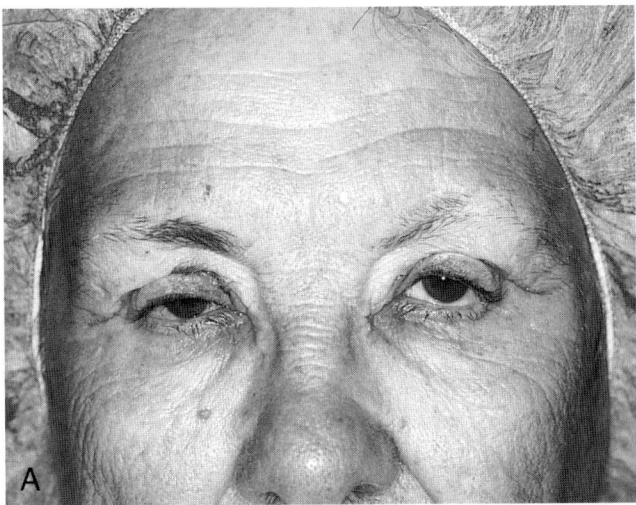

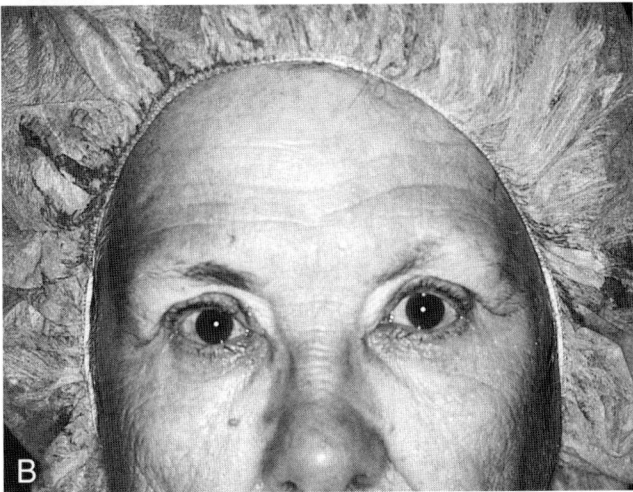

Figure 11.12. Pre- and postoperative photographs of a patient undergoing bilateral laser-assisted levator aponeurosis advancement.

aponeurosis from underlying Müller's muscle. Directing the beam posteriorly will result in a full-thickness eyelid defect, and may damage the eye. The levator aponeurosis and muscle may be advanced and sutured to the tarsal plate in the manner described above. Redundant muscle, aponeurosis, and septum are excised and discarded.

The wound is closed with running or interrupted 6-0 sutures. If a lid crease is to be reformed, it may be done now using standard techniques. The indications and methods for creating an eyelid crease extend beyond the scope of this chapter. Gross visual acuity (e.g., the ability of the patient to count fingers with each eye independently) is assessed before the patient leaves the operating room.

If the levator aponeurosis is too degenerated to hold a suture, the eyelid may be everted and 1% or 2% lidocaine solution *without epinephrine* injected subconjunctivally

above the tarsal plate, between conjunctiva and Müller's muscle. The eyelid is then returned to its normal anatomic position, and the power on the laser is decreased to 2 W. With inferior traction on the David-Baker clamp, dissection is carefully performed in a superior direction between conjunctiva and Müller's muscle all the way to the level of Whitnall's ligament, if necessary. Each arm of the 6-0 silk, double-armed suture is then passed through the Müller's muscle-levator complex, with Müller's muscle acting as a stent to help support the levator.

Postoperative management should include application of ice compresses continuously for the first 24–48 hours after surgery, elevation of the head (including sleeping on more than one pillow at night), and antibiotic ointment applied to the incisions daily 2–4 times until the sutures are removed. If necessary, lubricating ointments may be used during the day and at bedtime for the first several days after surgery to protect against exposure keratitis. Additional lubrication may be needed on an extended basis as the patient learns to retrain the eyelids to blink fully. Frequent and regular forcible closing of the eyes will facilitate ocular protection and lubrication. Avoiding bending, heavy lifting or exertion, and rubbing or manipulating the eyelids for at least 1 week is recommended. Contact lens wear may be resumed approximately 1–2 weeks after surgery. Sutures may be removed 6–10 days postoperatively.

Complications of Laser-Assisted Ptosis Surgery

Ptosis surgery may be unpredictable with any method. Some of the many factors that may affect the final outcome of ptosis repair include degree of ptosis, levator function, and the relative integrity of the levator aponeurosis. Any condition that impairs accurate intraoperative assessment of eyelid position will also make the results of ptosis repair less predictable: loss of orbicularis muscle tone, swelling of the eyelids and levator muscle, hemorrhage within Müller's muscle, stimulation of Müller's muscle by epinephrine in the anesthetic, and poor patient cooperation because of sedation, agitation, or discomfort (30).

The most common complication of laser-assisted ptosis surgery, as with standard ptosis repair, is over or under correction of the ptosis; management of this problem can be accomplished through standard techniques. A common consensus among experienced laser surgeons is that the results of ptosis repair are more predictable when the laser is used than when standard techniques are employed. This is perhaps from the decreased operating time, the decreased amount of intraoperative hemorrhage, clearer visualization of anatomic structures, or a combination of these factors. A comparative study has not been performed to assess this question in a prospective, controlled fashion.

Other complications of laser-assisted ptosis repair include all the complications of laser-assisted upper blepharoplasty (See Chapters 9, 14), and also: recurrence of ptosis, suture granuloma within the eyelid, superior rectus muscle damages, conjunctival prolapse, lash follicle damage with loss of lashes, eyelash ptosis, contour abnormalities, entropion or ectropion of the upper eyelid, lagophthalmos, ocular irritation resulting from erosion of tarsal sutures through the eyelid, adhesion between the conjunctiva of the superior palpebral and bulbar conjunctiva, and inadvertent excision of the levator aponeurosis (31).

ECTROPION

The lower eyelid is an important structure in the protection and maintenance of the eye. It offers a mechanical barrier, distributes the tear film evenly over the ocular surface with each blink, helps to guide the tear film towards the lacrimal drainage system, and acts in conjunction with the upper eyelid as the driving force for the lacrimal outflow system (32). Abnormalities of the lower eyelid that affect the ability to perform these functions must be corrected.

In its normal position the lower eyelid is firmly apposed to the globe. Rotation of the eyelid margin away from the eye is known as ectropion. Like ptosis, ectropion may also be classified by its pathophysiologic causes. The most common form is involutional, but cicatricial, paralytic, mechanical, and even congenital ectropion may occur. Involutional ectropion results when a combination of factors destabilizes the lower eyelid, allowing a gravitational effect to move the eyelid away from the globe (Figure 11.13). Factors involved in destabilization of the lower eyelid include weakness of the medial and/or lateral canthal ligaments, disinsertion of the lower eyelid retractors, and weakness of the orbicularis oculi muscle (33). Ectropion repair must address these destabilizing influences.

Preoperative Evaluation

Patients with lower eyelid involutional ectropion may present with complaints of tearing (epiphora), cutaneous

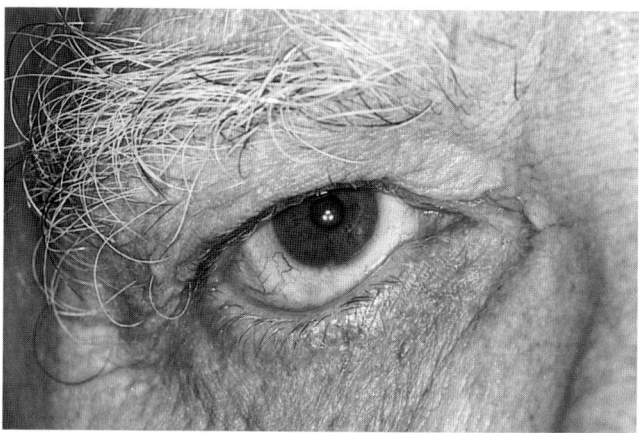

Figure 11.13. Moderately severe involutional ectropion. Lower eyelid function is severely compromised.

irritation, ocular foreign body sensation, and chronic redness of the bulbar and/or palpebral conjunctiva. The history should include specific inquiry regarding the presence of epiphora: situations in which tearing is most likely to occur, e.g., in downgaze (with exposure to wind or cold, etc.), prior eyelid or facial trauma or surgery, and a history of facial palsy or weakness.

As with any ophthalmic examination, visual acuity is tested and recorded before other diagnostic procedures are performed. The lower eyelid is assessed for laxity with the "pinch" or "snap" tests. To perform a pinch test the lid is grasped between the examiner's thumb and forefinger and pulled away from the globe. If the lid can be distracted more than 6 mm, then the eyelid is significantly lax (34). Alternatively, the snap test is performed by pulling the eyelid inferiorly and then quickly releasing it, observing the return of the lid to its initial position. If the lid returns promptly (in less than 5 seconds), laxity is not present. However, if ectropion is present, the lid will return slowly, may require one or more blinks to return, or may not return at all (35). Next, the lower eyelid should be observed for cicatricial changes, which usually occur in the anterior lamella as a result of actinic damage or prior surgery. The lower eyelid normally may be pushed superiorly until the entire cornea is covered. If cicatricial changes are present, the lid cannot be moved as far superiorly and, with superior traction, the entire cheek will be elevated. A cicatricial ectropion will be exaggerated by maneuvers that stretch the lower eyelid, such as gazing upward and opening the mouth. Finally, the ocular and conjunctival surfaces should be examined for the presence of keratinization or defects in the corneal or conjunctival epithelium.

As the most common involutional change responsible for the development of ectropion is laxity of the lateral canthal ligament, surgical efforts are most commonly directed toward tightening this structure. This was not always so as early surgical treatments (36–39) were directed toward other portions of the lower eyelid. Tenzel et al (40), and later Anderson and Gordy (41) advocated tightening the lower eyelid by creating a lateral canthal sling or a *lateral tarsal strip*. The tarsal strip was then advanced and fixed to the periosteum overlying Whitnall's tubercle (See chapter 1 for anatomic details). While this procedure is satisfying as it offers an anatomically correct solution to the problem of lateral canthal ligament laxity, it requires complete transection and subsequent reconstruction of the lateral canthal angle. This is undesirable as it not only requires additional time, but also increases the risk of functional or aesthetic complications. When the CO_2 laser is used as an incisional device, the tarsal strip procedure is easily performed as the complex anatomy may be readily visualized. However, division of the lateral commissure is still necessary. An alternative to the tarsal strip procedure is plication of the inferior limb of the lateral canthal tendon through a small CO_2 laser incision placed lateral to the lateral commissure while preserving the integrity of the lateral canthus (42). The lower lid may be shortened 5–7 mm with this procedure (43), making it useful for the treatment of mild-to-moderate cases of involutional ectropion. The lateral tarsal strip is a more powerful procedure that remains a procedure of choice to correct even severe involutional laxity and ectropion.

LASER-ASSISTED LATERAL CANTHAL TENDON PLICATION

Laser-assisted lateral canthal tendon plication may be performed in an office or operating room setting. Local anesthesia without intravenous sedation is usually adequate unless patients are extremely anxious. Two percent lidocaine with 1:100,000 epinephrine added may be used alone, or mixed 1:1 with 0.25–0.75% bupivacaine. One-to-two milliliters of local anesthetic is delivered through a 30-gauge needle to a single site overlying the lateral raphe, taking care not to engage the underlying orbicularis oculi muscle. The bolus of anesthetic is massaged into the tissue using digital pressure. An incision site measuring 0.5–1.0 cm is marked in the lateral raphe, extending to approximately 2 mm from the lateral commissure (Figure 11.14).

Ocular protection is provided by a laser-safe Jaeger plate placed between the globe and the lateral orbital rim. The CO_2 laser is set at 6 W in the continuous wave mode, or 10 W and 10 mJ/pulse in pulsed mode, using a focused delivery system that provides a beam no more than 0.2 mm in diameter. A smoke evacuator is employed, and standard laser safety precautions are observed. The incision is made with the handpiece held perpendicular to the skin, and is deepened until the periosteum covering the lateral orbital rim is visible. Hemostasis is achieved by defocusing the laser or by using bipolar cautery. The inferior limb of the lateral canthal ligament is identified and grasped at its insertion into the lower eyelid tarsus. With gentle traction on the tendon, the entire lid should move (Figure 11.15). The tendon is imbricated with a double-armed 4-0 suture of the surgeon's choice. Popular materials include polygalactin, polyester, polypropylene, and others. Needles should be strong and preferably half circle. Some common choices include S2 (Ethicon, Somerville, NJ), P2 (Ethicon), OPS5 (Ethicon, special order), and ME2 (Deknatel, Fall River, MA). Each arm of the double-armed suture is then passed through the periorbita overlying Whitnall's tubercle (Figure 11.16). The suture is tied temporarily and the lid position assessed as adequate before it is tied permanently. To prevent the 4-0 knot from

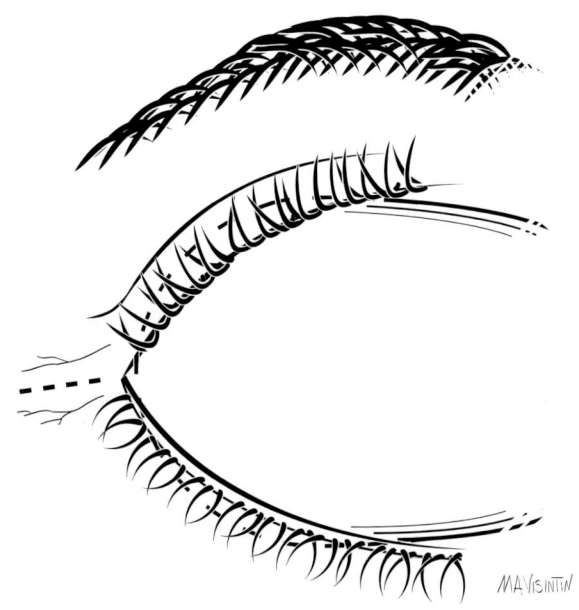

Figure 11.14. Proposed incision for laser-assisted lateral canthal tendon plication. The incision does not include the lateral commissure. (Figure adapted from unpublished drawings by Julie Woodward, MD.)

being easily palpable, the orbicularis oculi muscle is closed with 6-0 polygalactin buried sutures. The skin is closed with interrupted 6-0 sutures, using a permanent monofilament material. The visual acuity is again checked and recorded, and antibiotic ointment is applied to the wounds. A dressing or patch is usually not required (Figure 11.17).

Postoperatively ice packs are applied for 24–48 hours to decrease postoperative swelling. Antibiotic ointment is applied to the wounds daily 3–4 times until the sutures are removed in 5–7 days. Patients may note tenderness to palpation over the site of the fixation suture for

1–3 months after surgery. This usually resolves gradually but, should it persist, steroid injections or even suture removal may be required.

If upper eyelid surgery is being performed simultaneously, the inferior limb of the lateral canthal ligament may be approached through the lateral portion of upper eyelid defect, thus avoiding a separate skin incision.

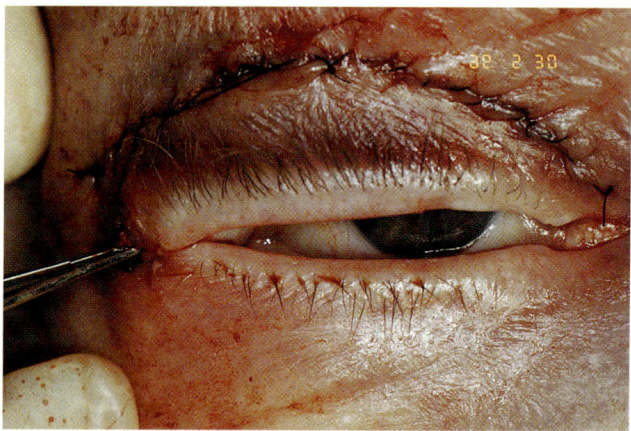

Figure 11.15. The upper and lower eyelids are distracted from the globe when traction is placed on the canthal ligament.

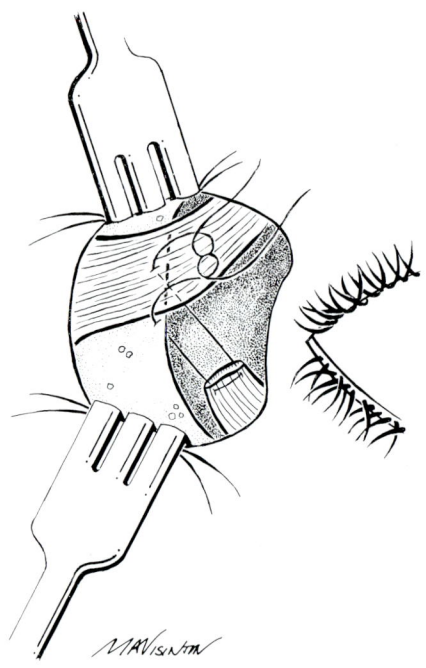

Figure 11.16. Schematic drawing demonstrating correct suture placement for lateral canthal tendon plication. (Figure adapted from unpublished drawings by Julie Woodward, MD.)

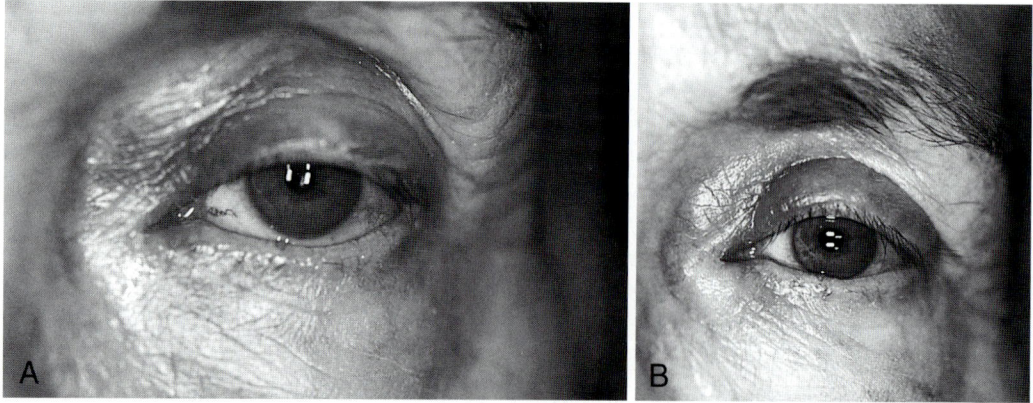

Figure 11.17. Mild involutional ectropion before and after laser-assisted plication of lateral canthal tendon.

CO₂ LASER-ASSISTED LATERAL TARSAL STRIP

The CO_2 laser-assisted tarsal strip procedure may be performed in either an office or an operating room setting. The preoperative evaluation is described above. The same local anesthetic agents described above may be used for the lateral tarsal strip procedure, but the injections should be administered into the lateral portion of the upper and lower eyelid margin as well as subcutaneously over the raphe.

With the laser set at 6 W in the CW mode, or 10 W and 10 mJ/pulse in ultrapulse mode, the procedure begins with division of the lateral commissure. With a metal Jaeger plate in position, the laser is used to make an incision 0.5–1.0 cm in length, dividing the lateral canthal ligament horizontally (Figure 11.18). The lateral end of the lower eyelid is grasped with a forceps and distracted from the globe, stretching the inferior limb of the ligament so that it may be easily palpated with the laser handpiece. The ligament is divided with the laser at or near its periosteal insertion site, allowing the lid to move freely. The amount of excess lid is estimated by pulling the lid laterally and slightly superiorly until an acceptable degree of tightening has been achieved.

An isolated strip of tarsus is then created. With the eyelid stretched, the laser is directed in a plane parallel to the tarsus, between the orbicularis muscle and tarsal plate. This dissection is expedited if the assistant uses a forceps to pull the anterior lamella in a direction perpendicular to the tarsus. The anterior surface of the tarsus is thus exposed and the unwanted anterior lamella is removed and discarded. The eyelid is held against a protective plate while the laser is used to make an incision along the inferior tarsal border, releasing the conjunctiva and lower eyelid retractors. The eyelid margin is removed using a focused beam to "graze" the top of the tarsus as it is held against the Jaeger plate. Finally, the laser is defocused to destroy the conjunctival epithelium on the posterior aspect of the tarsus. The lateral end of the tarsus is now free of all other tissues (Figure 11.19). The excess tarsus may be trimmed and discarded or left in place to be folded over the lateral canthal suture. The tarsal strip is imbricated with a double-armed 4-0 suture as described above (Figure 11.20). Again, each arm of the double-armed suture is passed through the periorbita overlying Whitnall's tubercle, and the suture is tied temporarily and adjusted until an acceptable eyelid position and contour have been achieved. The lateral commissure is reformed using a

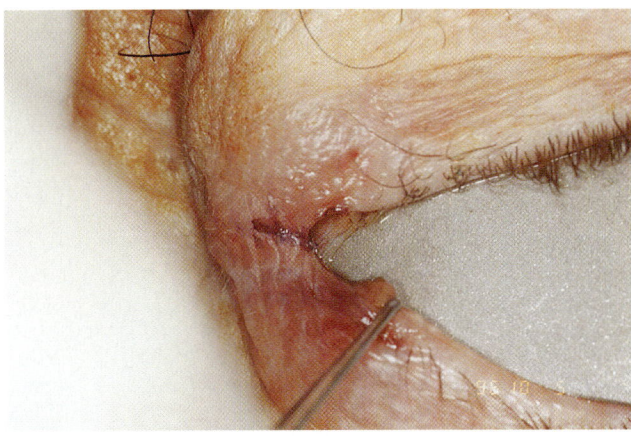

Figure 11.18. The lateral commissure has been divided with the laser.

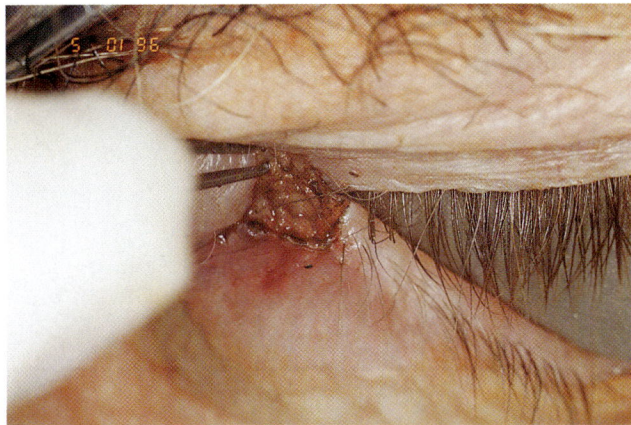

Figure 11.19. The tarsus has been freed of its attachments to surrounding structures.

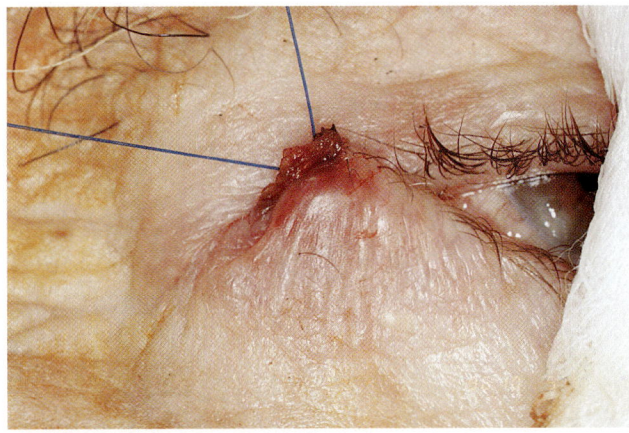

Figure 11.20. The excess tarsus has been resected and the tarsal strip has been imbricated with 4-0 polypropylene suture.

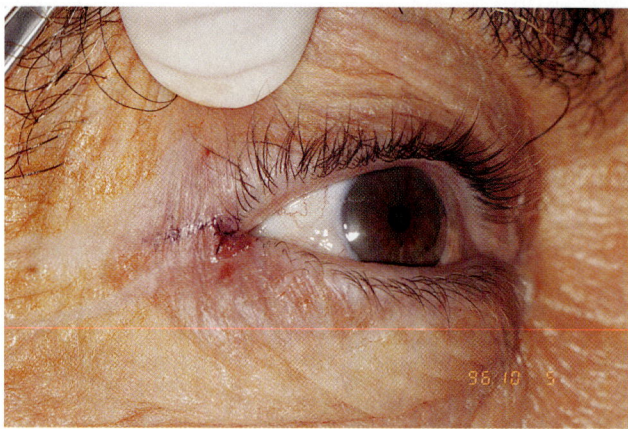

Figure 11.21. Appearance upon completion of the procedure. Ecchymosis and swelling are minimal.

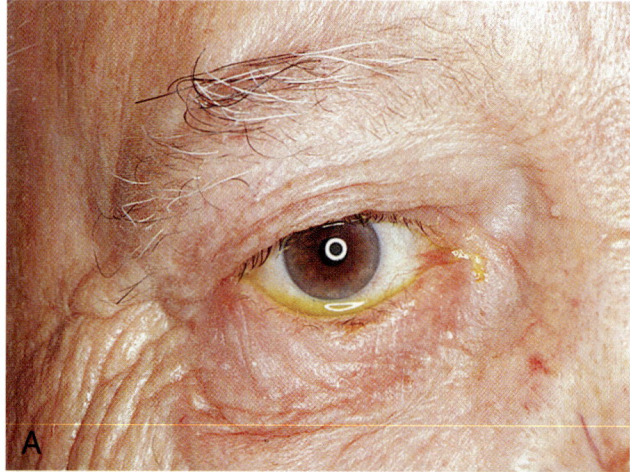

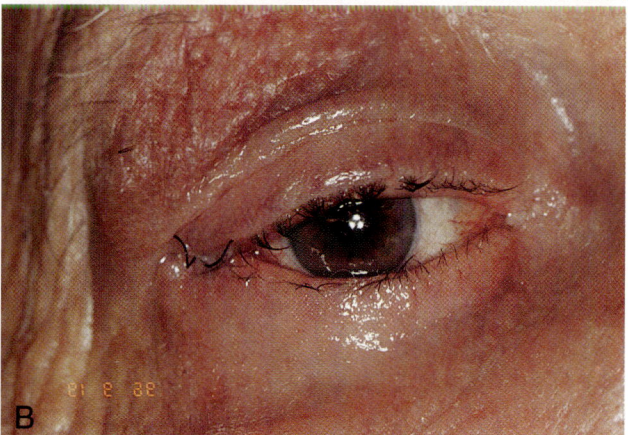

Figure 11.22. A, Before and **B,** 1 week after laser-assisted lateral tarsal strip ectropion repair. Only minimal swelling remains.

6-0 silk suture on a G1 micropoint needle (Ethicon). The orbicularis muscle and skin are closed as described above (Figure 11.21). Antibiotic ointment is applied to the wound and the same postoperative routine used following the plication procedure is followed. The lateral commissure suture is left in place for 14 days while the skin sutures may be removed 5-7 days postoperatively (Figure 11.22). Polygalactin sutures should not be used to form the canthal angle as wound dehiscence is more likely to occur.

Complications of laser-assisted canthal tendon plication or tarsal strip procedures may be divided into two groups: those related to the use of the laser, and those that are particular to ectropion repair. Laser-related complications of eyelid surgery are reviewed in Chapter 14 and will not be discussed here. Complications of the lateral canthal ligament plication and lateral tarsal strip procedures include aesthetic deformity, recurrence of ectropion, dehiscence of the tarsus from the periosteum, dehiscence of the lateral commissure, granuloma formation around the deep 4-0 suture, persistent pain in the lateral canthal region, formation of epithelial implantation cysts in the orbit, and incorporation of the lateral rectus muscle during the placement of the suture attaching tarsus to periorbita.

CICATRICIAL ECTROPION

Cicatricial ectropion most commonly occurs from of a shortage of lower eyelid skin resulting from mechanical trauma, thermal or chemical burns, severe actinic damage, or surgery. It may also result from scarring of the orbital septum, with fixation of the eyelid to the inferior orbital rim. This sometimes occurs after transcutaneous lower eyelid surgery in which the septum has been divided. Repair of cicatricial ectropion requires releasing the cicatrix and lengthening the foreshortened portion of the eyelid. In the case of mild skin shortage, a Z-plasty may be performed. Usually, full-thickness skin grafts harvested from the upper eyelid, retroauricular, supraclavicular, or preauricular regions, or the medial upper arm, are placed in the lower eyelid. Transposition of myocutaneous flaps from the upper eyelid to the lower eyelid may also be used in milder cases of cicatricial ectropion. The CO_2 laser has limited application in the harvesting of flaps or grafts, or in the preparation of their recipient beds, as it seals many of the small vessels crucial to the survival of the transplanted tissue. For this reason, a detailed description of cicatricial ectropion repair is beyond the scope of this text.

Mechanical ectropion occurs when a tumor mass causes the lower eyelid to be distracted from the globe (Figure 11.23). This is an unusual condition in Western society because of easy access to medical care. Treatment of mechanical ectropion is usually surgical excision of the offending lesion. The CO_2 laser may have a role in the debulking of vascular lesions, or even in performing full-thickness eyelid resections for the treatment of mechanical ectropion. If the laser is used to incise the eyelid margin and tarsus, the permanent sutures should be left in place at least 14 days before removal, slightly longer than the 10-14 days usually recommended when the laser is not used.

Paralytic ectropion occurs in the setting of a seventh cranial (facial) nerve palsy as a result of an inability of the orbicularis muscle to contract. The etiology of facial nerve palsy is multifactorial and has been reviewed elsewhere (44). In younger patients with good muscle tone, the lower eyelid may remain well apposed to the globe despite lack of orbicularis oculi innervation. In elderly patients, or those with preexisting laxity of the canthal tendons, the lower eyelid may become markedly ectropic with resulting exposure of the inferior portion of the globe and the inferior fornix. The surgical repair of paralytic ectropion is indicated when recovery of facial nerve function is not expected to occur, or when medical management of the exposed ocular surface with aggressive lubrication fails to maintain the integrity of the ocular surface. Surgical efforts are often directed at the medial and lateral canthal tendons, but suspension of the eyelid with fascia or other materials may also be required. The tarsal strip procedure described above is useful, but generally not sufficient to return the lower eyelid to an acceptable

position. The role of the CO_2 laser in the management of paralytic ectropion is limited to canthal ligament surgery.

Congenital ectropion is a rare condition of tissue deficiency in lower eyelid skin (45). Repair often requires skin grafting, and the CO_2 laser does not play a role in the care of these patients.

ENTROPION

Entropion of the lower eyelid is an in turning of the lid that places the keratinized eyelid skin and lashes against the globe, insulting the ocular surface. This condition may be associated with corneal ulceration and even irreversible visual loss. Entropion is traditionally classified into three categories: involutional, cicatricial, and congenital. Involutional entropion is by far the most common variant and the primary focus of this discussion. Cicatricial entropion occurs as a result of shrinkage or foreshortening of the posterior lamella of the eyelid (conjunctiva and lower eyelid retractors), and is usually caused by processes that produce injury or scarring of the conjunctiva. Examples of conditions that are known to cause cicatricial entropion include Stevens-Johnson syndrome, ocular cicatricial pemphigoid, trauma, chemical burns, advanced trachoma, membranous conjunctivitis, acne rosacea, and others. Surgical repair of cicatricial entropion may be accomplished by horizontal rotation of the eyelid in mild cases, but usually requires release of the cicatrix and placement of spacer grafts such as donor sclera, free tarsoconjunctival grafts, nasal septal cartilage with mucosa attached, auricular cartilage, and hard palate mucosa (46-50). Mucous membrane grafts may be used to cover the eyelid margin if it has become keratinized (51). Because of the need to maintain excellent vascularity of the graft beds, the CO_2 laser does not play an important role in the management of cicatricial entropion. Congenital entropion is a rare condition in which entropion is present at birth. It is felt to be caused by failure of the lower eyelid retractors to insert onto the tarsus (52). Congenital entropion may be treated by attaching the lower eyelid retractors to the inferior tarsal border, usually via transcutaneous approach. While the laser may be beneficial for this procedure, the condition is so uncommon that no information is available as to the healing of these wounds in a newborn infant.

Involutional entropion is thought to be caused by an instability of the forces that normally stabilize the lower eyelid. The anatomic factors commonly associated with involutional entropion include weakness or laxity of the

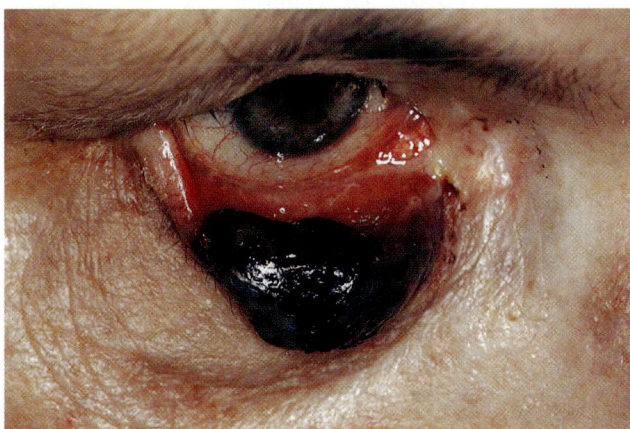

Figure 11.23. Mechanical ectropion caused by melanoma metastatic to eyelid.

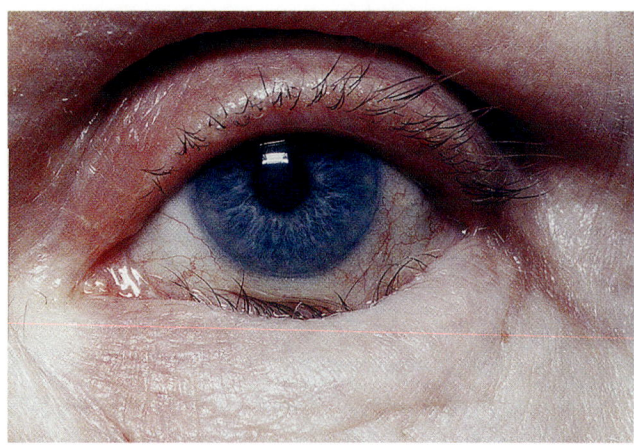

Figure 11.24. Involutional entropion with irritation of the ocular surface (surgeon's view).

canthal tendons, disinsertion of lower eyelid retractors, upward migration of the preseptal orbicularis onto the pretarsal orbicularis, and enophthalmos (53–55). As a result of these factors acting either independently or in concert, the lid rotates inward around a horizontal axis centered on the tarsus. The inward rotation brings the lashes and keratinized skin of the lower lid against the ocular surface (Figure 11.24). Correction of lower eyelid involutional entropion requires restoration of the balance of forces within the lower eyelid. Although a myriad of procedures has been proposed for accomplishing this goal, reinsertion of the lower eyelid retractors on the inferior tarsal border, repositioning the preseptal orbicularis muscle to prevent it from migrating superiorly, and tightening the canthal tendons when necessary, provides effective repair of lower eyelid entropion (56–59). Carbon dioxide laser techniques provide a bloodless field in which the lower lid structures can be easily identified and surgical goals can be quickly achieved.

Preoperative Evaluation

Patients presenting with lower eyelid entropion should be asked about the nature and duration of symptoms: changes in their vision (usually a decrease) occurring since the onset of symptoms, a history of eyelid trauma or surgery, chemical burns or exposure, chronic conjunctivitis, and acne rosacea. A history of travel to areas where trachoma is endemic may be pertinent if patients are found to have an unexplained cicatricial entropion.

The preoperative examination of a patient with entropion begins with measurement of the visual acuity. The eyelids are inspected for scarring or other evidence

of previous lid surgery. Laxity of the canthal tendons is assessed with the snap or pinch tests. A "fullness" of the lower eyelid 3–5 mm below the eyelashes may indicate upward migration of the preseptal orbicularis muscle to a position where it overrides the pretarsal orbicularis muscle. Upward movement of the preseptal orbicularis muscle may also sometimes be observed following forced closure of the eyelids. The conjunctival surface of the eyelid is examined under slit lamp magnification to rule out the presence of subconjunctival fibrosis or scarring. The bulbar conjunctiva is evaluated for signs of injection, scarring, or epitheliopathy. The cornea is examined before and after the application of dilute fluorescein solution, paying careful attention to the inferior cornea where epithelial defects caused by the entropic lower eyelid are most likely to be evident. The inferior fornix is assessed for depth and evidence of scarring or foreshortening.

Laser-Assisted Repair of Involutional Entropion

Endeavors to repair an involutional entropion should aim for correcting the underlying pathophysiologic mechanisms responsible for the imbalance within the eyelid. While many procedures have been described for entropion repair, plication of the lower eyelid retractors and repositioning the preseptal orbicularis oculi muscle is anatomically correct and is effective in the vast majority of cases. Eyelid laxity, if present, must be corrected, preferably by one of the techniques described above.

Reattachment of the lower eyelid retractors with repositioning of the preseptal orbicularis muscle may be performed in an office or an operating room setting. Local anesthesia may be achieved using 2% lidocaine with 1:100,000 epinephrine or as a 1:1 mixture with 0.25–0.75% bupivacaine. One-to-two milliliters of this solution is injected subcutaneously through a 30-gauge needle at a single site in the central portion of the eyelid, ensuring that the agent diffuses over the inferior tarsal border. The bolus of anesthetic is massaged into the tissue with digital pressure. Hyaluronidase may also be added to aid distribution of the anesthetic throughout the eyelid.

After the skin has been prepared and the patient draped (observing the usual laser safety precautions), the CO_2 laser is set at 6 W CW using a 0.2-millimeter focused delivery system. The globe is protected with a laser-safe Jaeger plate placed in the inferior cul de sac; the laser is used to make an incision parallel to the eyelid margin at the level of the inferior tarsal border measuring 2 cm in length (Figure 11.25). The medial extent of the incision is a point just lateral to the inferior punctum, and laterally the incision should blend in with a natural crow's feet line. Hemostasis is maintained with defocused laser or electrocautery, as needed. The preseptal orbicularis muscle is dissected from the underlying orbital septum using a combination of "sharp" dissection with the laser set at 3 W CW, and "blunt" dissection using the laser focus tip. The dissection is carried inferiorly to the level of the orbital rim. The power on the laser is then decreased to 2 W and the laser is used to separate the preseptal orbicularis muscle from its overlying attachment to skin. This dissection is aided if the assistant applies traction inferi-

orly on the lower eyelid so as to keep the lid stretched. If buttonholes are created, they should be repaired with 6-0 nylon interrupted sutures. This dissection is also carried to the level of the inferior orbital rim (Figure 11.26). With the Jaeger plate under the orbicularis muscle flap, the laser is used to make a full-thickness incision through the flap and parallel to the eyelid margin at the junction of the preseptal and pretarsal portions of the muscle. A rectangular-shaped section of the preseptal orbicularis muscle is resected with the laser set at 6 W, exposing the underlying orbital septum (Figure 11.27). The detached lower eyelid retractors are identified beneath the septum

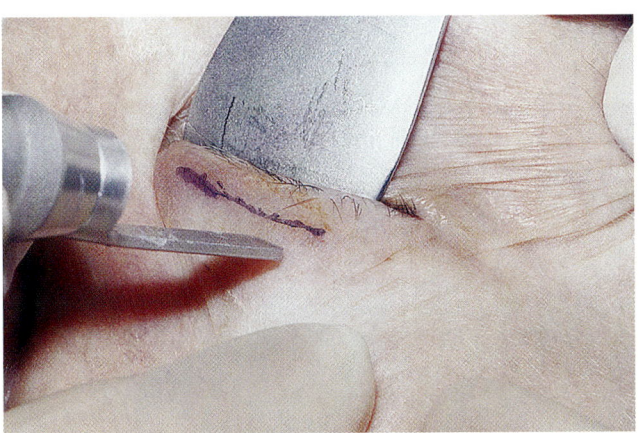

Figure 11.25. Incision for laser-assisted repair of CPF and orbicularis muscles (surgeon's view).

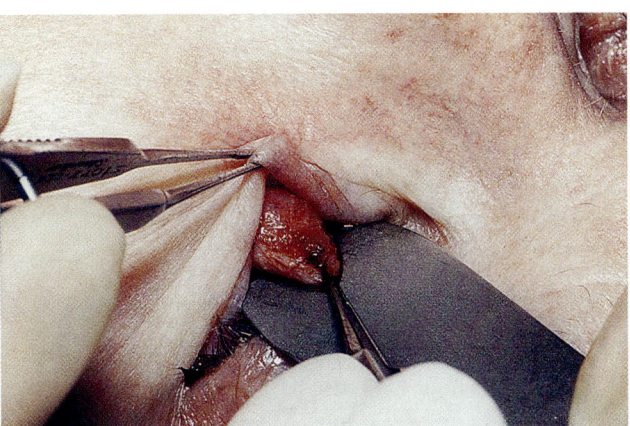

Figure 11.26. The orbicularis muscle has been isolated between the pretarsal area and the inferior orbital rim (surgeon's view).

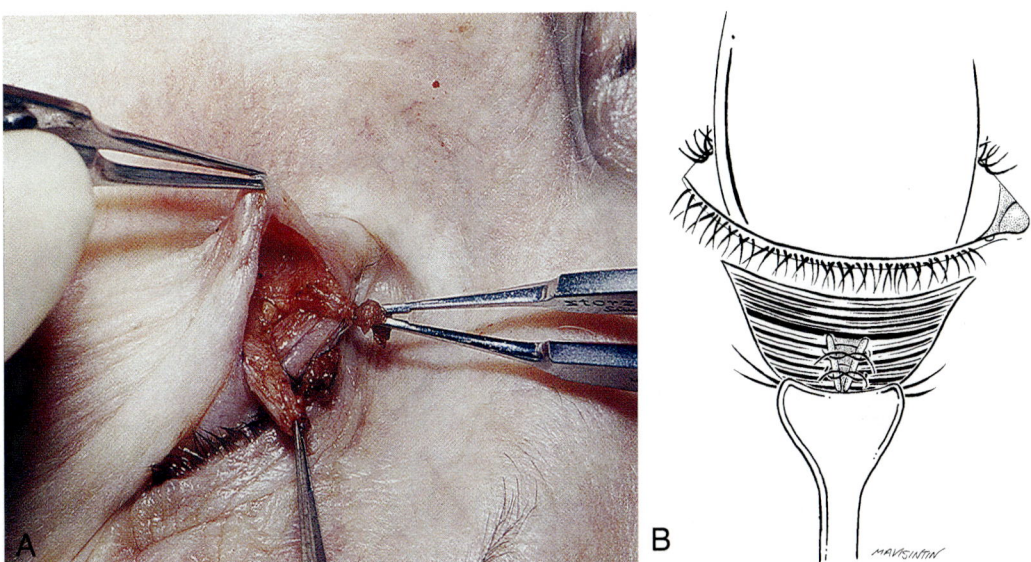

Figure 11.27. A. The laser is used to resect a portion of the preseptal orbicularis oculi muscle. **B.** Schematic drawing demonstrating closure of preseptal orbicularis oculi muscle with the pretarsal portion of the muscle left intact (surgeon's view). (Figure adapted from unpublished drawings by Julie Woodward, MD.)

and imbricated with 6-0 polygalactin suture in a mattress method. Asking the patient to voluntarily change gaze direction from up to down may enhance localization of the lower eyelid retractors and, in some cases, division of the orbital septum may be required (Figure 11.28). The 6-0 polygalactin suture is passed from the lower eyelid retractors to the inferior tarsal border, where it is tied (Figures 11.29 and 11.30). Several such sutures are placed along the length of the eyelid. The degree of eyelid margin rotation is controlled by the placement and tightness of the tarsal sutures. This is a powerful procedure that can produce a significant ectropion. The defect in the preseptal orbicularis muscle is closed with 6-0 polygalactin mattress sutures, helping prevent unwanted superior migration of the muscle. The superior edge of the pretarsal orbicularis muscle may be attached to the infe-

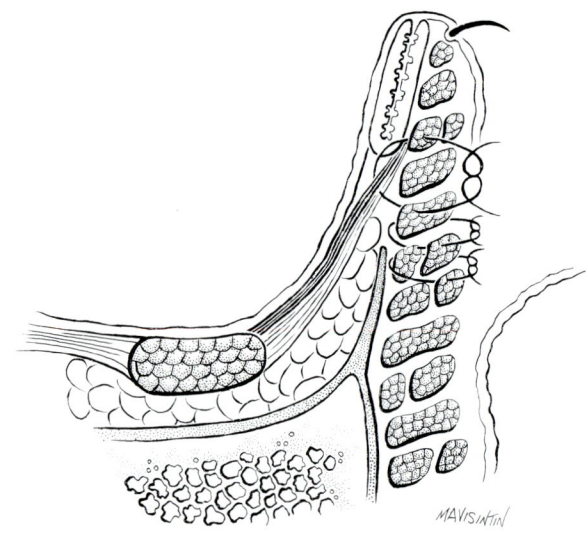

Figure 11.30. Sagittal view depicting correct placement of sutures for advancement of CPF and repair of orbicularis muscle defect. (Figure adapted from unpublished drawings by Julie Woodward, MD.)

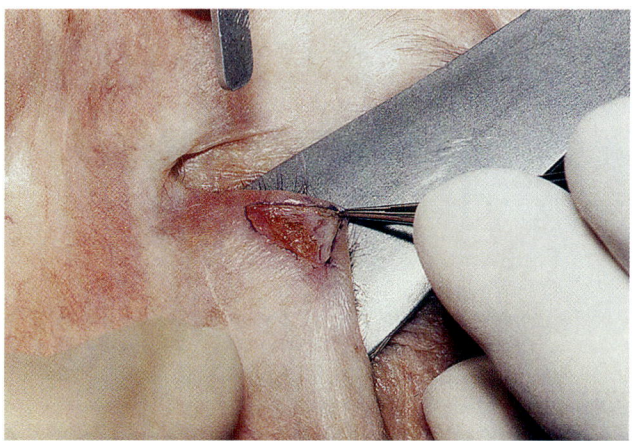

Figure 11.28. The lower eyelid retractor (CPF) is identified. The orbital fat may be either left undisturbed or resected.

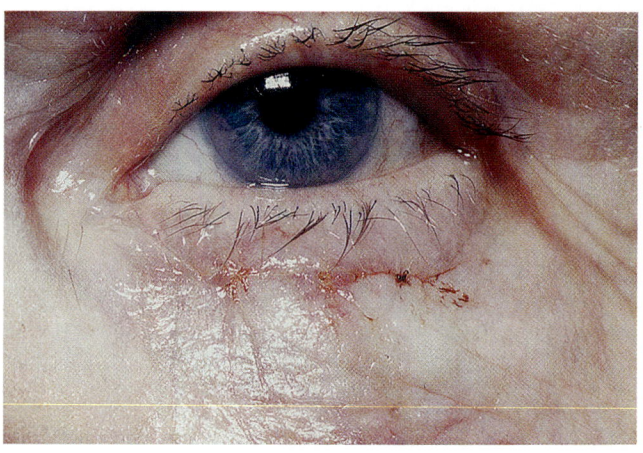

Figure 11.31. Appearance 1 week after surgery.

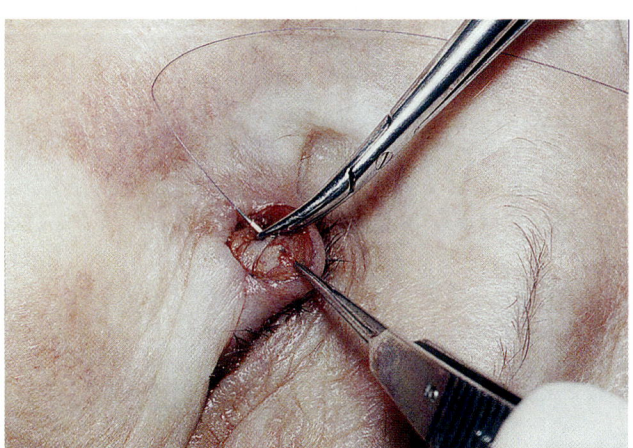

Figure 11.29. The CPF is advanced and sutured to the inferior tarsal border.

rior tarsal border with 6-0 polygalactin sutures and the skin closed with 6-0 sutures of the surgeon's choice (Figure 11.31). The visual acuity is measured and recorded in the immediate postoperative period.

The postoperative care of laser-assisted entropion repair is essentially the same as the postoperative ectropion repair described above. Topical antibiotic ointment is applied 2–3 times per day and lubricating ointment is used as needed. The skin sutures are removed in 5–7 days.

The complications of laser-assisted entropion repair include all of those complications associated with laser-assisted incisional surgery as outlined in Chapter 14. Complications specifically related to this procedure may include under correction, overcorrection (ectropion), suture granuloma, buttonholing of the skin with the laser, wound dehiscence, incorporation of the orbital septum in the retractor-tarsal suture producing lower lid retraction, infection, recurrence of entropion, and damage to the globe. With careful attention to surgical technique, these problems may largely be avoided.

REFERENCES

1. Sano K. Trigemino-oculomotor synkinesis. Neuralgia 1959;1:29–51.
2. Dortzbach RK, Sutula FC. Involutional blepharoptosis. A histopathological study. Arch Ophthalmol 1980;98:2045–2049.
3. Beard C. Ptosis, 3rd ed. St. Louis: CV Mosby, 1981.
4. Shore JW, McCord CD. Anatomic changes in involutional blepharoptosis. Am J Ophthalmol 1984;98:21–27.
5. Baker SS. Carbon dioxide laser ptosis surgery combined with blepharoplasty. Dermatol Surg 1995;21:1065–1070.
6. Beard C. The surgical treatment of blepharoptosis: a quantitative approach. Trans Am Ophthalmol Soc 1966;64:401–487.
7. Berke RN. Results of resection of the levator muscle through a skin incision in congenital ptosis. Arch Ophthalmol 1959;61:177–201.
8. Fasanella RH, Servat J. Levator resections for minimal ptosis: another simplified operation. Arch Ophthalmol 1961;65:493–496.
9. Jones LT, Quickert MH, Wobig JL. The cure of ptosis by aponeurotic repair. Arch Ophthalmol 1975;93:629–634.
10. Anderson RL, Beard C. The levator aponeurosis. Arch Ophthalmol 1977;95:1437–1441.
11. Anderson RL, Dixon RS. Aponeurotic ptosis surgery. Arch Ophthalmol 1979;97:1123–1128.
12. Paris GL, Quickert MH. Disinsertion of the aponeurosis of the levator palpebrae superior muscle after cataract extraction. Am J Ophthalmol 1976;81:337–340.
13. Older JJ. Levator aponeurosis disinsertion in the young adult: a cause of ptosis. Arch Ophthalmol 1978;96:1857–1858.
14. Older JJ. Levator aponeurosis surgery for the correction of acquired ptosis. Ophthalmology 1983;90:1056–1059.
15. Carroll RP. Cautery dissection in levator surgery. Ophthalmic Plast Reconstr Surg 1988;4:243–247.
16. Wilkes TDI, Adams DF. Involutional (senile) ptosis. Geri Ophthalmol 1986;2:14–22.
17. Wilkins RB, Patipa M. The recognition of acquired ptosis in patients considered for upper-eyelid blepharoplasty. Plast Reconstr Surg 1982;70:431–434.
18. Baker SS, Muenzler WS, Small RG, Leonard JE. Carbon dioxide laser blepharoplasty. Ophthalmology 1984;91:238–243.
19. Wesley RE, Bond JB. Carbon dioxide laser in ophthalmic plastic and orbital surgery. Ophthalmic Surg 1985;16:631–633.
20. Gregory RD. Letter to the editor. Ophthalmology 1985;92:52A.
21. Mittleman H, Apfelberg DB. Carbon dioxide laser blepharoplasty: advantages and disadvantages. Ann Plastic Surg 1990;24:1–6.
22. Flaharty PM, Anderson RL. Lasers in oculoplastic surgery. In: Benson WE, Marshall J, Spaeth GL, eds. Annual of ophthalmic laser surgery. Philadelphia: BC Decker, 1991.
23. David LM, Sanders G. CO_2 laser blepharoplasty: a comparison to cold steel and electrocautery. J Dermatol Surg Oncol 1987;13:110–114.
24. Baker SS. Carbon dioxide laser upper lid blepharoplasty. Am J Cosmetic Surg 1992;9:141–145.
25. Morrow DM, Morrow LB. CO_2 laser blepharoplasty: a comparison with cold steel surgery. J Dermatol Surg Oncol 1992;18:307–313.
26. Baker SS, Glaser DA. Periorbital and Facial Laser Applications. Missouri: Medical Video Production, 1996.
27. David LM, Baker SS. David-Baker Eyelid Retractor. Am J Cosmetic Surg 1992;9:147–148.
28. Sevel D. Ptosis and underaction of the superior rectus muscle. Ophthalmol 1984;91:1080.
29. von Noorden GK. Burian-von Noorden's binocular vision and ocular motility: theory and management of strabismus, 3rd ed. St. Louis: CV Mosby, 1985:66–69.
30. Putnam JR, Nunery WR, Tanenbaum M, McCord CD Jr. Blepharoptosis. In: McCord CD Jr, Tanenbaum M, Nunery WR, eds. Oculoplastic surgery, 3rd ed. New York: Raven Press, 1995:192–193.
31. Enzer YR, Shorr N. Medical and surgical management of chemosis after blepharoplasty. Ophthal Plast Reconstr Surg 1994;10(1):57–63.
32. Bergin DJ. Anatomy of the eyelids, lacrimal system, and orbit. In: McCord CD Jr, Tanenbaum M, Nunery W, eds. Oculoplastic surgery, 3rd ed. New York: Raven Press, 1995:75–77.
33. Jones LT. The anatomy of the lower eyelid and its relations to the cause and cure of ectropion. Am J Ophthalmol 1961:66:111.
34. Hill JC. Analysis of senile changes in the palpebral fissure. Trans Ophthalmol Soc UK 1975;95:49.
35. Bosniak SL, Zilkha MC. Ectropion. In: Nesi FA, Lisman RD, Levine MR, eds. Smith's ophthalmic plastic and reconstructive surgery, 2nd ed. St. Louis: Mosby, 1997:290.
36. Snellen H. Suture for ectropion. Congr Int Ophthalmol 1862;236.

37. Ziegler SL. Galvanocautery puncture in ectropion and entropion. JAMA 1909;53:183-186.
38. Kuhnt H. Beitrage zur operationen augenheilkunder. Jena, Germany: G. Fischer, 1883:45-55.
39. Bick MW. Surgical management of orbital tarsal disparity. Arch Ophthalmol 1966;75:386.
40. Tenzel RR, Buffam FV, Miller GR. The use of the "lateral canthal sling" in ectropion repair. Can J Ophthalmol 1977;12:199-202.
41. Anderson RL, Gordy DD. The tarsal strip procedure. Arch Ophthalmol 1979;97:2192-2196.
42. Baker SS, Pham RTH. Lateral canthal tendon suspension using the carbon dioxide laser: a modified technique. Dermatol Surg 1995;21:1071-1073.
43. Dutton JJ. Atlas of clinical and surgical orbital anatomy. Philadelphia: WB Saunders, 1994:116.
44. May M. Facial paralysis, peripheral type: a proposed method of reporting. Laryngoscope 1970;80:331.
45. Cahill KV, Buerger GF, Sheppard JD. Ectropion of the lower eyelid. In: Hornblass AH, ed. Oculoplastic, orbital and reconstructive surgery. Baltimore: Williams & Wilkins, 1988;1:370-377.
46. Bartley GB, Kay PP. Posterior lamellar eyelid reconstruction with a hard palate mucosal graft. Am J Ophthalmol 1989;107:609-612.
47. Silver B. The use of mucous membrane from the hard palate in the treatment of trichiasis and cicatricial entropion. Ophthal Plast Reconstr Surg 1986;2:129-131.
48. Shorr N, Christenury JD, Goldberg RA. Tarsoconjunctival grafts for upper eyelid cicatricial entropion. Ophthalmic Surg 1988;19:316-320.
49. Tenzel RR, Miller GR, Rubenzik R. Cicatricial upper lid entropion treated with banked scleral graft. Arch Ophthalmol 1975;93:999-1000.
50. Lyon DB, Dortzbach RK. Entropion, trichiasis, and distichiasis. In: Dortzbach RK, ed. Ophthalmic plastic surgery: prevention and management of complications. New York: Raven Press, 1994:31-48.
51. McCord CD, Chen WP. Tarsal polishing and mucous membrane grafting for cicatricial entropion, trichiasis and epidermalization. Ophthalmic Surg 1983;14:1021-1025.
52. Tse D, Anderson RL. Aponeurosis disinsertion in congenital entropion. Arch Ophthalmol 1983;101:436-440.
53. Sisler HA, Labay GR, Finaly JR. Senile ectropion and entropion. A comparative histopathological study. Ann Ophthalmol 1976;8:319-322.
54. Jones LT. The anatomy of the lower eyelid and its relation to the cause and care of entropion. Am J Ophthalmol 1960;49:29-36.
55. Martin RT, Nunery WM, Tanenbaum M. Entropion, trichiasis, and distichiasis. In: McCord CD Jr, Tanenbaum M, Nunery W, eds. Oculoplastic surgery, 3rd ed. New York, Raven Press: 1995:221-248.
56. Jones LT, Reeh MJ, Wobig JL. Senile entropion: a new concept for correction. Am J Ophthalmol 1972;74:327-329.
57. Hargis JL. Inferior aponeurosis vs. orbital septum tucking for senile entropion. Arch Ophthalmol 1973;89:210-213.
58. Wheeler JM. Spastic entropion corrected by orbicularis transplantation. Trans Am Ophthalmol Soc 1938;36:157-162.
59. Bracup DH. Modified Wheeler orbicularis overlap procedure for senile entropion. Ophthalmic Surg 1979;10:35-40.

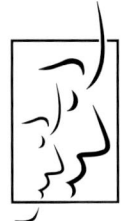

Chapter Twelve

Laser-Assisted Rejuvenation of the Upper and Lower Face

Cynthia Weinstein

LASERS IN UPPER FACIAL REJUVENATION

Introduction

The aesthetic surgeon is increasingly challenged to achieve improved surgical results with lower postoperative morbidity. Advances in laser technology and minimally invasive surgical instrumentation and techniques allow these goals to be met with increasing effectiveness. The current approach to facial rejuvenation uses a combination of techniques including endoscopic forehead lifting, laser-assisted blepharoplasty and rhytidectomy, and laser skin resurfacing.

AGING OF THE FACE

Facial changes associated with aging include gravitational descent of tissues, solar elastosis, herniation of orbital fat, and excessive contraction of facial muscles. The lateral portion of the eyebrows (which is not well supported by the occipitofrontalis muscle), and the lower face ("jowls") are particularly sensitive to the effects of gravity. Herniation of orbital fat in the upper and lower eyelids produces a tired, aged appearance and may occur idiopathically in young patients, or because of age-related weakening of the orbital septum in older individuals. Sun damage to the skin is cumulative, ultimately leading to solar elastosis with destruction of dermal collagen and elastic fibers, dyspigmentation, wrinkling, and laxity of the skin (See Chapter 3 for a more detailed discussion of actinic damage). These changes are most evident in the periorbital and perioral regions and on the cheeks, but also appear on the forehead. Muscular activity leads to dynamic movement lines, especially in the glabella, forehead, and lateral periorbital regions. Hyperkinetic facial lines often appear more prominent if the overlying skin is extensively damaged.

FACIAL REJUVENATION

Ideals of beauty are established by societal norms, which are often reflected in fashion magazines. These norms vary from culture to culture, often evolve with time, and must be recognized by the aesthetic surgeon. Today, most Western societies' ideals include smooth, unblemished skin that does not sag, high, arched, eyebrows, upper eyelids with a well-defined crease and a platform to apply makeup, smooth lower eyelids and a sharply defined jaw line (1, 2).

The Evolution of Surgical Techniques

Surgical rejuvenation of the face has traditionally required extensive surgical procedures capable of producing excellent results, but carried significant morbidity and were not always used appropriately. For example, elevation of the eyebrows and rejuvenation of the forehead was traditionally performed though long coronal or pretrichial incisions. Although these procedures were highly effective, their public acceptance was poor because of concerns about scarring, scalp numbness, alopecia, excessive medial brow elevation with a subsequent "startled" appearance, unwanted increases in the eyebrow-hairline distance, and the perception that these were major operations (3, 4). Similarly, upper eyelid blepharoplasty is an excellent procedure for treating dermatochalasis and herniated orbital fat. However, failure to recognize a superimposed eyebrow ptosis will produce worsened brow ptosis, crowding of the eyelid-eyebrow complex, and an unacceptable aesthetic result. Traditional transcutaneous lower eyelid blepharoplasty is known to produce an ectropion or scleral show in some patients, even when surgery is performed well and precautions (such as suspension of the orbicularis oculi muscle to the lateral orbital rim) are taken (5). Surgical rejuvenation of the lower face is another procedure traditionally perceived as dangerous, but may now be accomplished with increased success and decreased morbidity.

To avoid some problems associated with traditional facial rejuvenation techniques, an improved understanding of facial aesthetics and new surgical approaches has been developed. The coronal and pretrichial brow lifting procedures have been largely replaced by the endoscopic forehead lift. This procedure has become increasingly popular as it offers the advantages of smaller incisions and lower postoperative morbidity while producing a natural result. The rationale behind this operation is adjusting the eyebrow position by altering the relationship between the elevator and depressor muscles of the eyebrow and forehead, without increasing the eyebrow-hairline distance (6–8). As discussed in Chapter 2, eyebrow elevation occurs through the action of the frontalis muscle, while brow depression occurs through the actions of the orbicularis oculi, depressor supercilia, corrugator, and procerus muscles. If the brow depressors can be inactivated and the underlying periosteum released, the unopposed action of the occipitofrontalis muscle will elevate the brow to a higher and more youthful position. While this operation offers significant advantages over open techniques, it is less effective in elevating and fixating the lateral third of the eyebrow, which is unaffected by the occipitofrontalis muscle (9). Although the corrugator and procerus muscles are often regarded as the major depressors of the eyebrow, the effect of the orbic-

ularis oculi muscle as a significant factor in brow depression must be recognized. The orbicularis oculi muscle is largely unaffected by the traditional endoscopic browlift procedure. Furthermore, if significant dermatochalasis is present in the upper eyelids, the browlift procedure alone will not produce an acceptable aesthetic result without concomitant upper blepharoplasty.

The ideals of upper facial rejuvenation are often best met via a combination of surgical and laser techniques. The combined approach recommended today may include laser blepharoplasty, minimal incision forehead lifting, transblepharoplasty resections of "frown" muscles, and cutaneous laser resurfacing. Each of these procedures addresses one or more of the changes associated with aging of the upper face. Laser blepharoplasty and transblepharoplasty resection of frown muscles allow excess skin and fat to be removed from the upper eyelid, permit the resection of the frown muscles, namely the depressor supercilia portion of the orbicularis oculi and the corrugator supercilia muscles under direct visualization, and provide easy access to the periosteum of the orbital rim, precluding the need for work at a distant site under a flap (10–16).

Indications for the Combined Approach to Upper Facial Rejuvenation

Many candidates are eligible for the combined upper facial rejuvenation procedure. Those who would benefit most are often older than the age of 50. Males are often better candidates for the combined approach as fewer and smaller incisions in the scalp are placed where the hair may be receding. While males may not tolerate the prolonged erythema of CO_2 laser resurfacing as readily as females, Er:YAG resurfacing as a good option remains for them. Patients with high foreheads and thus a long brow to hairline distance may benefit from the "shrinkage" of skin that may occur following CO_2 laser resurfacing; those with severe lateral brow ptosis benefit from the permanent fixation of the lateral brow. Other candidates for this procedure are those patients who have brow ptosis in addition to excess skin and fat on the upper eyelid, and/or severe actinic damage.

Preoperative Assessment

Many patients believe that their upper facial aging and tired appearance are caused by excess skin on the eyelids alone. They attribute the hooded appearance to loose skin, and rarely realize that in fact, brow descent has led to the "crowded" appearance of the eye region. If a brow lift is suggested, patients are not only surprised, but frequently shy away from such a procedure. The patient's ability to decide may be enhanced by computer imaging, which can display the expected result following blepharoplasty, browlifting, or a combination of both procedures (with or without concomitant laser skin resurfacing). If a digital imaging system is unavailable, manual elevation of the eyebrows and eyelids may be useful while the patient looks into a hand-held mirror (Figure 12.1A and B).

Marking the Patient

The success of the combined approach to upper facial rejuvenation is entirely dependent on proper placement of preoperative markings. Marks are made in the scalp, the upper eyelid, and on the forehead. Five incisions are usu-

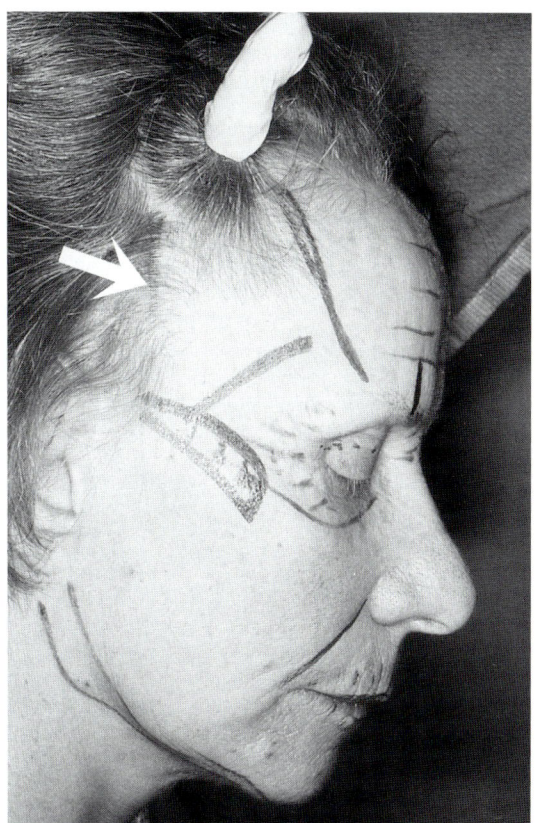

Figure 12.2. The temporal incision is aligned with the lateral orbital rim and the ala of the nose (arrow).

ally marked on the scalp: 2 in the temporal region, 2 paramedian, and 1 in the midline. The temporal incisions are made parallel and 1 cm posterior to the temporal hairline. The incision should be bisected by the extension of a line drawn from the ala of the nose to the lateral canthal angle (Figure 12.2). Paramedian incisions are made obliquely, in line with the ala of the nose and the mid pupil. The central incision is made vertically in the midline. Each incision is approximately 2 cm long. The upper eyelid incision is marked in the standard method for upper eyelid blepharoplasty (see Chapter 9). The brow may be manually elevated to its approximate postoperative position so that an excessive amount of skin will not be removed from the eyelids. The approximate locations of important surgical landmarks are marked on the eyebrow and forehead to help the surgeon maintain correct orientation and preserve vital structures during the procedure. Supraorbital and supratrochlear neurovascular bundles are marked in relation to the eyebrow. The supraorbital nerve emerges from the supraorbital notch or foramen before coursing into the forehead to supply sensation to most of this region (Figure 12.3). The supraorbital notch, when present,

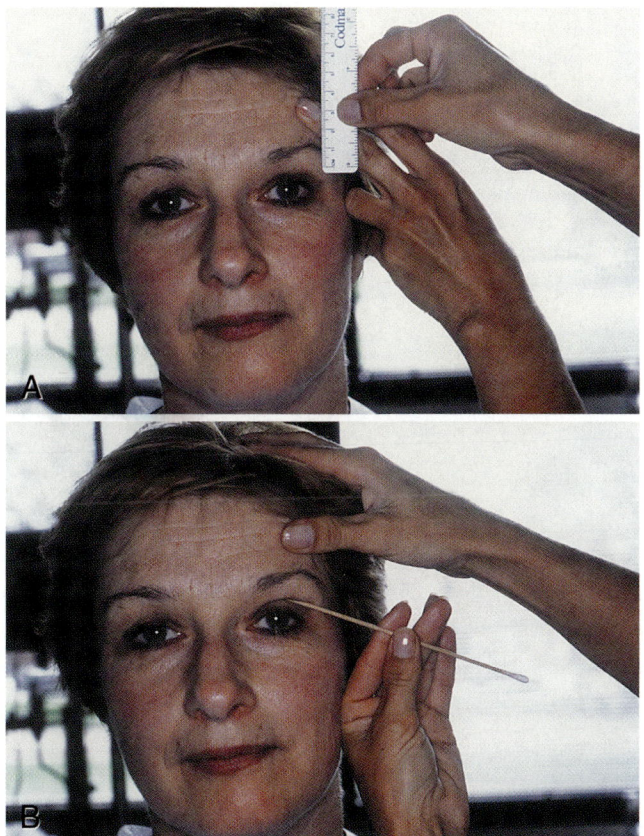

Figure 12.1. A. Manual demonstration of lateral brow lift. **B.** Manual demonstration of combined blepharoplasty and lateral brow lift.

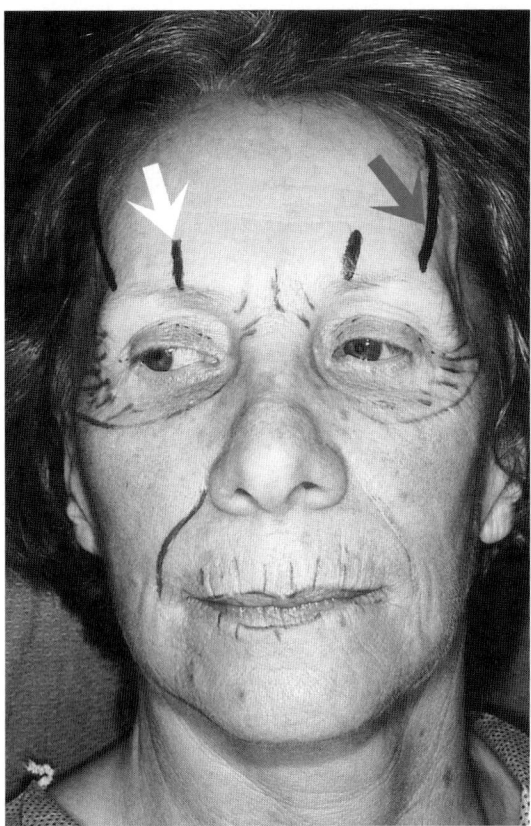

Figure 12.3. Important landmarks for the supraorbital nerve (white arrow), and the temporal crest (dark arrow).

is readily palpable. Medial to the supraorbital nerve is the supratrochlear nerve, which supplies sensation to a small area on the medial forehead. The frontal branch of the facial nerve is perhaps the most important structure in the forehead and temple. It travels superficially in the superficial temporalis (temporoparietal) fascia through the temporal region above the malar arch. A nerve trajectory is approximated by a line drawn from the tragus of the ear to the lateral aspect of the eyebrow (Figure 12.4). The temporal crest is also marked, indicating the transition from the central forehead pocket, where the dissection will be in the subperiosteal plane, to the temporal pocket, where the dissection will be between the superficial and deep temporalis fascia (Figure 12.3).

Anesthesia

Although general anesthesia is favored by many surgeons, regional nerve blocks and direct local infiltration, in combination with intravenous sedation, is often adequate. A regional blockade of the supraorbital and supratrochlear

nerves may be achieved by injecting approximately 1cc of anesthetic in the region of each supraorbital notch. Local anesthetic is injected directly into the eyelid and scalp incision sites, along the malar arch, and into the subperiosteal plane, to provide hemostasis with anesthesia. The preferred choice of anesthetic agents is a combination of 2% lidocaine containing 1:200,000 epinephrine and 0.5% bupivacaine, mixed in a 3:1 lidocaine to bupivacaine ratio. The injection is administered using 25-gauge or 27-gauge needles, and approximately 20 cc of mixture is required.

The Procedure

The eyelid portion of the procedure is performed first. The globe is initially protected using an anodized Baker-David clamp, and the eyelid incisions are made with the carbon dioxide laser in continuous wave (CW) mode setting at 5 W. The predetermined amount of skin and orbicularis muscle are removed, the septum incised, and fat pads removed, as described in Chapter 9. An incision is

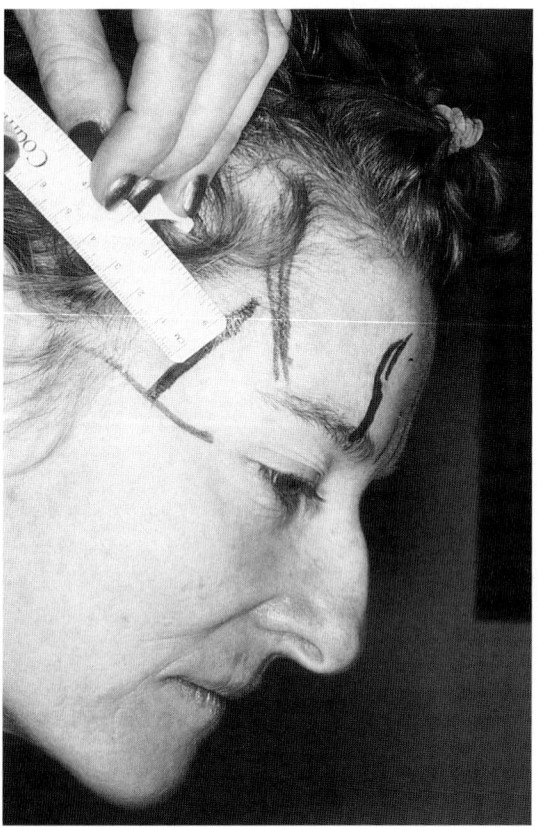

Figure 12.4. The frontal branch of the facial nerve is marked (pointed by the ruler).

then made with the laser set at 5 W CW in the infrabrow subcutaneous tissue and carried through the periosteum of the orbital rim. The medial aspect of the incision will quickly reveal the depressor supercilia portion of the orbicularis oculi muscle, which is paler in color than the corrugator muscle. This muscle may be readily ablated under direct visualization, using the carbon dioxide laser set at 5 W CW. The corrugator supercilia muscle lies immediately behind the depressor supercilia, and may be easily identified as it is deeper red in color than the surrounding orbicularis oculi muscle. Multiple branches of the supratrochlear nerve may be identified coursing through the corrugator muscle, and an effort should be made to preserve these nerves as the corrugator is ablated. Once the corrugator has been carefully resected, the supraorbital neurovascular bundle may be seen in the subperiosteal space, posterior and lateral to the muscle's origin. The neurovascular bundle should be avoided. The procerus muscle lies medial to the corrugator: it may also be incised or ablated if clinically indicated (Figure 12.5). The laser is then used to make an incision through the tissues overlying the orbital rim until the periosteum is exposed from the supraorbital neurovascular bundle to the lateral orbital rim. Dissection is now directed superiorly, using the carbon dioxide laser to incise the periosteum across the full extent of the superior orbital rim. Care must be taken to avoid entering the supraperiosteal plane as bleeding will occur. Once the incision is complete, a periosteal elevator is used to open the subperiosteal space superiorly to the scalp margin. Laterally, the dissec-

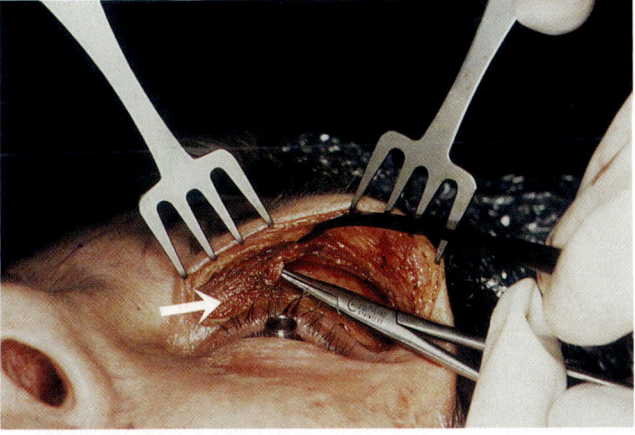

Figure 12.5. An incision is made superiorly to identify the depressor supercilia and corrugator muscles (white arrow). The supraorbital nerve is lateral and posterior to these muscles, and lies below the periosteum (artery forceps point to the nerve).

tion must be carried only as far as the temporal crest, where the superficial and deep temporalis fascias fuse with the periosteum (see Chap 2 for a more detailed description of the anatomy of the temporal region). Dissecting beyond the temporal crest from a medial to lateral direction may result in entry into the wrong plane, with subsequent injury to the frontal branch of the facial nerve. Virtually the whole central forehead may be released through the eyelid incision. Once complete release has been achieved, this pocket is packed with gauze soaked in dilute epinephrine solution (1:200,000), and attention is turned to the scalp. The goal of the next portion of the procedure is to create a pocket between the superficial and deep layers of temporalis fascia, which is then connected with the previously created central pocket, thus freeing the eyebrows and entire forehead. To reiterate, the temporal compartment of the forehead must be dissected before further dissection of the central compartment to avoid injury to the frontal branch of the facial nerve. A temporal incision is made with a #15 Bard Parker blade; the laser should not be used as thermal damage to the hair follicles and peri-incisional alopecia will result. The incision is carried down to the level of the deep temporalis fascia, a thick, shiny-white structure that lies directly over the temporalis muscle. The loose areolar plane between the superficial and deep temporalis fascia is bluntly dissected inferiorly to the lateral orbital rim and medially to the temporal crest. The frontal branch of the facial nerve lies above the plane of dissection, and therefore should be well protected. Even with the help of an endoscope, the nerve can rarely be seen. Blunt dissection is also carried out posteriorly and past the orbital rim to join with the previous eyelid dissection. The temporal crest is released by sweeping a periosteal elevator in a temporal-to-nasal direction, allowing the temporal compartment and central compartments to join in the subperiosteal plane. Once the temporal pocket has been completely dissected, the blade is used to make an incision in the previously marked paramedian sites. These incisions are carried down to bone, and a periosteal elevator is introduced and used to release the periosteum: posteriorly to the occiput, and anteriorly to 2 cm above the orbital rim. This joins the previous dissection from the eyelid. The endoscope may be introduced at this point, to ensure complete periosteal release to the level of the orbital rim. A central incision may also be made if medial brow ptosis or horizontal lines at the nasal root are being addressed, but is otherwise unnecessary.

Once the eyelid and scalp dissections are complete, the forehead and brow must be fixed into position. Much debate exists concerning the best method of forehead fixation (17). Undoubtedly, adequate release of the periosteum is very important in obtaining long-lasting forehead elevation. Fixation of the lateral brow is especially important as brow ptosis is usually more marked laterally than medially. Furthermore, the sole brow elevator, the occipitofrontalis muscle, does not extend laterally to the temporal crest and thus exerts little effect on the lateral brow. As the lone source of support for the lateral brow must be provided intraoperatively, a sturdy, permanent suture such as 2-0 or 3-0 nylon is used to fix the lateral eyebrow to the temporalis muscle. The suture is passed via the temporal incision, from the subcutaneous tissue immediately under the lateral eyebrow posteriorly, where it is placed through the deep temporalis fascia and part of the temporalis muscle. The degree of lateral brow elevation can be varied by adjusting the placement and tension on the suture. Fixation of the arch of the eyebrow is achieved via the paramedian incision. Either screw fixation with a Mitek Anchor or a 2.0 mm Tacit Anchor (Ethicon, Somerville, NJ), or a similar device, is used to anchor the brow in position. One advantage of using Mitek fixation screws is that they may be left in position permanently. A subcutaneous permanent suture, such as 2-0 Ethibond (Ethicon, Somerville, NJ), is passed through the anchoring screw and the anterior aspect of the paramedian incision and permanently left in place. The position of the fixation device compared with the anterior aspect of the incision will determine the amount of brow elevation. Fixation of the medial brow can be achieved through the central incision if medial brow ptosis is present. Elevation of the medial brow should be performed carefully to avoid producing an unnatural appearance. Wound closure may be according to the surgeon's preference. The scalp incisions are closed with skin staples, and the eyelid incision is closed with permanent sutures.

Once the forehead has been elevated, and sufficient eyelid skin and fat excised, the skin is resurfaced with either a carbon dioxide or Er:YAG laser. If significant actinic damage is present and full face resurfacing is being performed, the carbon dioxide laser is chosen. Alternately, if wrinkling is milder, localized resurfacing is being performed, or the patient is male, the Er:YAG is preferred. If a segmental treatment is performed, the forehead and periorbital areas are treated. Segmental treatments should not be performed on patients with significant actinic damage. Laser resurfacing may be performed in the standard manner because of the excellent vascular supply of the forehead.

The end point of treatment with the Er:YAG laser differs from that sought when the carbon dioxide laser is used. Because of the high coefficient of absorption of water for Er:YAG laser energy, treatment with this laser produces far less coagulative necrosis than the carbon dioxide laser. Consequently, the true skin architecture is more readily visible, especially if magnification is used. Once the papillary dermis is entered, collagen bundles seem regular, as do the appendages. Pinpoint bleeding may occur. Once the reticular dermis is entered, collagen bundles appear more haphazard, the follicles wider, and splotchy bleeding may occur. The skin contraction noted with carbon dioxide laser skin resurfacing does not occur when the Er:YAG is used. Instead, with aggressive treatment, wrinkle lines may be seen to disappear, as a result of the truly ablative properties of Er:YAG lasers (18) (Figures 12.6A-D to 12.8A and B).

Postoperative Care

Postoperatively, all patients receive broad-spectrum antibiotics until the resurfacing wounds have healed. Antiviral agents must be used in patients with a history of *Herpes simplex* and in some areas are considered standard of care for any patient undergoing skin resurfacing. A short course of oral steroids may be administered to help reduce postoperative edema. The resurfaced skin may be treated with either an open or a closed dressing technique until reepithelialization is complete. A compression dressing is placed on the forehead; drains are not required. Postoperative care for the eyelids is as outlined in Chapter 9. Skin staples are removed on approximately postoperative day 7.

Once the skin has fully reepithelialized, an ultraviolet-A blocking sunscreen containing titanium dioxide is introduced. A tinted sunscreen will provide even greater protection from UV-A light. An oil-free, nonirritating moisturizer and cleanser are also introduced to avoid contact irritant and allergic dermatitis and postoperative acne. All patients receive a prophylactic bleaching preparation when reepithelialization has occurred, usually between days 10 and 14. Patients with Fitzpatrick skin types 1, 2, and 3 use hydroquinone 2%, with or without glycolic acid, beginning alternate nights for the first week, and then every night for 4–6 weeks. Patients with skin type 4 are treated with hydroquinone 2%, kojic acid 2%, and glycolic acid 18%. This combination is available in a mixture known as Pigment Gel Forte (Physician's Choice).

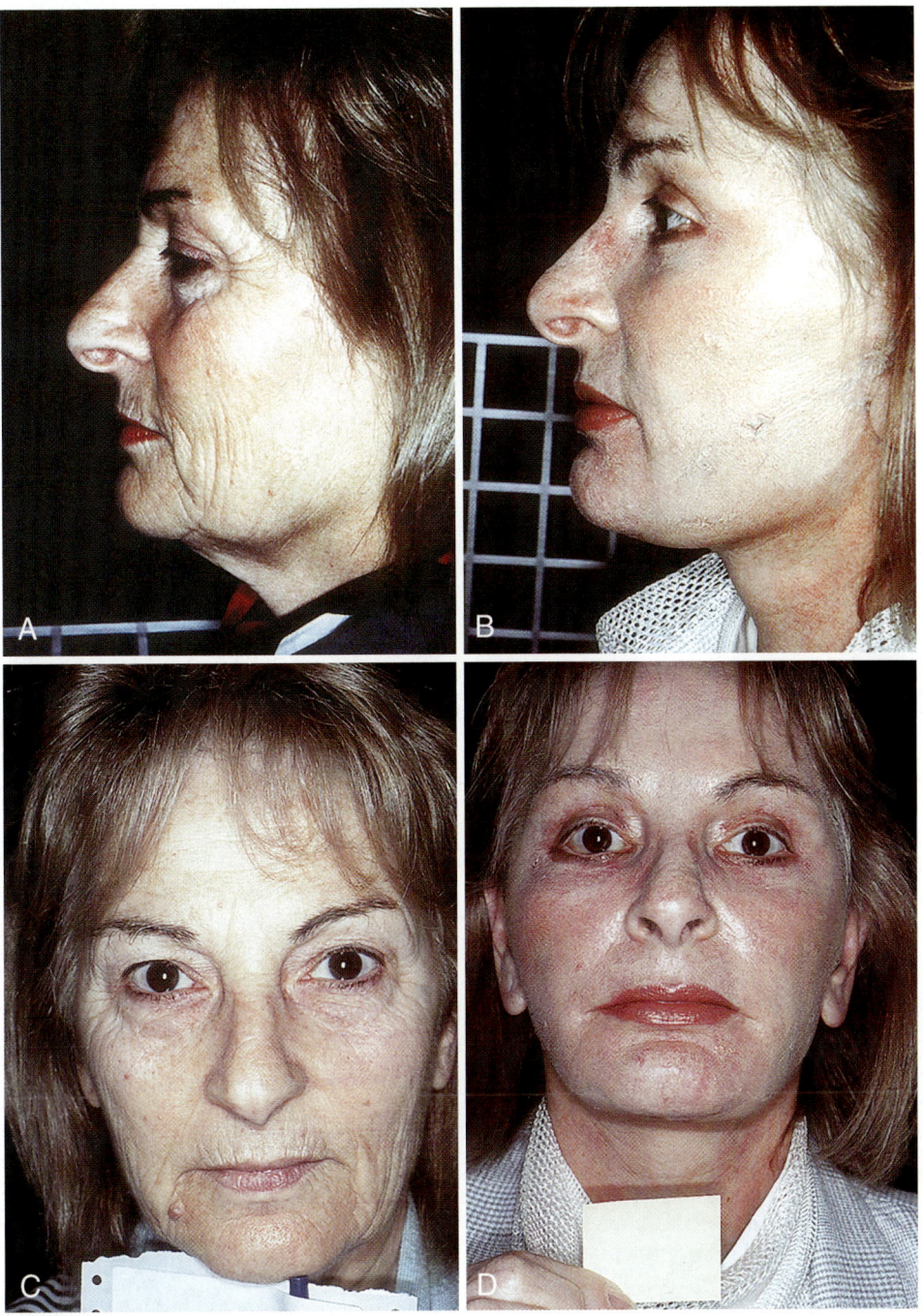

Figure 12.6. A. 58-year-old female before laser-assisted brow, face, and neck lift, laser-assisted upper and lower blepharoplasty, and full face Er:YAG laser skin resurfacing. A scanning handpiece was used with the following parameters: Flu-ence = 15 J/cm² on forehead, periorbital, perioral, and central cheek regions, and 10 J/cm² on the lateral cheek; number of passes = 2–3. **B.** Results after 3 weeks. **C.** Frontal view, pre-operatively. **D.** Frontal view, 3 weeks postoperatively.

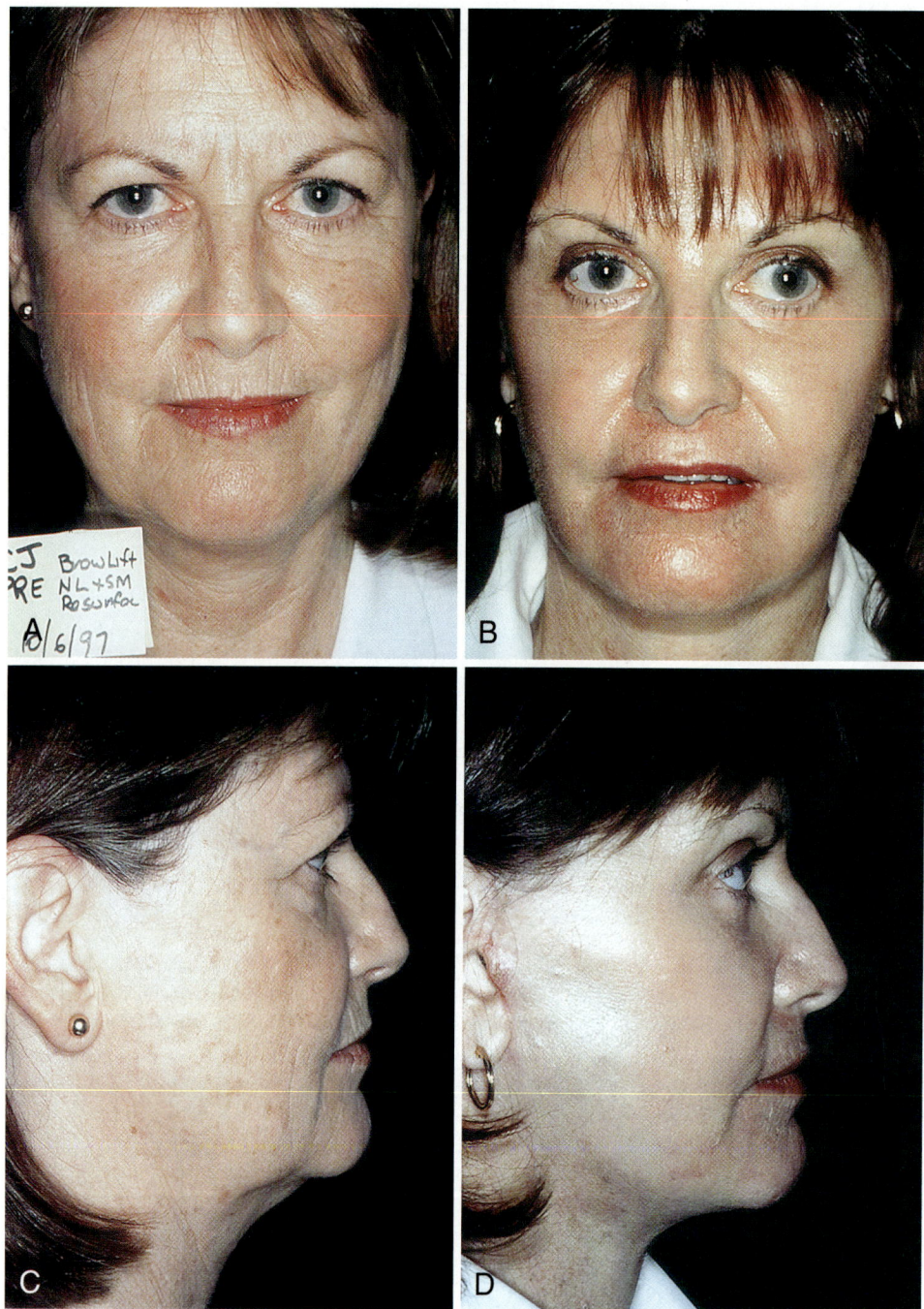

Figure 12.7. A. 56-year-old female before laser-assisted face and neck lift, laser-assisted upper and lower blepharoplasty, and full face Er:YAG laser skin resurfacing. A scanning handpiece was used with the following parameters: Fluence = 15 J/cm² on the forehead, periorbital, perioral, and central cheek regions and 10 J/cm² on the lateral cheek; number of passes = 2–3. **B.** Results 3 weeks post operatively. **C.** Profile view, preoperatively. **D.** Profile view, postoperatively.

Patients with Fitzpatrick skin types 5 and 6 require 2.5% hydroquinone, with 0.05% retinoic acid. Sometimes breakthrough pigmentation occurs, requiring stronger bleaching preparations. This is more likely to occur following carbon dioxide laser resurfacing (19).

Complications

As with all newer techniques, complications decrease once experience is gained. Care must be taken to understand and respect the anatomy of the forehead and

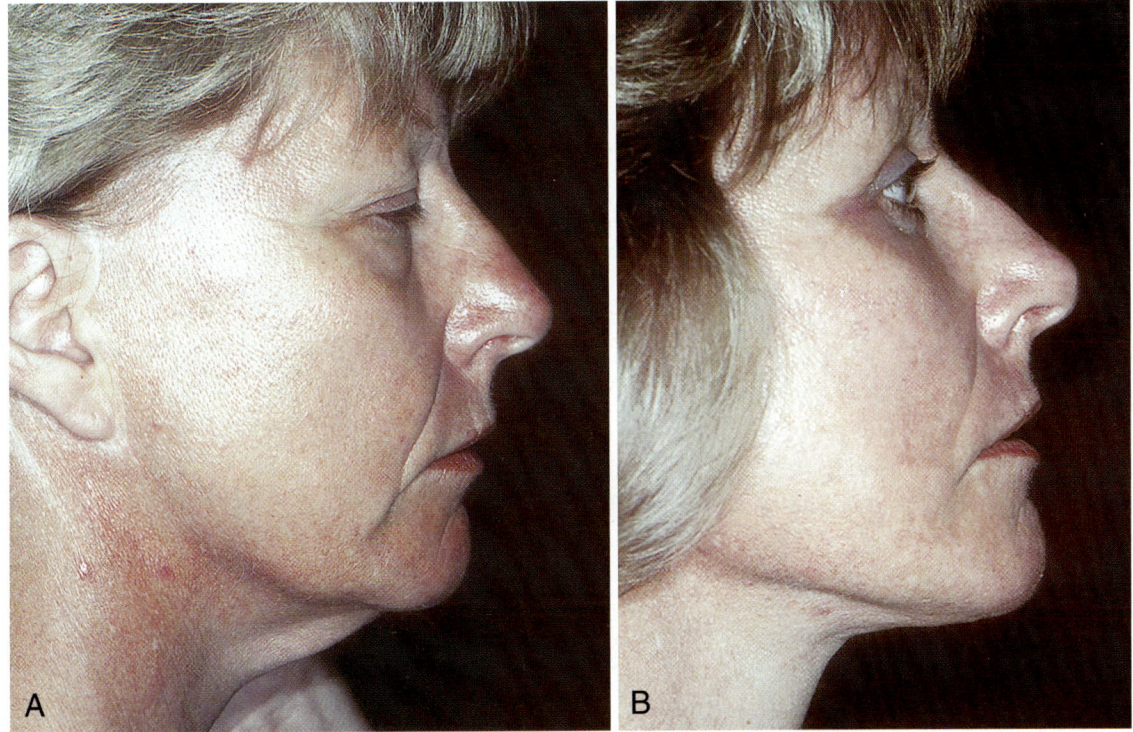

Figure 12.8. A. 55-year-old female before laser-assisted face and neck lift, and CO_2 laser skin resurfacing of the forehead, perioral, periorbital, and central cheek regions.
B. Results 6 weeks postoperatively.

temporal region (see Chapter 2). The supraorbital and supratrochlear nerves may be injured with resection of the frown muscles, particularly the depressor supercilia of the orbicularis oculi and the corrugator muscles. The supraorbital neurovascular bundle may be directly visualized and should be spared without difficulty: fibers of the supratrochlear nerve run through the corrugator muscle and are susceptible to injury. Preservation of these fibers will avoid bothersome numbness of the forehead. Inadequate resection of the brow depressors may result in failure to eliminate, or recurrence of, deep glabellar and forehead lines. The balance between adequate resection and injury to the nerve must be carefully maintained. As the muscles are resected under direct visualization, the nerves should be clearly visible and thus somewhat easy to protect. While injury to sensory nerves is undesirable, injury to the frontal branch of the facial nerve can have devastating consequences. Injury may occur with partial or complete transection or simply as a result of intraoperative traction or manipulation. To avoid this complication, dissection in the temporal region must be performed below the plane of the temporoparietal fascia, and the temporal pocket should always be connected with the central pocket by dividing the temporal crest from a lateral to medial direction. Asymmetry of the eyelids and brows may be avoided by marking patients in both a supine and upright position preoperatively, and by sitting patients up intraoperatively. Complete periosteal release and adequate fixation are also important for symmetry. Recurrent brow ptosis is most likely to occur laterally where support for the brow is minimal. Every effort should be made to secure the lateral brow firmly to the temporalis muscle using a permanent suture. Excessive eyelid skin resection, especially when aggressive brow elevation is planned, can result in lagophthalmos, keratitis, and even visual loss. Hematoma formation under the flap is uncommon when the laser is used to resect and ablate the brow depressors. Drains are generally not required. Several large veins, which may be seen well with the endoscope, may be present in the region of the temporal crest. If present, these veins should be closed with a bipolar cautery before their division. Hair loss may occur if the laser is used to make scalp incisions, or if excessive friction develops from manipulation of the endoscope. Scalp incisions should therefore not be made with the laser, and endoscopic protectors may be used to reduce trauma to the wound edges caused by the endoscope itself. If hair loss does occur, hair transplantation may be helpful. Infection may occur after any surgical or skin resurfacing procedure. With adequate antibiotic prophylaxis and good sterile technique, this complication is unlikely. The complications of skin resurfacing are well known and are discussed in detail in Chapter 7. Necrosis of the flap is very rare, but may occur if excessively deep laser resurfacing is performed. As the blood supply to the forehead is so rich, and the dissection is performed in a deep avascular plane, endoscopic forehead lifting may be successfully combined with laser resurfacing.

Conclusion

The combination of laser blepharoplasty, endoscopic forehead lifting, and laser skin resurfacing addresses all the components of upper facial aging. The use of lasers can advance both the incisional and resurfacing aspects of this procedure.

LASERS IN LOWER FACIAL REJUVENATION

Introduction

Manifestations of aging in the lower face are represented in the skin and in the relationship of the subcutaneous tissues to the overlying skin and underlying muscle. The clinical and histopathologic changes associated with age and actinic damage are detailed in chapters 3, 5, and 6. Subcutaneous tissues become inelastic and sag under gravitational influence, producing heavy nasolabial folds, jowling, and loss of a clearly defined jaw line (20). While rejuvenation of the skin may be readily accomplished with skin resurfacing techniques, repositioning of subcutaneous tissues to rejuvenate the facial structure requires rhytidectomy.

LASERS IN RHYTIDECTOMY

Although the CO_2 laser has gained wide acceptance in periorbital incisional surgery, it has not been as useful an adjunct to rhytidectomy. When used to incise nonhair-bearing skin, the laser often produces aesthetically unacceptable scars; when used in hair-bearing skin, peri-incisional alopecia results (see Chapter 13). While subcutaneous dissection may be performed with the laser, this is more tedious than a traditional approach. If a deep plane lift is being performed (21), the laser may be used to enhance the SMAS dissection. Typical parameters include

a power setting of 5 W CW with a beam no more than 0.2 mm in diameter. The dissection should not proceed beyond the anterior border of the parotid gland to avoid injury to the facial nerve. Occasionally power settings as high as 8–10 W may be required. The laser should not be used in the sub-SMAS plane inferior to the parotid gland.

Skin Resurfacing and Rhytidectomy

Skin resurfacing and rhytidectomy are complementary procedures: the former addresses the skin, the latter addresses the deeper facial structures. Using CO_2 techniques, skin resurfacing was either avoided entirely or performed only lightly because of concerns about wound healing and skin necrosis, especially in the lateral cheek where the blood supply is more tenuous.

The Er:YAG laser produces only a minimal amount of residual thermal damage and has been used successfully at the time of rhytidectomy. In contrast to the CO_2 laser, the Er:YAG is used as aggressively as necessary to produce the desired clinical result, even over the lateral cheek. Computer-driven scanning handpieces are used with a square pattern and 30% overlap of spots. The laser is set at 20 Hz and the fluences used are approximately 15 J/cm^2 over the medial cheeks and 10 J/cm^2 over the lateral cheeks. Two-to-three passes are usually made over the medial cheeks and no more than 2 passes should be made over the lateral cheeks. The orientation of the laser handpiece is changed after each pass to avoid producing a "printed" appearance when the wounds heal.

The Er:YAG laser is also used in the perioral region to efface rhytids. The scanning handpiece is used with a frequency of 20 Hz, 30% overlap of spots, and a fluence of 15 J/cm^2. Three-to-four passes are usually required. Note that the color changes typical of CO_2 resurfacing are not produced by the Er:YAG laser. Surgical endpoints are judged by the elimination of wrinkles or the appearance of the reticular dermis. When viewed under surgical loupe magnification, the papillary dermis has a light pink color and a regular sponge-like appearance with small follicular orifices. In contrast, the reticular dermis has a more coarse and irregular appearance. Postoperative care following skin resurfacing performed concomitantly with rhytidectomy corresponds with the regimens discussed above and in Chapter 6. The rate of epithelialization does not seem to be delayed when Er:YAG resurfacing and rhytidectomy are performed concomitantly.

Precautions

As the ablation threshold for soft tissue is approximately 5 J/cm², the novice laser surgeon should start with more conservative energy settings. Similar conservative measures should also be taken when treating smokers, diabetics, severe hypertensives, or other patients expected to be at increased risk for compromised wound healing. Laser resurfacing may be inappropriate at the time of rhytidectomy when treating high-risk patients. Clinical data are needed to define the relative safety of treating these patients.

Combined CO₂ and Er:YAG Techniques for Skin Resurfacing

When full face skin resurfacing is performed with the CO₂ laser, the amount and duration of postoperative erythema may be reduced by treating the entire face with 1–2 passes of the Er:YAG laser after the CO₂ treatment is complete. The concept behind this maneuver is to capitalize on the greater soft tissue absorption of Er:YAG energy by ablating some of the thermally damaged tissue left behind by the CO₂ laser. The benefits of this combination have not been quantified, but qualitatively, postoperative erythema appears to be significantly reduced.

CONCLUSION

Lasers play an important role in upper and lower facial rejuvenation. While less valuable as an incisional device in rhytidectomy than in periorbital surgery, newer lasers may be used to safely resurface the skin at the time rhytidectomy is performed. Combining CO₂ and Er:YAG techniques may reduce the amount and duration of postoperative erythema.

REFERENCES

1. Weinstein C. Endoscopic forehead lifting, laser blepharoplasty, transblepharoplasty corrugator resection, and laser resurfacing. J Dermatol Surg. In press.
2. Weinstein C. Endoscopic forehead lift. In: Coleman W, et al, eds. Cosmetic surgery skin. St. Louis: Mosby, 1997;27:421–427.
3. Connell BF, Lambros VS, Neurohr GH. The forehead lift: techniques to avoid complications and produce optimal results. Aesthetic Plast Surg 1989;13:217.
4. Core GB, Vasconez LO, Askren C, et al. Coronal face lift with endoscopic techniques. Plast Surg Forum 1992;1515:227.
5. Carraway JH, Mellow CG. The prevention and treatment of lower lid ectropion following blepharoplasty. Plast Reconstr Surg 1990;85:971.
6. Ramirez OM. Endoscopic techniques in facial rejuvenation. An overview: part 1. Aesthetic Plast Surg 1994;18:141–147.
7. Isse NG. Endoscopic facial rejuvenating: endoforehead, the functional lift: case reports. Aesthetic Plast Surg 1994;18:21.
8. Liang M, Narayanan K. Endoscopic ablation of the frontalis and corrugator muscles—a clinical study. Plast Surg Forum XV, 1992:54.
9. Weinstein C. In: Coleman W, Lawrence N, eds. Endoscopic forehead lifting combined with laser resurfacing. Laser Resurfacing, 1997. In press.
10. Knize DM. Transpalpebral approach to the corrugator supercilia and procerus muscles. Plast Reconstr Surg 1995;95:52–60.
11. Weinstein C. Ultrapulse carbon dioxide laser rejuvenation of facial wrinkles and scars. Am J Cosm Surg 1997;14:3–11.
12. Weinstein C, Alster TS. In: Alster TS, Apfelberg DG, eds. Skin resurfacing with high energy, pulsed carbon dioxide lasers. Cosmetic laser surgery. New York: Wiley & Sons. 1996;9–27.
13. Weinstein C. In: Coleman WP, Hanke WC, et al, eds. Carbon dioxide laser resurfacing. Cosmetic surgery of the skin, 2nd ed. St. Louis: Mosby. 1997;11:152–175.
14. Lask GP, Keller G, Lowe NJ, et al. Laser skin resurfacing with the silk touch flash scanner for facial rhytids. J Dermatol Surg 1995;21:1021–1024.
15. Lowe NJ, Lask GP, Griffin ME, et al. Skin resurfacing with the UltraPulse carbon dioxide laser. J Dermatol Surg 1995;21:1025–1029.
16. Weinstein C, Roberts TL. Aesthetic skin resurfacing with the high energy ultrapulsed CO₂ laser. Clin Plast Surg 1997;24:379–405.
17. Gallaher T, Glover AE, et al. An outer table suspension technique for endoscopic browlift. Aesthetic Plast Surg 1997;21:262–264.
18. Weinstein C. Scanning Erbium:YAG lasers for skin remodeling. J Dermatol Surg 1998. In press.
19. Weinstein C, Ramirez OM, Pozner JN. Post operative care following laser resurfacing: avoiding pitfalls. Plast Reconstr Surg 1998. In press.
20. Owsley JQ. Aesthetic facial surgery. Philadelphia: WB Saunders, 1994:28–31.
21. Hamra ST. The deep plane rhytidectomy. Plast Reconstr Surg 1990;86:53.

Chapter Thirteen

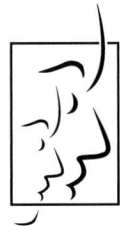

Laser-Assisted Hair Transplantation

Walter P. Unger

Laser hair transplantation began in the Fall of 1993 when Dr. Laurence David and the author began a series of studies utilizing a new UltraPulse laser developed by Coherent Medical Inc (Palo Alto, CA). This laser produces high-energy pulses that are delivered in very brief bursts with intervals between them of less than 695 ms (the thermal relaxation time of skin).

Photomicrographs of incisions made to the depth of superficial subcutaneous tissue showed zones of thermal damage that were less than 70 μ wide at the level of the hair matrix. Hair follicles—whether original or previously transplanted—lying adjacent to an incision made by this laser, could be expected to be spared injury with such narrow zones of thermal damage. In addition, the blood supply to the grafts that would be inserted in these incisions could reasonably be expected to be adequate for survival of graft hair follicles. A series of studies were carried out using this laser and several different hand pieces over a period of several years. The results of the first study involving 10 patients were reported in 1994 (1). It revealed that hair survival in grafts placed into laser-prepared slits, when compared to those placed into conventionally prepared sites in contralateral but otherwise similar locations, was better in 4 of 10 patients, equal in 5 patients, and produced less hair yield in 1 patient. In addition, hair growth occurred earlier in the "laser grafts" in five patients. The author then began studying increasing numbers of grafts each time satisfactory hair growth oc-

curred in previous studies in which smaller numbers were employed. Each study also involved different hand pieces and varying levels of laser energy, power, and time settings. In all the studies, hairs were again counted in grafts transplanted into laser-prepared and scalpel-prepared sites in similar but contralateral locations in the subject's recipient area and were recounted 5 months later. In contrast to what was found in the initial study, there was a delay in hair regrowth rather than accelerated hair regrowth at the laser sites with larger numbers of grafts. On the other hand a more "even" and, therefore, more natural looking distribution of hair was seen in the laser prepared areas when they were compared to the conventionally treated "control" sites (2, 3).

Why Use a Laser for Hair Transplanting at All?

Laser surgery has the obvious advantages of complete control of bleeding in the recipient area, as well as control of the depth of ablation. It is important to note, however, that although all bleeding can be eliminated by increasing the energy (millijoules) of the laser, the goal should not be the absence of all blood. A small amount of bleeding increases the likelihood that the grafts are getting adequate and rapid revascularization. Blood also acts as a "biologic glue," holding the grafts in place and orientated correctly; however, adequate control of bleeding in the recipient area can also be accomplished by other means, such as higher concentrations of epinephrine and better operative technique. The latter also can ensure proper depths of incision sites. Less bleeding and ideal depths of incisions are, therefore, not compelling reasons for buying an expensive machine and learning a new technique. The advantage foreseen as a consequence of using a laser was the production of wider slits that would avoid the compression of slit grafts normally seen when slit sites are prepared with a scalpel. The darker, coarser, and/or more dense the hair, the more potential there is to produce dense, dark lines of hair that are at least as unsightly as is seen with round grafting. In addition, with scalpel slit grafting, no alopecic or potentially alopecic skin is being eliminated as the sites are being prepared and, in addition, the surface area of skin is actually being increased. Therefore, if one is moving the same amount of donor tissue, slit grafting does not produce the same hair density as round grafting will. On the other hand, round grafting tends to look "pluggier." Lastly, because a 0.5 to 1 mm wide graft is being squeezed into a narrow slit when that slit is being made with a scalpel blade, there is an increased opportunity for graft elevation or depression.

All three of these potential drawbacks of conventional slit-grafting—compression, decreased density and graft elevation, or depression—are avoided if the linear recipient site can be made 0.5 to 1 mm wide, for example, by using a laser to ablate tissue in a line. It is important to stress that no cosmetic advantage can be expected if the laser is used to make round recipient sites. The only potential advantages are noncosmetic and include a) decreased bleeding and, therefore, more rapid preparation of sites; b) elimination of the necessity to remove the plug from the recipient site; and c) less chance of a plug being inadvertently left in the hole and buried when a graft is placed over it, resulting in an epidermal cyst.

The author has used both the Coherent UltraPulse and the Sharplan Silktouch (Sharplan Lasers, Allendale, NJ) laser for producing round holes and slits. Initial studies with the Sharplan laser to produce slits instead of round holes were not cosmetically successful and were reported elsewhere (3). The Coherent laser was abandoned for round holes for reasons described below.

TECHNIQUE

The technique of hair transplanting with regard to planning, anesthesia, and donor area preparation is the same as that used in conventional hair transplanting. They are reviewed briefly below.

Planning

It is important to try to estimate the long range donor/recipient area ratio when deciding what proportion of the area of male pattern baldness (MPB) one can reasonably hope to treat. The hairline ideally should begin and end where one expects the *ultimate* anterior-superior most points of the temporal hair will be. These two points should be joined to a midline point that is chosen so that the hairline runs more or less parallel to the ground when viewed laterally or alternately begins where the top of the head begins to flatten out (4, 5). In most patients, it is wise to transplant not only clearly alopecic or thinning areas, but to also transplant through hair-bearing areas that reasonably can be expected to eventually become bald. This minimizes the likelihood of having to "chase" an enlarging bald area (Figure 13.1). In a minority of patients, it is more appropriate to create only an "isolated frontal forelock" (6, 7) making no attempt to attach a midline transplanted "island" of hair to the adjacent temporo-parietal areas (Figure 13.2). In general, one also should not attempt to treat the whole developing bald area without using alopecia reduction (AR) or planning to use AR in the future. The younger the patient, the more important it is to follow this general rule (4).

At present, the author prefers to reserve laser transplanting for individuals with alopecic or nearly alopecic recipient areas. Evaluation of the results of laser trans-

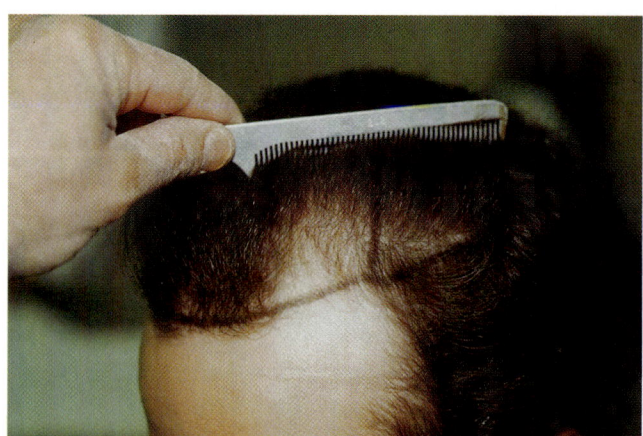

Figure 13.1. In many patients, an area of persisting hair is present superior to the anterior temporal area that, on close inspection, shows thinning that is strongly suggestive of future loss. A typical example of such a triangular-shaped area is outlined in black crayon in the photograph. It should be transplanted at the same time as the more obviously bald areas more anteriorly and medially, in order to avoid constantly "chasing" an enlarging area of alopecia.

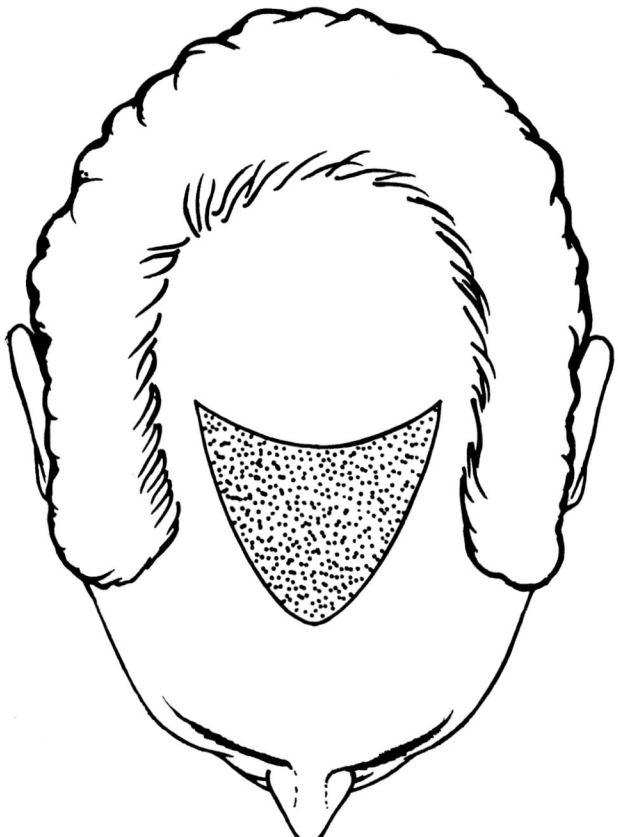

Figure 13.2. A schematic drawing of one variant of an isolated frontal forelock.

planting, which is still ongoing by the author, is more difficult if hair is present in the recipient area; in addition, existing hair is destroyed as the laser ablates lines of tissue. Thus, treating hair-bearing areas with the laser results in less hair for the first 3 months, rather than more. This does not occur when scalpel slits or needle holes are made between existing hairs. It is important to note, however, that hair-bearing areas initially treated with conventional micrografting and slit grafting, in order to conserve any original hair, may be treated with laser transplanting at a later date when more of the persisting hair between the previously transplanted grafts has been lost with the progression of MPB. Ultimately, such individuals could be treated with a mixture of laser transplanting and conventional transplanting.

Although a substantial majority of alopecic patients can expect to have better cosmetic results in laser treated areas, a significant minority will produce no better and sometimes worse results (see also below) (8). Therefore, the author, with the patient's concurrence, will often treat only a limited area of the recipient area with the laser dur-

ing the first session, while the majority of the site is treated conventionally. Waiting 5 to 6 months allows both the doctor and patient to assess the difference in the postoperative course and results in conventionally and laser-treated areas. Subsequent treatment is then decided depending on what has occurred.

Anesthesia

Patients receive 15 to 20 mg oral Diazepam 30 minutes before surgery to minimize anxiety, as well as lidocaine toxicity (9). Oxycodone may also be added to reduce pain. The anesthetic solution for the donor area consists of 5.0 mL 2% lidocaine without epinephrine, 0.4 mL fresh epinephrine 1/1000, and 100 cc normal saline. Usually, between 70 to 100 cc of this mixture is infiltrated slowly using a single injection site and an 18 × 3.5 inch spinal needle (10). Before infiltrating this "tumescent" solution, a field block in the donor area is produced using 1% lidocaine with 1/100,000 epinephrine buffered with 50 milliequivillents per liter of sodium bicarbonate. Buffering lidocaine markedly decreases pain during infiltration of the field block (10, 11).

In the recipient area, a similar field block is produced with buffered lidocaine, but in this location a 2% solution of lidocaine is used. Superior to the buffered field block, unbuffered 2% lidocaine with 1/50,000 epinephrine is injected to produce another field block. Areas that have been treated with buffered lidocaine will bleed more profusely than those treated with unbuffered solutions (10). A solution of 1/50,000 epinephrine (without lidocaine) is used in the balance of the recipient area. The author does not use tumescent anesthesia in the recipient area because of the difficulty of accurately estimating the spacing of grafts once the distention caused by the tumescent anesthesia has resolved, and the increased likelihood of "losing" a graft beneath the surface of the skin. Tumescent anesthesia in the recipient area also might cause more postoperative edema.

The Donor Area

A "safe" donor area for most patients under the age of 80 has been established in a study of persisting rim hair in 328 men aged 65 to 79 years of age (Figure 13.3) (12). Grafts are taken from this area using a quadruple- or quintuple-bladed knife on excised strips of skin, each of which is 2.0 to 3.0 mm wide (13). The strips are carefully sectioned into grafts containing 1 to 6 hairs each. A donor

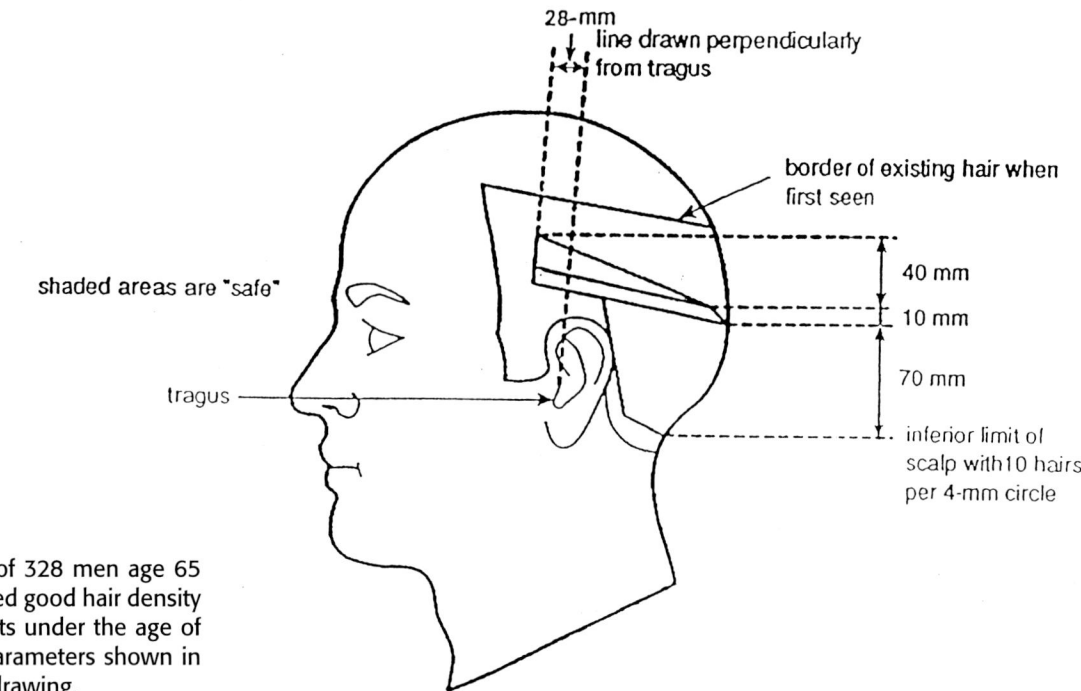

Figure 13.3. A study of 328 men age 65 years and older revealed good hair density in over 80% of patients under the age of 80 years within the parameters shown in the above schematic drawing.

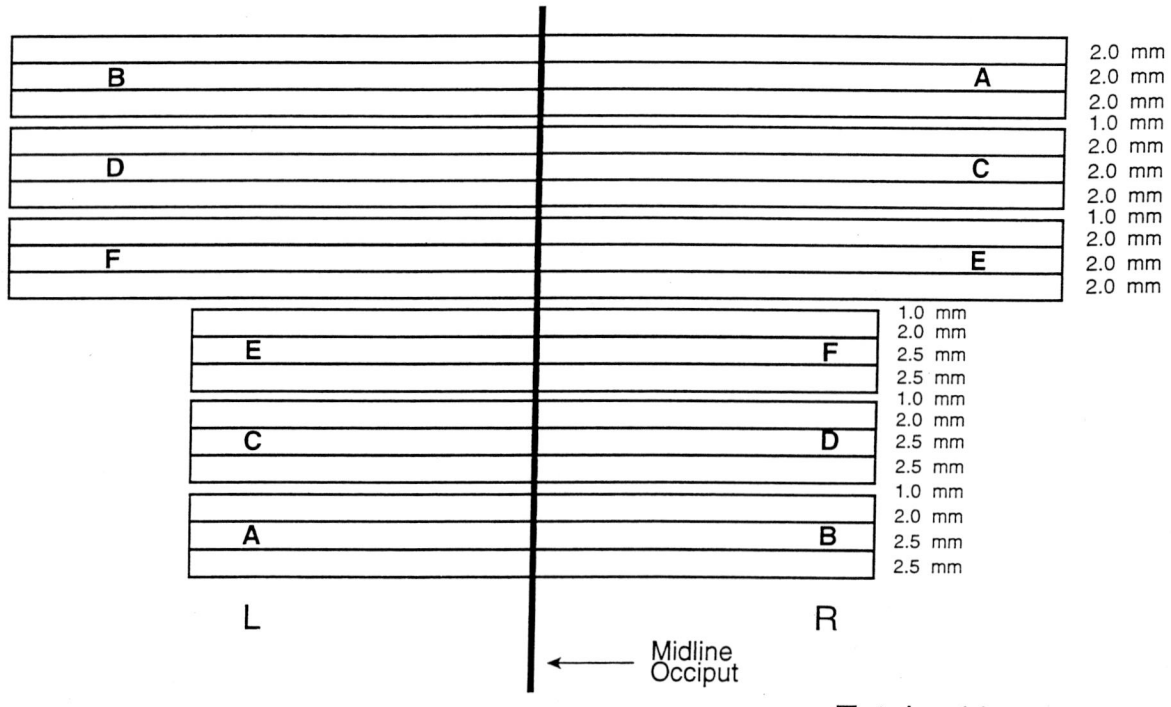

Figure 13.4. The schematic drawing shown demonstrates the organization of the donor area for strip harvesting sessions of micrografts and minigrafts. **A, B, C, D, E,** and **F** represent donor strips excised in sessions 1, 2, 3 ,4, 5 and 6, respectively. The 1 mm gap between each of the session areas represents a typical 1 mm wide band of scar from the previous session(s), which is excised as part of subsequent ones. This donor area is well within the parameters of the "safe donor area" shown in Figure 13.3.

area running from the left to right ear that is only 44 mm high can, in most patients, produce six sessions of 350 to 400 slit grafts and 200 micrografts per session (Figure 13.4). Large bleeding vessels are cauterized before closing the wound in a single layer using a single layer running suture, usually 2-0 Supramid on a CL-20 needle.

Two different areas in the donor area are used so grafts contain hair of varying textures and color (Figure 13.4). Finer hair in the inferior occipital area and temporal area, for example, is advantageous for producing very soft hairlines and the center of the whorl of the crown. Coarser and/or denser hair more superiorly in the occipital and parietal areas is more suitable for creating greater density in the remainder of the recipient area. Subsequent donor areas are excised immediately superior or inferior to the scars from previous sessions. The old scars are excised as part of the new "donor strip" so that no matter how many procedures are carried out, only two usually very fine donor site scars are produced. As indicated earlier, in most patients, it is rare to be unable to obtain enough donor material from the occipito-parietal temporal areas for six or *more* sessions.

The Recipient Area

It is important to spread the grafts as evenly as possible over the recipient area, while at the same time using an irregular or random pattern. Both help to create the most "natural" looking hair distribution after each surgery. The following four parameters are recommended to achieve this "organized disorganization." Grafts in session one should be a) 2 to 3 mm apart (2 mm for conventional and 3 mm for laser transplantation), b) 1 mm anterior or posterior to their neighboring grafts, c) angled, and d) the direction of incision should follow the angle and direction of any remaining original hair in that area (14). Learning how to consistently accomplish these four goals is a difficult and time-consuming process that will often distinguish the novice from the veteran surgeon. A distinct advantage of using a laser for hair transplanting is that it is possible to attach a computer driven "scanner" to move the laser beam in a very accurate and consistent fashion, as described above. This enables a relative novice to produce results similar to a veteran surgeon. At present, Coherent has a scanner available that will produce three slit sites at 45° (in most recipient areas, hair usually exits at approximately this angle), that incorporate the three other parameters (Figure 13.5). The potential exists for much larger areas, indeed the entire recipient area, being

Representative Example of Pattern Adjustments

Mode	Slit						Mode	Hole			
	16 spots/mm			22 spots/mm							
Pattern Number	1	2	3	4	5	6	Pattern Number	1	2	3	4
Graphic Representation							Graphic Representation				

The pattern push buttons control the shape of the incisions.

Representative Example of Size Adjustments

Mode	Slit			Mode	Hole		
Size Number	1	5	9	Size Number	1	5	9
Graphic Representation				Graphic Representation			
Approximate Slit Length (millimeters)	2.0	3.0	4.0	Approximate Hole Diameter (millimeters)	0.4	1.2	2.0

The size push buttons control the slit length or hole diameter.

Representative Example of Density Adjustments

Mode	Slit			Mode	Hole		
Density Number	1	5	9	Density Number	1	5	9
Graphic Representation				Graphic Representation			
Approximate Slit Spacing (millimeters)	3.0	2.5	2.2	Approximate Hole Spacing (millimeters)	4.0	3.0	2.0

In slit mode, the density push buttons are used to select horizontal spacing between slits. In hole mode, the density push buttons are used to select horizontal and vertical spacing between spots. The density push buttons have no affect on single slit or single hole patterns (i.e., pattern family 1).

©Coherent, Inc. February 1996   0625-154-01 Rev 85

Figure 13.5. A schematic drawing of the various patterns produced by the UltraPulse pattern generating scanner. (Photo courtesy of Coherent Laser Inc.)

treated in a similarly systematic way. A new, exciting "Redfield Slot Punch" (Redfield Corporation, Montvale, NJ) is now available that will produce recipient sites very similar to those created by a laser, but it does not offer the inherent advantage of a scanner attachment.

During session two, the slits should be made midway between those of the first session. In session three, for the present, it is recommended that conventional slit grafting or "slot" grafting with the Redfield Slot Punch be used to fill the spaces between previously transplanted grafts (Figure 13.6). Three sessions of conventional slit grafting will usually produce excellent cosmetic results, if characteristics are particularly good—for example fine and/or

Figure 13.6. A schematic drawing of the spacing and pattern of slits recommended for laser transplanting. The laser slits are produced with a 0.2 mm spot in focus and results in a wound that is approximately 0.5 mm wide. The distance between adjacent slits is 3 mm. Slits are 1 mm anterior or posterior to their nearest neighbors. The ablating angle and direction should mimic that of the original hair in the area.

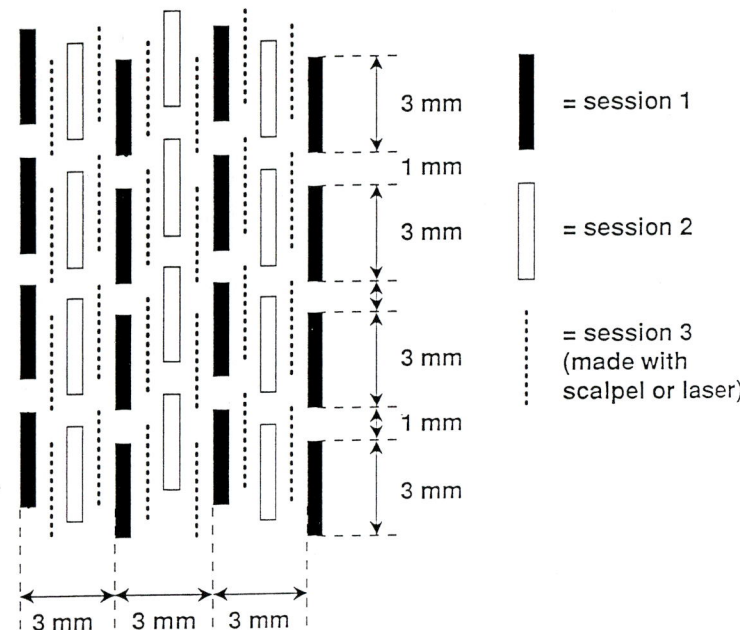

3 mm

1 mm

3 mm

3 mm

1 mm

3 mm

3 mm   3 mm   3 mm

∎ = session 1

▢ = session 2

⋮ = session 3 (made with scalpel or laser)

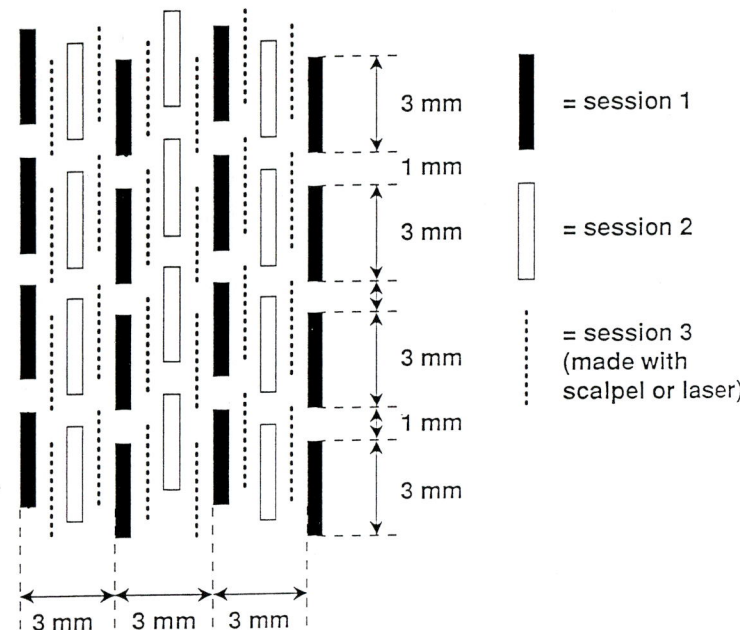

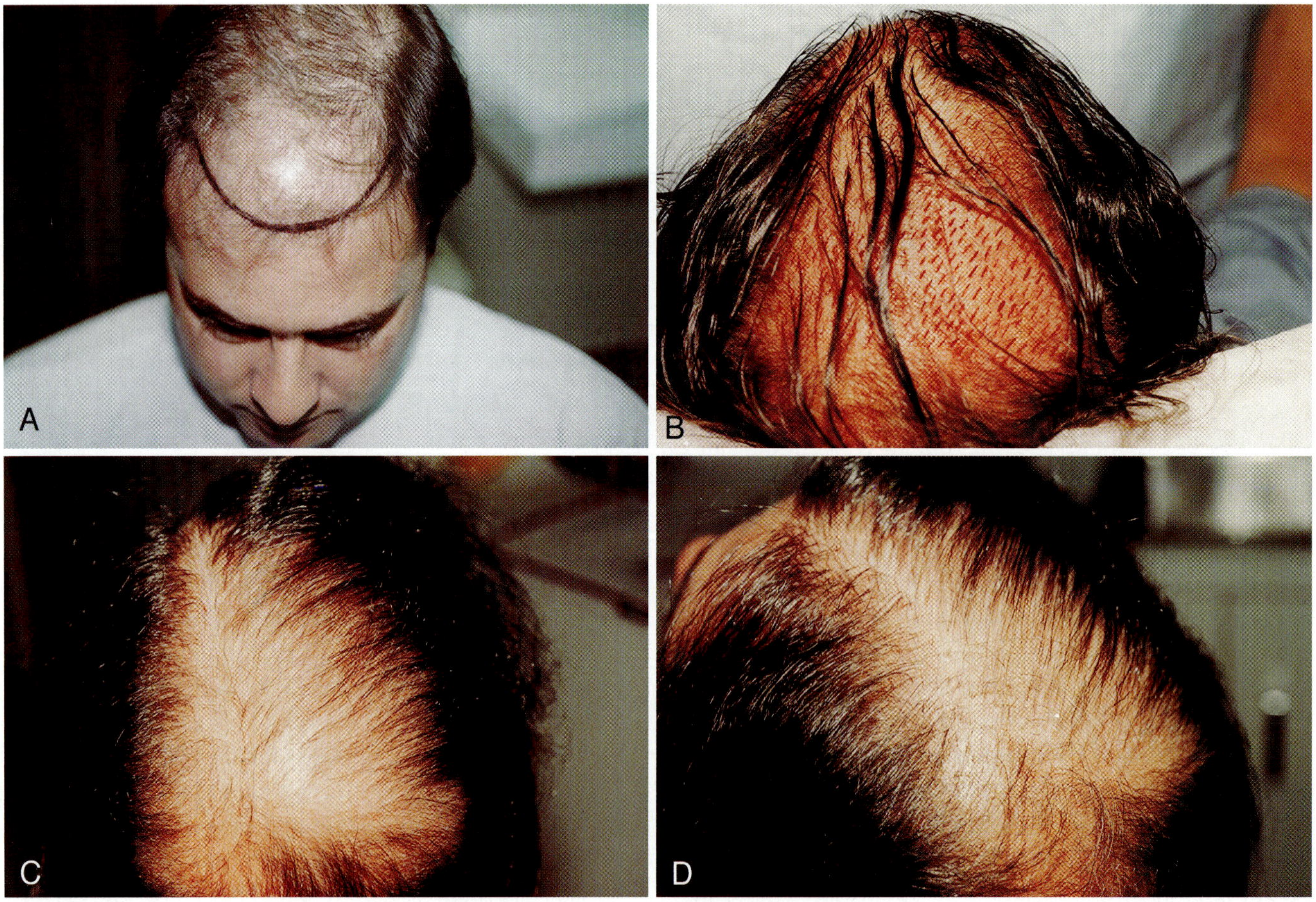

A

B

C

D

Figure 13.7. A. Before treatment. **B.** Intraoperative photo showing 110 laser slit sites on the right side of the midline frontal area, and a similar number of scalpel slit sites on the left side. Hair from two earlier conventional transplants can be seen growing more anteriorly. **C.** The same area as seen in **B**, 9 months later. Note the denser and more even distribution of hair on the laser- treated side. Clinically the results in the zone treated with only a single session of hair trans- planting looked so natural that the patient and his wife thought that it had never been treated until they were shown the "before" photographs. **D.** Another view from the left side of the study area, demonstrating greater hair density on the laser side as well as some mild "compression" of hair on the scalpel prepared side, which probably would not have been noticed if the laser treated side was not available for comparison.

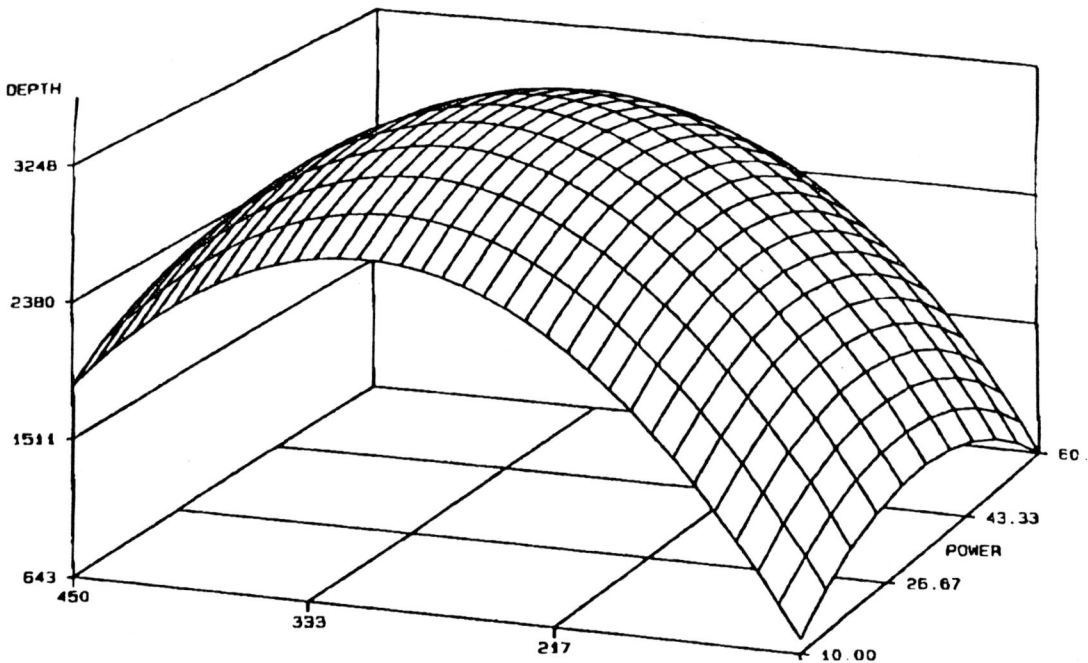

Figure 13.8. A schematic drawing of the findings in 500 patient biopsies using the UltraPulse laser with the pattern generator set at Pattern 4 and various millijoule and watt parameters. The optimal settings appear to 300 millijoules and 40 to 60 watts. (Photo courtesy of Coherent Laser Inc).

light colored and/or dense hair—even a single session may produce a satisfactory result in some patients (Figure 13.7). Because the postoperative crusting overlying the grafts is somewhat greater and longer-lasting when a laser is used and because hair growth also usually occurs later than is seen with conventional transplanting (see below), a conventionally prepared hairline zone anterior to laser prepared areas is recommended. Keeping the surface of the recipient area moist with saline as the sites are ablated, in order to minimize surface heat and thermal injury, greatly reduces postoperative crusting. It is also worth noting that because there is no need to worry about graft compression, one can more often use larger minigrafts, with, for example, 5 to 6 hairs instead of 3 to 4 hairs each.

The graph shown in Figure 13.8 is a summary of the histologic findings in over 500 biopsies of laser slits carried out in four centers using a variety of millijoule and watt settings. These results indicate that the optimal settings for ideal depth of incision and minimal adjacent thermal damage appear to be 300 millijoules and 40 to 60 watts when using the Coherent UltraPulse CO_2 laser with its scanner set at "Pattern 4." This pattern produces lines that are 3 mm long, created with 22 0.2 mm collimated spots laid down in a *nonsequential* order (Figure 13.9). The line is produced in less than 0.5 seconds

and is approximately 0.2 mm deep. Zones of thermal damage are 50 to 70 microns wide at the level of the hair matrices. The author has also produced excellent cosmetic results utilizing "Pattern 1" (16 spots per 3 mm line), 300 millijoules, and 12 to 15 watts. Regardless of the

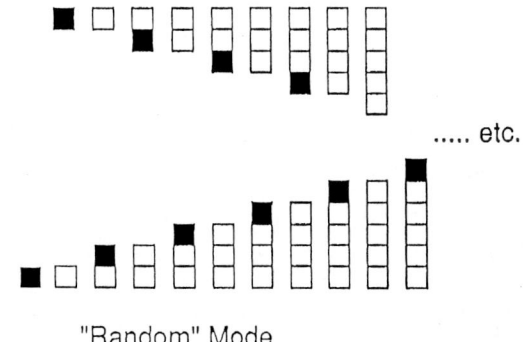

"Random" Mode

Figure 13.9. Using the UltraPulse laser in Pattern 4, the ablating spot skips from one end of the preselected line length to the other end, then back to just inside the first spot before returning to just inside the spot on the other end of the line, and so on, until the last pulse occurs at the midpoint of the line. This "random" ablation pattern results in longer intervals between adjacent spots than a sequential pattern would and, therefore, produces less thermal damage. (Each black square denotes an ablating spot on that line, while each open square denotes a previously ablated spot.)

pattern selected, and whatever the millijoule and watt settings, the initial line should be made and then a test graft inserted into that site to see if it fits properly without protruding or falling beneath the surface of the skin. Millijoule and watt settings can thereafter be adjusted accordingly.

As indicated earlier, a Sharplan handpiece designed to create lines for slit grafts has been tried and was found to be unacceptable. This is because the beam of light is not collimated and lines of equal depth can only be produced with the handpiece held perpendicular to the skin. This results in hairs growing perpendicularly, rather than at their more usual approximately 45° angle. For those patients or physicians who prefer round minigrafts to slit grafts, however, the Sharplan CO_2 laser with Flashscanner attachment can be used to create a round hole by rapidly moving of the spot in a spiral fashion (Figure 13.10). The author assessed 48 patients with this machine and concluded that optimal settings for the "minus size," which produces a round hole approximately 0.8 mm in diameter, are 0.1 to 0.15 seconds and 50 to 80 watts. Other authors have reported good results with similar settings (15, 16). (Once again settings must be adjusted for each patient using "test" grafts.) Zones of thermal damage that are approximately 50 microns wide at the level of the hair matrices can be made rapidly with these settings. The author prefers to use the Sharplan laser instead of the UltraPulse laser for making round holes, because the holes produced by the former are more or less of equal depth throughout the entire hole, whereas holes made with the UltraPulse are more saucer-shaped (Figure 13.11).

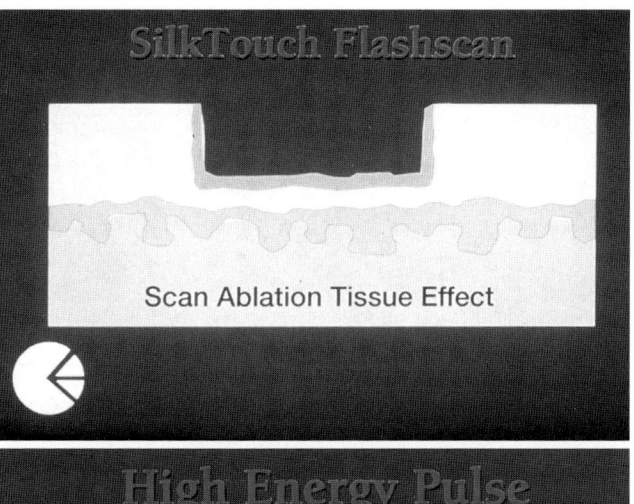

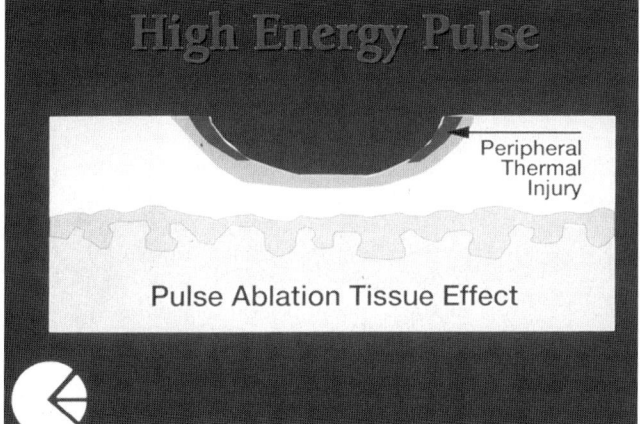

Figure 13.11. A. The Sharplan laser produces a round defect of equal depth throughout the entire hole. **B.** Pulse ablation produces a saucer-shaped base to the hole. (Photos courtesy of Sharplan Laser Inc.)

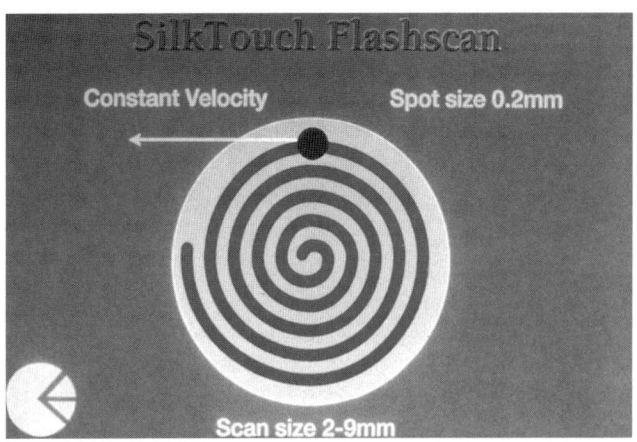

Figure 13.10. The Silktouch Flashscanner uses an ablating spot that is rapidly moved in an enlarging spiral to produce a round hole. (Photo courtesy of Sharplan Laser Inc.)

The most promising new laser for hair transplanting is the Erbium:YAG (Er:YAG) laser. Theoretically, the amount of thermal damage created with this laser should be as little as 1/10 that created by the CO_2 laser because of its much shorter absorption length. Some of the less desirable side effects of using the CO_2 laser for hair transplanting—such as increased crusting over the first 1 to 2 postoperative weeks and hair growth occurring approximately 4 to 6 weeks later than that seen with conventional transplanting—should be much improved with the Erbium laser because of its narrower zones of thermal damage. Inevitably, other lasers will be developed that are more user-friendly or otherwise better for hair transplanting.

The author has used the UltraPulse CO_2 laser for the past 4 years in 357 patients. In 285 of the 357 patients, cosmetic results were superior on the laser treated side.

Sixty-nine of the studied patients had equivalent cosmetic results, while 3 of the earliest patients had worse cosmetic results (8). Because a) of the ablation of existing hair, b) of more postoperative crusting, c) of delayed growth, and d) superior results are inconsistent, the author is not comfortable with recommending laser transplanting as the treatment of choice for all patients at this time. The author continues to view laser transplanting as a promising but still investigational form of treatment. It is, however, not simply a marketing tool, although it has been widely used for this purpose. To view it this way is to ignore the advantages of nearly bloodless ablation of tissue and superior cosmetic results in most patients undergoing laser-slit grafting when compared to conventional slit grafting or round minigrafting (Figures 13.12

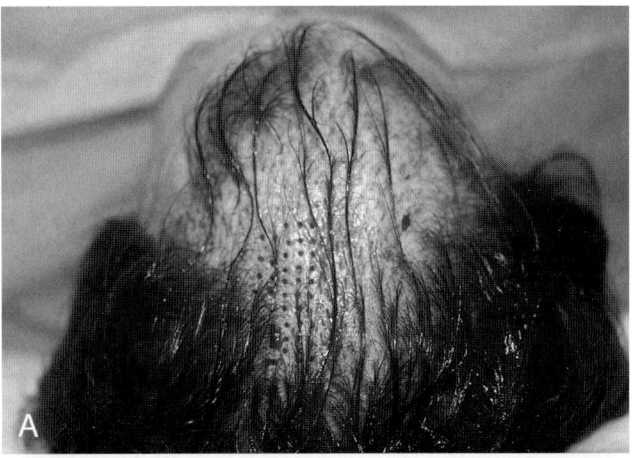
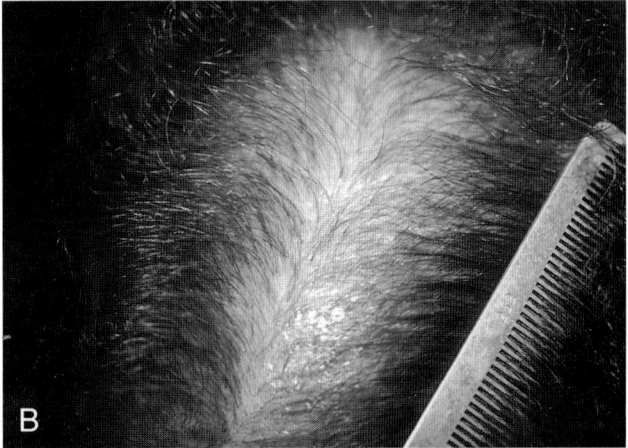
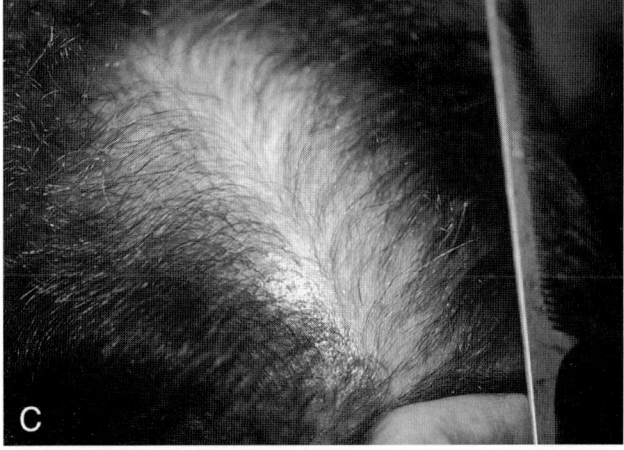

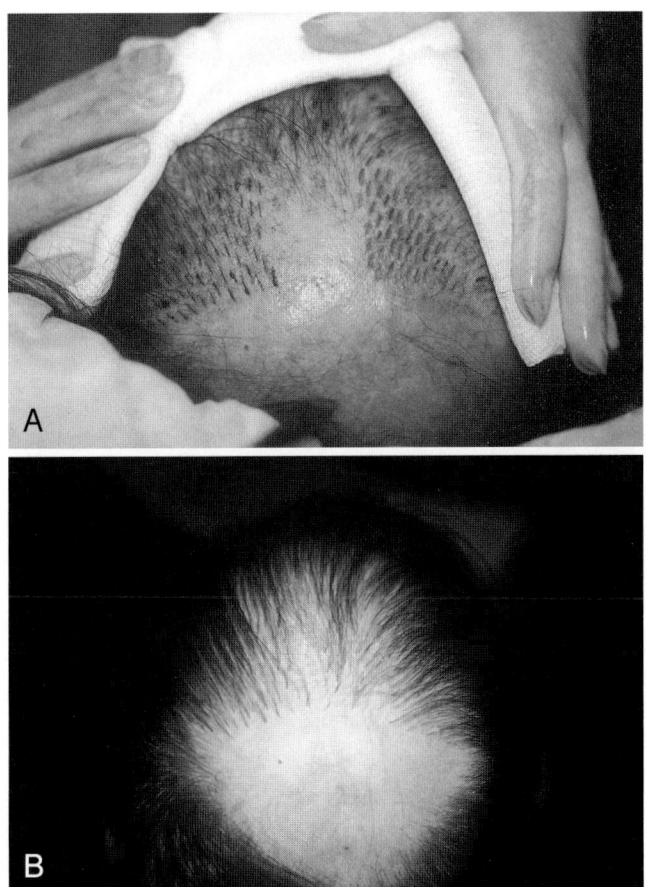

Figure 13.12. A. Fifty laser slits have been made on the right side of the recipient area. Fifty "control" scalpel slits are shown on the left side. Each site was filled with a graft containing 5 to 6 hairs. **B.** Nine months later, the laser-treated side shows less compression with a more evenly spread, denser looking growth of hair than the conventionally treated side.

Figure 13.13. A. Fifty conventionally produced 2 mm round recipient sites are shown on the left side and serve as a "control" for 50 laser-produced slit sites on the right side. Each site was filled with a graft containing 5 to 6 hairs. **B.** Nine months later, the laser-treated side shows a more evenly spread, more natural looking growth of hair than the slightly pluggier looking conventionally prepared side. The darker the hair, the more obvious the difference in plugginess becomes. **C.** A different viewing angle. This photo was taken at the same time as the photo shown in **B**.

and 13.13). In my opinion, there is no doubt that laser-assisted hair transplantation will play an important role in the future of hair transplant surgery.

Graft Insertion and Bandaging

If recipient sites have been properly prepared, then the grafted hair will be directed and angled in the same direction and angle as the original hair at that site. It is important that the grafts be handled gently, that they sit flush with the surrounding skin, and that no hairs are accidentally trapped beneath them. Baciguent ointment is applied in both the recipient and donor areas. The recipient area is then covered with Telfa and an overnight pressure bandage is applied (17). The next morning, the patient returns to have his bandage removed. There is usually very little bleeding when the laser has been used; however, any blood that is present can be gently washed away with hydrogen peroxide. The patient's hair is then carefully washed, blown dry, and styled.

POSTOPERATIVE COURSE

Patients are advised to apply Baciguent ointment three times daily to both the recipient and donor areas for 1 week. This is important because a small amount of superficial de-epithelization occurs around each laser site, making the area more prone to secondary infection, which could affect hair yield. It is also helpful in accelerating healing and decreasing the amount of postoperative crusting over the grafts. If Baciguent or another antibiotic ointment is used regularly, most or all of the crusts will have fallen off the grafts in 14 or fewer days. Sutures are removed from donor sites in 7 to 10 days.

As indicated earlier, when 75 or more grafts have been transplanted, hair regrowth will usually occur 2 to 6 weeks later at laser-prepared areas than what is normally seen with conventional slit grafting (2, 3). Applying a 3% Minoxidil solution twice daily for the first 5 postoperative weeks is recommended to counter-balance the effect of sealing blood vessels by the laser. Topical Minoxidil will result in vasodilation of intact blood vessels and may help to shorten the dormant period.

Patients are given acetaminophen with 60 mg codeine (Tylenol #3), oxicodone (Percocet), and 50 mg meperidine hydrochloride (Demerol) to take as required for postoperative pain. Few patients use anything more than Tylenol #3 and usually only for the first 24 to 48 hours.

Aside from a slightly increased tendency to develop postoperative infection due to laser-induced adjacent de-epithelization, all complications that can occur with conventional transplanting may also occur with laser transplanting but are equally infrequent. The reader is referred elsewhere for a summary of them (18).

REFERENCES

1. Unger W, David L. Laser hair transplantation. J Dermatol Surg Oncol 1994;20:515–521.
2. Unger W. Laser hair transplantation II. J Dermatol Surg Oncol 1995;21:759–765.
3. Unger W. Laser hair transplantation III. J Dermatol Surg Oncol 1995;21:1047–1055.
4. Unger WP, Knudsen R. General principles of recipient site organization and planning. In: Unger W, ed. Hair transplantation. 3rd ed. New York: Marcel Dekker Inc, 1995:105–158.
5. Unger WP. What's new in hair replacement surgery. In: Whiting DA, ed. Dermatologic clinics. Philadelphia: WB Saunders, 1996;14:4783–4802.
6. Marritt E, Dzubow L. The isolated frontal forelock. Dermatol Surg 1995;21:523–538.
7. Beehner ML. The frontal forelock concept in hair transplantation. Am J Cosm Surg 1997;14:125–132.
8. Unger WP. Laser hair transplanting 1997. Am J Cosm Surg 1997;14:143–148.
9. de Jong RH, Heavener J. Diazepam prevents and aborts lidocaine convulsions in monkeys. Anesthesiology 1971;41(3):226–230.
10. Unger W. Anethesia in hair transplantation. In: Unger W, ed. Hair transplantation. 3rd ed. New York: Marcel Dekker Inc, 1995:165–181.
11. McKay W, et al. Sodium bicarbonate attenuated pain on skin infiltration with lidocaine with or without epinephrine. Anesth Analg 1987;66:572–574.
12. Unger W. Delineating the "safe" donor area for hair transplanting. Am J Cosm Surg 1994;11:239–243.
13. Unger W. The donor site in hair transplantation. In: Unger W, ed. Hair transplantation. 3rd ed. New York: Marcel Dekker Inc, 1995:183–214.
14. Unger W. The recipient area in hair transplantation. In: Unger W, ed. Hair transplantation. 3rd ed. New York: Marcel Dekker Inc, 1995:215–322.
15. Villnow M, et al. Laser assisted hair transplanting. In: Stough D, Haber R, eds. Hair replacement, surgical and medical. St Louis: Mosby, 1995:365–370.

16. Avrom M. The role of the laser in hair transplantation. Annual meeting of the International Society of Hair Restoration Surgery, Nashville, 1996.

17. McKeown M. Preparation and insertion of grafts. In: Unger W, ed. Hair transplantation. 3rd ed. New York: Marcel Dekker Inc, 1995:331–348.

18. Unger W. Complications of hair transplantation. In: Unger W, ed. Hair transplantation. 3rd ed. New York: Marcel Dekker Inc, 1995:363–374.

Chapter Fourteen

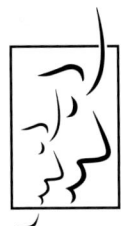

Complications of Laser Incisional Surgery and Laser-Assisted Blepharoplasty

Harvey P. Cole III and Brian S. Biesman

Complications of laser-assisted surgery may be related to either the specific procedure performed or the use of the laser itself. This chapter focuses on the prevention and management of some of the complications associated with laser-assisted blepharoplasty and other laser incisional procedures.

Problems may arise even before surgery is performed. While not harmful in a physical sense, these problems reflect negatively on the physician and the practice. Most are related to inadequate patient education and poor preoperative communication between the patient, the physician, and the office staff. In such situations, patients may develop inaccurate expectations of postoperative results, an unclear understanding of surgical risks, or may not follow preoperative instructions properly. Printed material containing clear and concise information describing the surgical procedure, special preoperative instructions, the need for ancillary testing, postoperative care, and informed consent should be provided to all patients. If unanswered questions remain, another consultation should be considered.

INTRAOPERATIVE COMPLICATIONS

Intraoperative complications of incisional laser surgery may be related to laser safety violations, laser misuse, loss of anatomic orientation, and, when working in the orbit, hemorrhage. These problems may be avoided if sound safety measures and surgical techniques are observed. All standard laser safety precautions should be observed when performing laser-assisted blepharoplasty or other laser incisional procedures. Please see Chapter 1 for a more detailed discussion of laser safety principles and protective devices.

Proper use of the laser decreases the risk of intraoperative complications. One of the most common errors committed by the novice user is failing to keep the laser focused as an incision is made. As shown in Chapter 1, as the distance the laser is held from the tissue increases, the power density of its beam decreases exponentially and the zone of irreversible thermal damage becomes larger. We studied this phenomenon by comparing the histopathologic effects of focused versus defocused CO_2 laser energy on human eyelid skin. The Coherent UltraPulse (Coherent Medical, Palo Alto, CA) laser with a 0.2 mm beam diameter was used as an energy source. To eliminate the surgeon-dependent variables, the eyelid tissue was mounted on a device that moved the tissue at constant linear velocity while the laser handpiece was held in fixed position by a freestanding clamp. We found that the incision produced when the beam was focused was surrounded by a zone of thermal damage measuring approximately 115 microns on each side of the wound. When the beam was defocused a distance of 2 cm, the incision was too superficial to be clinically useful, while the zone of thermal damage became substantially larger (Figure 14.1A and B). Defocusing a lesser distance created smaller increases in the zone of thermal damage (1).

Laser burns outside the intended surgical field may be produced if a laser safe backstop is not in place when incisions are made. If the burn involves only the skin (as is usually the case), the wounds are generally superficial and heal without adverse sequelae, although temporary hyperpigmentation may occur. Managing these wounds requires regular application of topical antibiotic ointment until healing is complete.

Inadvertent laser burns of other structures, including the eyelashes, can also occur during blepharoplasty or other eyelid surgery. Typically, only the cilia themselves are burned and will regrow without incident; however, this process may require weeks to months and, thus, is a source of concern. Burns to the lash follicle may produce

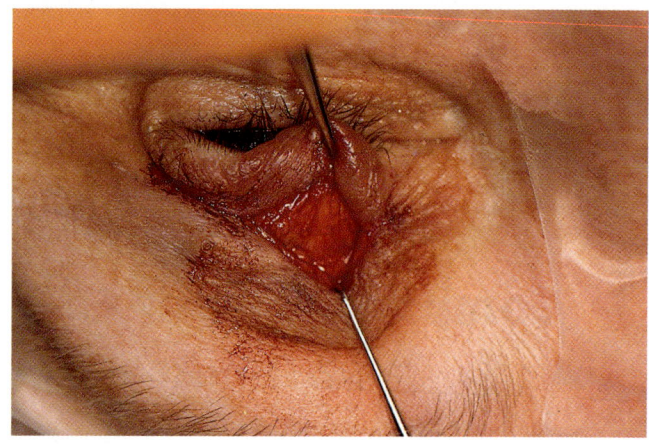

Figure 14.2. Levator aponeurosis infiltrated by fat. Note its dull appearance.

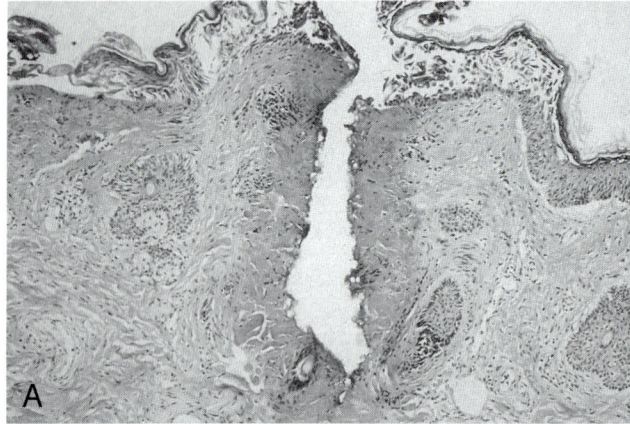

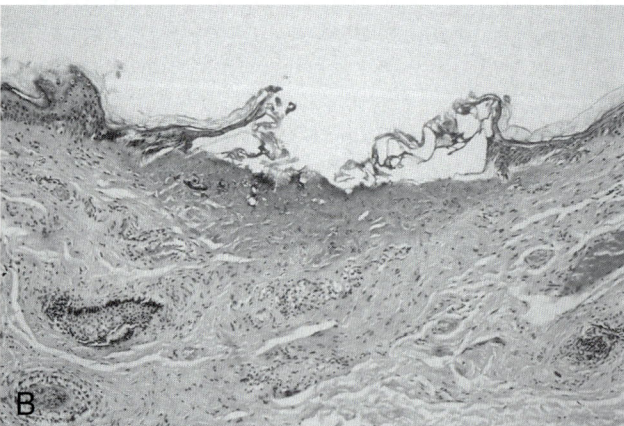

Figure 14.1. A. Incision made with a focused 0.2 mm CO_2 laser beam in eyelid skin. Note the absence of hemorrhage and the zone of surrounding thermal damage. **B.** The same laser defocused 2 cm. The resulting incision is shallow and the zone of thermal damage is much larger. The identical power setting was used to create both incisions.

permanent loss of cilia, a condition that may only be treated with transplantation (2).

Inadvertent burns of the eye itself is a true emergency. Laser burns of the globe may be detected by direct visualization, softening of the globe, or both. In the event this should occur, the procedure should be aborted and emergent ophthalmic consultation obtained (3). In the presence of a perforating ocular injury, even minimal pressure on the globe can produce retinal or choroidal detachment, intraocular hemorrhage, and even loss of intraocular contents and permanent blindness.

As discussed in Chapter 8, laser incisional surgery requires visual (as opposed to tactile) feedback to properly identify tissue planes. This is especially important in the eyelid, a thin but complex structure composed of seven layers. Familiarity with some important anatomic relationships facilitates the identification of tissue planes within the eyelid. Additional information regarding the surgical anatomy of the eyelid may be found in Chapters 2 and 9.

The central fat pad in the upper eyelid is an important landmark that should be identified whenever upper eyelid ptosis or blepharoplasty surgery is performed. It occupies the space between the levator aponeurosis and the orbital septum, and may be balloted anteriorly where it is easily visible if gentle pressure is applied to the globe (4). In cases where the levator aponeurosis has undergone an involutional process known as fatty degeneration, the aponeurosis loses its glistening white appearance and may be confused with the preaponeurotic fat pad (Figure 14.2). Unsuspecting surgeons have inadvertently resected the levator aponeurosis, creating a full thickness eyelid defect. Should this occur, immediate re-pair of the remaining levator should be accomplished with 6-0 silk or polyglactin suture is necessary to prevent postoperative ptosis (5, 6). Secondary repair of these in-juries is difficult due to the presence of scar tissue that develops rapidly within the eyelid.

The lacrimal gland may be encountered during upper eyelid surgery if involutional changes, inflammation, or trauma cause it to prolapse from its usual position in the superior lateral orbit. In extreme cases, the gland will mi-grate into the central portion of the eyelid where it has been mistaken for preaponeurotic fat and resected (7). This distinction should not be difficult to make as the glandular tissue is normally firm and white or gray in color while the preaponeurotic fat is softer and has a yel-low color.

Transconjunctival lower eyelid surgery can be somewhat confusing to the surgeon accustomed to the external approach. Structures vulnerable to injury dur-ing transconjunctival lower eyelid surgery include the orbital septum, skin, canthal tendons, the lacrimal sys-tem, the inferior oblique and inferior rectus muscles, and even the globe. Just as the preaponeurotic fat pad is a useful landmark in upper eyelid surgery, there are lower eyelid structures that may be used as visual guides to help the surgeon remain oriented to the location of vital structures.

The orbital fat removed during transconjunctival blepharoplasty is bound posteriorly by the lower eyelid retractors (CPF) and anteriorly by the orbital septum. The cut edge of the CPF is identified at the beginning of the case to define the posterior limit of the dissection. The central and nasal fat pads are then identified. These fat pads are separated by the inferior oblique muscle, which may or may not be easily visible in the wound. Injury to the inferior oblique muscle must be avoided; if the mus-cle does not present itself, a diligent search, as suggested by some surgeons, should not be performed.

The inferior orbital rim is another important land-mark in transconjunctival lower eyelid surgery. It marks the insertion site of the orbital septum, a structure that should be preserved to prevent scarring and eyelid re-traction. If a laser-safe retractor is placed immediately be-hind the orbital fat as it is resected, injury to the orbital septum should be avoided (Figure 14.3). Failure to direct the laser against a protective device can even result in full thickness eyelid burns. Should this occur, the skin should be repaired with permanent sutures. Suturing the orbicu-laris oculi muscle is not necessary and, as a general rule, the orbital septum should never be closed (8–13).

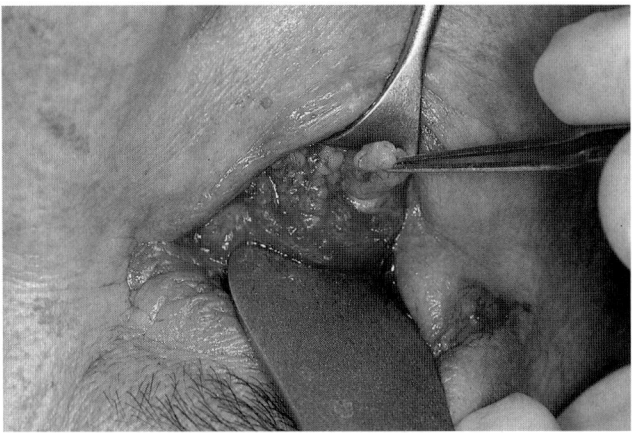

Figure 14.3. A laser-safe instrument should always be placed behind the tissue as it is incised with a laser.

Other Intraoperative Complications of Blepharoplasty

Injury to the extraocular muscles may occur during ble-pharoplasty. As indicated above, the inferior oblique mus-cle may appear in the surgical field during lower eyelid blepharoplasty. Should this occur, the muscle should not be manipulated as its connective tissue sheath could be disrupted. Injury to this protective sheath predisposes the area to the subsequent development of adhesions be-tween the muscle and the surrounding orbital fat, a con-dition that produces bizarre and disabling diplopia, which may be incurable. This is not to be confused with the temporary diplopia and pupillary dilation resulting from injection of an anesthetic agent into the inferior oblique muscle, in which case the symptoms resolve once the anesthetic effect has dissipated. Injury to the inferior rec-tus, superior rectus, and superior oblique muscles has been reported following blepharoplasty surgery, but only rarely. Damage to extraocular muscles has not been specifically related to use of the laser (14–18).

Perhaps the most common complication of lower eyelid transconjunctival blepharoplasty is incomplete ex-cision of the lateral fat pad (19–21). Although considered a single pad by anatomists, it usually is found to have two distinct portions surgically (22, 23). As described in Chap-ters 2 and 10, the anterior portion lies adjacent to the cen-tral and nasal fat pockets and the posterior lateral portion tightly adheres to the CPF. The posterior-lateral portion of the lateral fat is easily overlooked resulting in the appear-ance of an unsightly bulge below the level of the lateral canthal tendon. This fat pad may be easily removed if an incision is made in a plane parallel and just anterior to the lower eyelid retractor in the most lateral part of the eyelid.

Orbital hemorrhage is a potentially serious complication of blepharoplasty surgery that may occur either intraoperatively or in the immediate postoperative period. If unrecognized or improperly managed, orbital hemorrhage can lead to blindness resulting from interruption of blood flow to the optic nerve head and/or eye secondary to elevated intraorbital pressure. If intraorbital pressure does not become significantly increased, there is essentially no risk of blindness (Figure 14.4A and B).

Hemostasis must be maintained meticulously throughout the blepharoplasty procedure. Once the orbital septum has been opened, even bleeding from the orbicularis oculi muscle can produce a sight-threatening orbital hemorrhage. While the CO_2 laser will simultaneously divide and seal the majority of the vessels encountered during blepharoplasty surgery, bleeding may still occur if larger vessels are divided. Defocusing the laser beam 2 to 6 mm

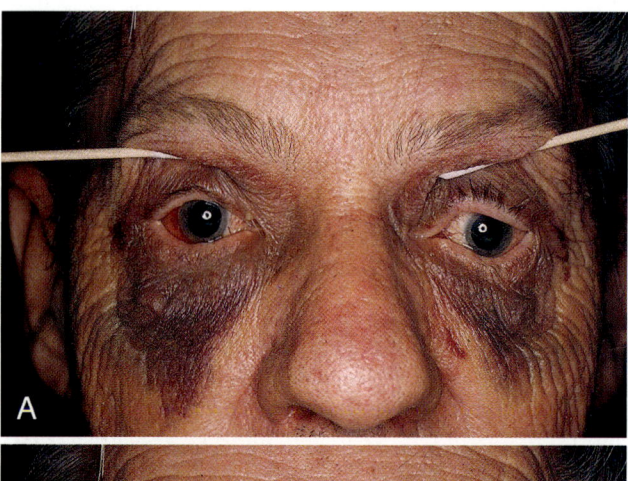
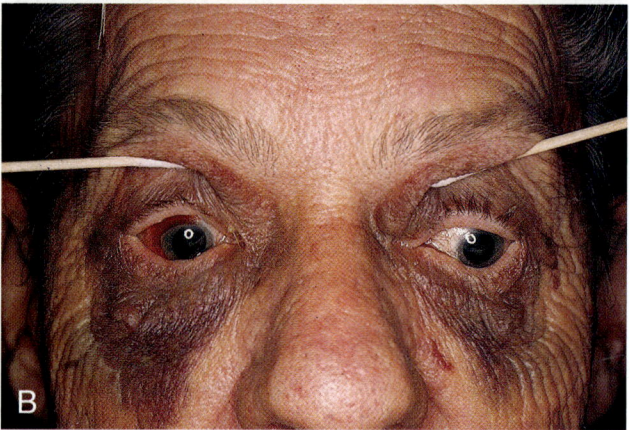

Figure 14.4. A, B. Bilateral orbital hemorrhage. Note the decreased movement of the right eye as the patient gazes to the left. The intraocular pressures were normal and this patient was managed conservatively.

is effective in cauterizing most of the vessels encountered during blepharoplasty, but electrocautery should always be available. Bipolar, rather than unipolar, cautery is recommended to avoid channeling current to the posterior orbit where it has been theorized that spasms of the central retinal or posterior ciliary arteries or direct damage to the optic nerve may result (24). Posterior channeling of current does not occur when bipolar cautery is used.

Orbital hemorrhage also may be produced when tractional forces exerted on the anterior orbital fat are conducted to the posterior orbit via the orbital connective tissue network. Vessels deep within the orbit may be torn and, as access to these vessels is limited, the bleeding may be difficult to control. This complication may be avoided if the orbital fat pads are handled gently. If an orbital hemorrhage is noted intraoperatively, efforts should be made to locate the source.

Vessels in the medial fat or the orbicularis muscle are the most common sources of hemorrhage during upper lid surgery, while bleeding during lower lid surgery usually arises from either the fat or the cut edge of the lower lid retractors. Hemorrhage from the wound edges is easily managed. If hemorrhage occurs within an orbital fat pad, then the pad containing the suspected source of the hemorrhage should be gently grasped and brought into the surgical field where it may be more easily inspected and cauterized. Hemostasis is achieved with judicious use of the bipolar cautery (25–29).

Complications Occurring After Laser-Assisted Blepharoplasty

Complications after laser-assisted blepharoplasty are quite uncommon. Orbital hemorrhage is potentially the most devastating complication, as it may lead to blindness. Fortunately, the incidence of this problem has been estimated at 0.01% or less. Even if an orbital hemorrhage occurs, prompt and proper management can usually prevent visual loss.

Despite a meticulous surgical technique, retrobulbar hemorrhage may occur several hours postoperatively. The importance of clear written and verbal communication with the patient and their caretaker cannot be overemphasized. The information provided must include the signs and symptoms of orbital hemorrhage and instructions to contact the physician immediately if a hemorrhage is suspected.

The signs and symptoms of postoperative orbital hemorrhage include proptosis, orbital and eyelid swelling, periorbital ecchymosis, moderate to severe orbital pain, nausea, vomiting, decreased vision, diplopia, limitation of extraocular movements, and, in some cases, bleeding from the wounds. If a hemorrhage originates in the posterior orbit, pain and decreased vision may be present even before the eyelids appear ecchymotic.

When evaluating a patient with a suspected postoperative orbital hemorrhage, the visual acuity should be assessed promptly because emergent intervention is indicated if optic nerve function has been compromised (29, 30). If the visual acuity is decreased due to optic nerve dysfunction, therapeutic intervention is directed for decreasing intraorbital pressure. The first step is to open the surgical wound, evacuate any hematoma present, and identify the source of the bleeding. If diffuse oozing is present, absorbable gelatin (Gelfoam, Upjohn, Kalamazoo, MI), oxidized cellulose (Surgicel, Johnson and Johnson Medical, Arlington, TX), microfibrillar collagen hemostat (Avitene, MedChem Products, Inc, Woburn, MA), or other hemostatic agents may be briefly applied. These agents should not be left within the orbit at the conclusion of the surgical procedure. Mannitol may be used to help promote orbital decongestion, and systemic steroids may be administered to help reduce edema. Additional treatment measures include elevating the head of the bed, applying ice compresses, controlling blood pressure, and using diuretics. Canthotomy, cantholysis, and vertical splitting of the eyelid are used to manage increased intraorbital pressure if surgical wounds are not present (31). Clinical scenarios where these maneuvers may be useful include carotid-cavernous sinus fistula, posttraumatic hemorrhage, and hemorrhage into an orbital tumor or vascular lesion. Bony decompression rarely is required (32).

If a small hematoma subsequently reaccumulates it may be drained after several days through a stab wound made directly over the most prominently distorted area (33). Small hematomas require several weeks to resolve and, during this time, the eyelid may remain indurated and swollen. The temptation to administer steroid injections to treat slowly resolving hematomas should be resisted since the risk of complications may outweigh the potential benefits.

Preventative measures that may reduce the risk of orbital hemorrhage include discontinuing use of aspirin and nonsteroidal anti-inflammatory medications for at least 10 days before surgery, taking appropriate intraoperative precautions, and administering antiemetic agents as needed postoperatively to avoid valsalva maneuvers. Patients should be instructed to avoid flying for at least several days so as to avoid exposure to potentially significant changes in atmospheric pressure, which may precipitate an orbital hemorrhage.

Nonhemorrhagic postoperative complications of laser-assisted transconjunctival blepharoplasty include excessive swelling and lymphedema, entropion, and subconjunctival collection of a straw-colored fluid. Postoperative swelling may be minimized by limiting the amount of laser energy used. Each orbital fat pad should be resected in "en bloc" fashion and the use of defocused laser energy for the purposes of "shrinking," "contouring," or "sculpting" orbital fat should be avoided. Postoperative entropion may be avoided by pulling the eyelid margin superiorly at the end of each case; the wound edges must not be allowed to overlap. A small percentage of patients will present for the first postoperative visit with complaints of mild foreign body sensation and irritation. Upon inspection of the inferior cul-de-sac and bulbar conjunctiva, a subconjunctival collection of amber colored fluid will be present (Figure 14.5). The nature of this fluid is not known, but it may represent the equivalent of a seroma. This condition is self limiting but if the fluid extends to the corneal limbus, the normal pattern of tear film distribution may be temporarily altered. Significant corneal thinning has been noted in at least one case. If ophthalmic ointment is used postoperatively, cysts containing subconjunctival ointment may develop. Allergic reaction to topically applied ointments can produce severe orbital inflammation and may even mimic cellulitis (Figure 14.6).

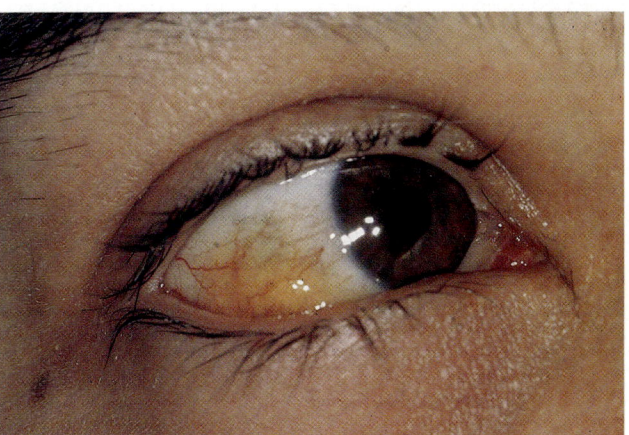

Figure 14.5. Patient presented with complaints of ocular irritation at 1 week follow up after laser-assisted lower blepharoplasty. The subconjunctival straw-colored fluid filled the inferior fornix and extended to the corneal limbus. It resolved in 1 week with the use of topical steroid antibiotic ophthalmic drops.

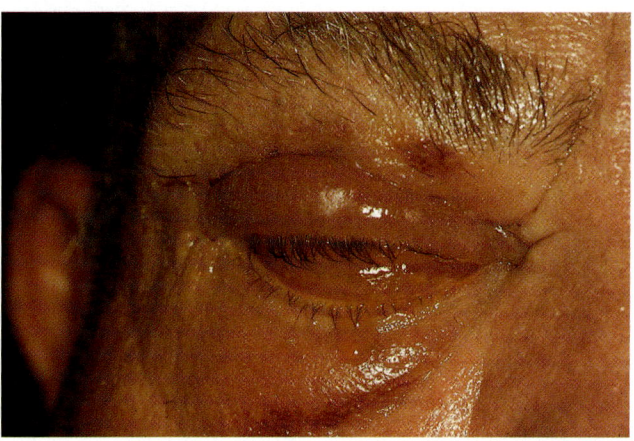

Figure 14.6. Allergic reaction to topical antibiotic ointment applied after blepharoplasty surgery.

Unacceptable scarring of the cutaneous incision in the upper eyelid has been reported (34). This problem has been attributed to inflammation at the wound edges caused by excessive thermal damage, absorbable sutures, or both. Thermal damage may be minimized by using a laser that produces a high-frequency, pulsed beam with a diameter no greater than 0.2 mm and by keeping the beam in focus at all times. If an eyelid wound assumes an elevated and irregular appearance, initial management should involve massaging a weak topical steroid ointment into the wounds two the three times daily for no longer than 2 weeks. Super potent steroids (e.g., Temavate) should not be used on the eyelids since thinning of the eyelid skin, cataracts, and glaucoma may develop (35). Slight elevation of the wound in the immediate postoperative period is common and should be differentiated from hypertrophic scarring, a rare problem. Should a hypertrophic scar develop, triamcinolone 1 to 10 mg/mL may be injected into the scars at weekly intervals as dictated by clinical response. Low concentrations are used initially with higher concentrations administered as needed. The number of injections into the delicate eyelid skin should be limited. The 585 nm pulsed dye laser has been used to treat hypertropic scarring in other areas, but the role of this device in managing eyelid scarring is not clear. The final character of a hypertrophic wound will not be apparent for at least 6 to 8 months following the initial surgery and, therefore, any contemplated surgical revision should be deferred for at least this period of time. Er:YAG laser resurfacing of eyelid scarring may help (36, 37).

Wound dehiscence may occur following any surgical procedure. Wounds created by a continuous wave laser will not have the same tensile strength as a similar cold steel wound for 3 to 6 weeks (38). To compensate for the delayed healing of a laser wound, sutures are left in place for 7 to 10 days, twice the length of time necessary following a cold steel wound. Logic suggests that the incidence of wound dehiscence may be higher following laser blepharoplasty, but this has not been demonstrated clinically. If wound dehiscence does occur, it may be managed with adhesive steri-strips and increased lubricant if the dehiscence is less than 1 mm wide and 3 to 5 mm long. If the dehiscence is larger, the wound edges should be freshened with standard instruments and resutured in the ideal anatomic position. Despite the concerns that have been raised about the increased incidence of wound infection and dehiscence, these complications have not been recognized with an increased frequency following laser blepharoplasty (39).

Many well-known complications of blepharoplasty surgery occur independently of the device used to make incisions. Lower eyelid ectropion may result whenever the orbital septum is violated or eyelid laxity is not corrected. Symptoms of dry eyes or ocular surface exposure, such as foreign body sensation, redness, epiphora, and inability to wear contact lenses, may occur after any blepharoplasty procedure (40). Patients with an underlying dry eye condition should be identified preoperatively and, in these cases, care should be taken to minimize the amount of skin and orbicularis muscle removed to minimize impairment of the eyelid closure. Lymphedema may also occur after blepharoplasty surgery. Many surgeons believe that it is more common if large amounts of laser energy or cautery are applied intraoperatively, but this has yet to be conclusively demonstrated. Cicatricial entropion may develop following any transconjunctival procedure, but this is rare. Persistent chemosis is a well-known complication of blepharoplasty surgery, but has not specifically been reported after laser-assisted blepharoplasty (41). While some surgeons claim that postoperative swelling, pain, and ecchymosis are less following laser blepharoplasty than after blepharoplasty performed with standard techniques, others have disagreed (42). Injuries to the lacrimal system should not be produced with either technique. Any lower eyelid transcutaneous incision may become erythematous and/or elevated (Figures 14.7 and 14.8).

Lagophthalmos is the term applied to the condition in which the eyelids fail to close completely (Figure 14.9). A small amount of lagophthalmos is not unusual in the immediate (days 2 to 5) postoperative period due to edema of the upper eyelid skin and orbicularis muscle. All patients should be advised of this possibility preoperatively and instructed to use lubricating drops (artificial tears) and ointment for the first 1 to 2 weeks after surgery. When performing upper blepharoplasty surgery, skin and muscle removal should be planned with respect to the relationship between eyelid structure and function. Rather than measuring the amount of tissue to excise, the surgeon should measure the amount needed to maintain proper eyelid function and excise the excess. Compromise of the ocular surface due to insufficient blinking, permanent lagophthalmos, or a combination of these factors can lead to chronic ocular irritation, decreased vision, and even blindness.

If overly aggressive removal of upper eyelid skin should occur, vertical augmentation with a skin graft may be required to restore an appropriate relationship between the eyelids and globe, a disappointing and frustrating procedure for a patient who initially sought aesthetic improvement of their appearance. If a skin graft is re-

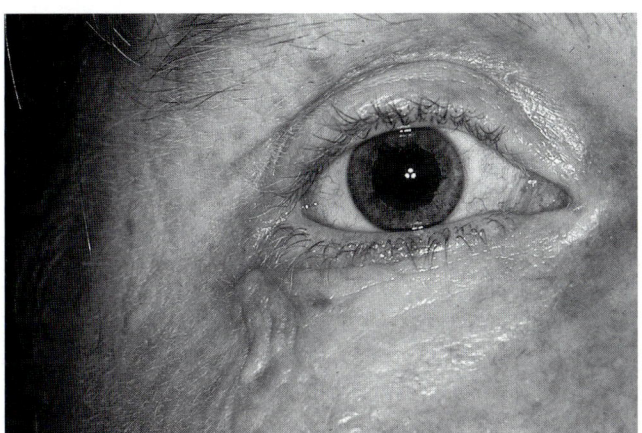

Figure 14.7. Hypertrophic scar following lower eyelid external blepharoplasty.

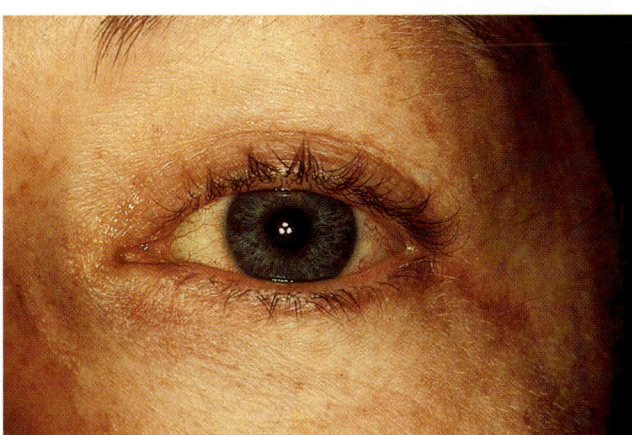

Figure 14.8. Erythematous scar more than 1 year after external lower blepharoplasty. The erythema did not respond well to topical steroids or pulsed dye laser treatment.

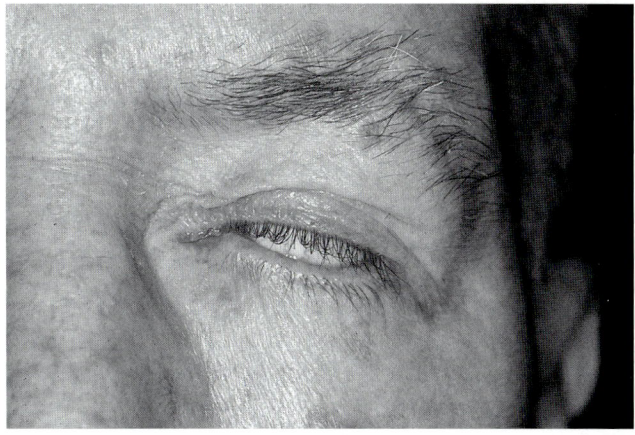

Figure 14.9. Lagophthalmos due to lower eyelid cicatricial ectropion.

quired for proper health of the ocular surface, every effort should be made to maintain a satisfactory aesthetic result. Placing the graft between the base of the lashes and the lid crease will minimize its visibility when the eyelids are open. Laser skin resurfacing may be performed several months after surgery to improve the aesthetic result. The CO_2 laser should not be used to harvest the graft or prepare the recipient bed due to the need to maintain excellent vascularity of these tissues.

If a cicatricial ectropion is produced in the lower eyelid, skin grafting may sometimes be avoided by elevating the midface through a combined eyelid and lateral canthal approach (Figure 14.10).

Blepharoplasty Revision

Before undergoing surgery, each patient should understand that it is normal to experience a self-image transition phase following facial surgery and that a minimum of 3 months must be allowed before the surgical result may be accurately assessed. Most surgical revisions should be postponed until at least 6 months after surgery to allow completion of the wound healing process.

Postoperative revision of surgery performed by another surgeon should be approached with caution. The care of an unhappy blepharoplasty patient should not be divided between two surgeons and is best left to the primary surgeon. In the event that secondary surgery is indicated, the goals and limitations of the planned procedure should be clearly defined and understood by both parties. Some surgeons require patients to sign a waiver releasing the operating surgeon from responsibility for the results of the initial surgery and stating that the

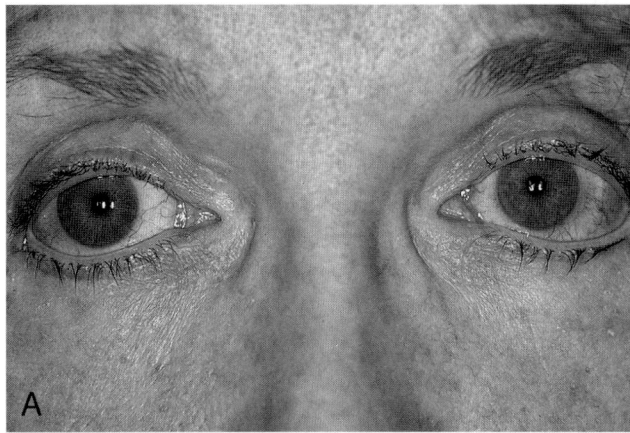

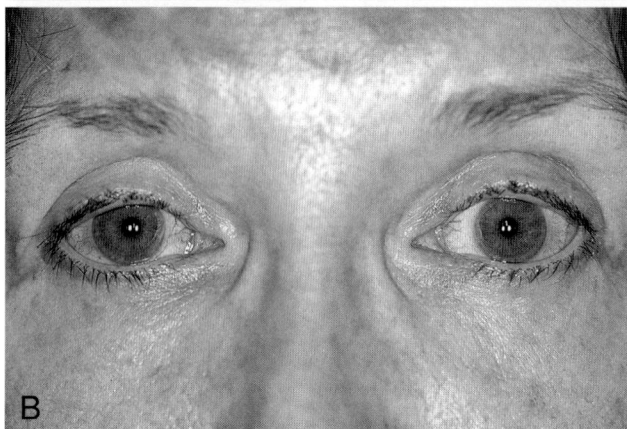

Figure 14.10. A. Lower eyelid ectropion after external lower blepharoplasty. **B.** Improved functional and aesthetic eyelid position after elevating the midface through a combined eyelid and lateral canthal approach.

results of secondary or tertiary procedures intended to achieve aesthetic and/or functional goals is not guaranteed. Excellent communication remains the best tool for dealing with these difficult situations.

REFERENCES

1. Biesman BS, Baker SS, Khan J, et al. Effects of defocused carbon dioxide laser beam on human eyelid tissue. Presented at the ASOPRS Annual Meeting, San Francisco, October 1997.
2. Seckel BR. Blepharoplasty: avoidance and treatment of complications. In: Aesthetic laser surgery: a text and videotape atlas. Boston: Little, Brown and Company, 1996:117.
3. Biesman BS. Safe use of the carbon dioxide laser in blepharoplasty surgery. Plast Reconstr Surg 1997;99: 275-277.
4. Clemente CD. Anatomy: a regional atlas of the human body. Baltimore: Urban & Schwarzenberg, 1981:Fig. 591.
5. Baker SS, Muenzler WS, Small RG, Leonard JE. Carbon dioxide laser blepharoplasty. Ophthalmology 1984;91: 238-244.
6. Baker SS. Carbon dioxide laser ptosis surgery combined with blepharoplasty. Dermatol Surg 1995;21: 1065-1070.
7. Lemke BN, Lucarelli MJ. Anatomy of the ocular adnexa, orbit and related facial structures. In: Nesi FA, Lisman RD, Levine MR, eds. Smith's ophthalmic plastic and reconstructive surgery. 2nd ed. St. Louis: Mosby, 1997: 18-19.
8. Zarem HA, Resnick JL. Expanded applications for transconjunctival lower lid blepharoplasty. Plast Reconstr Surg 1991;88:215-220.
9. Edgerton MT Jr. Causes and prevention of lower lid ectropion following blepharoplasty. Plast Reconstr Surg 1972;49:367-373.
10. McCord CD, Shore JW. Avoidance of complications in lower lid blepharoplasty. Ophthalmology 1983;90: 1039-1046.
11. McCord CD, Moses JL. Exposure of the inferior orbit with fornix incision and lateral canthotomy. Ophthalmic Surg 1979;10:53-63.
12. Shorr N, Cohen MS. Cosmetic blepharoplasty. Ophthalmol Clin North Am 1991;4(1):17-33.
13. Baylis HI, Long J, Groth M. Transconjunctival lower eyelid blepharoplasty. Ophthalmology 1989;96:1027-1032.
14. Hayworth RS, Lisman RD, Muchnick RS, Smith B. Diplopia following blepharoplasty. Ann Ophthalmol 1984;16:448-451.
15. Harley RD, Nelson LB, Flanagan JC, Calhoun JH. Ocular motility disturbances following cosmetic blepharoplasty. Arch Ophthalmol 1986;104:542-544.
16. Jameson NA, Good WV, Hoyt CS. Fat adherence simulating inferior oblique palsy following blepharoplasty. Arch Ophthalmol 1992;110:1369.
17. Wesley RE, Pollard ZF, McCord CD Jr. Superior oblique paresis after blepharoplasty. Plast Reconstr Surg 1980; 66:283-286.
18. Putterman AM. Diplopia following transconjunctival blepharoplasty: report of a case. Presented at the ASOPRS Spring Meeting, Williamsburg, VA, May 1995.
19. Doxanas MT. Minimally invasive lower eyelid blepharoplasty. Ophthalmology 1994;101:1327-1332.
20. Putterman AM. The mysterious second temporal fat pad. Ophthal Plast Reconstr Surg 1985;1:83-86.
21. Palmer FR III, Rice DH, Churukian MM. Transconjunctival blepharoplasty. Complications and their avoidance: a retrospective analysis and review of the literature. Arch Otolaryngol Head Neck Surg 1993;119:993-999.

22. Lemke BN, Lucarelli MJ. Anatomy of the ocular adnexa, orbit and related facial structures. In: Nesi FA, Lisman RD, Levine MR, eds. Smith's ophthalmic plastic and reconstructive surgery. 2nd ed. St. Louis: Mosby, 1997:55.

23. Barker DE. Dye injection studies of intraorbital fat compartments. Plast Reconstr Surg 1977;59:82.

24. Callahan MA. Prevention of blindness after blepharoplasty. Ophthalmology 1983;90:1047-1051.

25. Goldberg RA, Marmor MF, Shorr N, Christenbury JD. Blindness following blepharoplasty: two case reports, and a discussion of management. Ophthalmic Surg 1990;21:85-89.

26. Stasior OG. Blindness associated with cosmetic blepharoplasty. Clin Plast Surg 1981;8:793-795.

27. Putterman AM. Temporary blindness after cosmetic blepharoplasty. Am J Ophthalmol 1975;80:1081-1083.

28. Rafety FM. Transient total blindness during cosmetic blepharoplasty. Ann Plast Surg 1979;3:373.

29. Hislop WS, Dutton GN. Retrobulbar haemorrhage: can blindness be prevented? Injury 1994;25:663-665.

30. Hargarden M, Goldberg SH, Cunningham D, et al. Optic neuropathy following simulation of orbital hemorrhage in the nonhuman primate. Ophthal Plast Reconstr Surg 1996;12:264-272.

31. Yung CW, Moorthy RS, Lindley D, et al. Efficacy of lateral canthotomy and cantholysis in orbital hemorrhage. Ophthal Plast Reconstr Surg 1994;10:137-141.

32. Liu D. A simplified technique of orbital decompression for severe retrobulbar hemorrhage. Am J Ophthal 1993;116:34-37.

33. Baker TJ, Gordon HL, Stutzin JM. Surgical rejuvenation of the face. St. Louis: Mosby, 1996:492.

34. Wesley RE, Bond JB. Carbon dioxide laser in ophthalmic plastic and reconstructive surgery. Ophthalmic Surg 1985;16:631.

35. Newell FW, Ernest JT. Diseases and injuries of the eye. In: Ophthalmology: principles and concepts. 3rd ed. St. Louis: Mosby, 1974:313-344.

36. Alster TS. Laser treatment of hypertrophic scars, keloids, and striae. In: Alster TS, ed. Dermatologic clinics. Philadelphia: WB Saunders, 1998. In press.

37. Dierickx C, Goldman MP, Fitzpatrick RE. Laser treatment of erythematous/hypertrophic and pigmented scars in 26 patients. Plast Reconstr Surg 1995;95: 84-90.

38. Hall RR. The healing of tissues excised by a carbon-dioxide laser. Br J Surg 1971;58:222-225.

39. Glassberg E, Babapour R, Lask G. Current trends in laser blepharoplasty: results of a survey. Dermatol Surg 1995; 21:1060-1063.

40. Jelks GW, Jelks EB. Preoperative evaluation of the blepharoplasty patient: bypassing the pitfalls. Clin Plast Surg 1993;20:213-223.

41. Enzer Y, Shorr N. Medical and surgical management of chemosis after blepharoplasty. Ophthal Plast Reconstr Surg 1994;10:57-63.

42. Mittelman H, Apfelberg DB. Carbon dioxide laser blepharoplasty—advantages and disadvantages. Ann Plast Surg 1990;24:1-6.

Index

Page numbers in *italics* denote figures; those followed by a t denotes tables.